AMERICAN
HEALTH$CARE

How the healthcare industry's scare tactics have screwed up our economy – and our future.

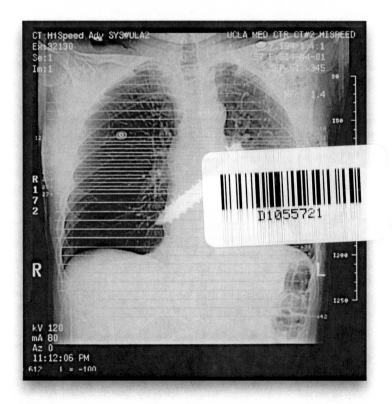

RICHARD YOUNG, M.D.

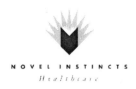

NOVEL INSTINCTS
Healthcare

NOVEL INSTINCTS PUBLISHING
6008 Ross Avenue
Dallas, Texas 75206
www.novelinstincts.com

The opinions in this book are those of the author and do not reflect those of Novel Instincts, its employees and its vendors.

www.HealthScareonline.com

Born to Be Wild Words and Music by Mars Bonfire. Copyright (c) 1968 UNIVERSAL MUSIC PUBLISHING, A Division of UNIVERSAL MUSIC CANADA, INC. Copyright Renewed. All Rights in the United States Controlled and Administered by UNIVERSAL MUSIC CORP. All Rights Reserved. Used by Permission. Reprinted by Permission of Hal Leonard Corporation

All other graphics, tables and charts are original creations of the author unless noted.

ISBN: 978-0-9726007-7-4
Cataloging information: 1. Healthcare 2. Medical Issues 3. Medicine

Library of Congress Control Number: 2012930710

Printed in the United States of America.
10 9 8 7 6 5 4 3 2 1

IMPORTANT NOTICE – PLEASE READ

The information in this book is for educational and entertainment purposes only and is NOT a substitute for qualified medical or professional evaluation, guidance or treatment. The author and publisher specifically disclaim any and all liability related to the use of this book.

Every effort has been made to ensure the accuracy of the information contained herein; however, no claims are made by the author or publisher regarding either the book's completeness or its accuracy. Readers are urged to conduct their own relevant research and to consult appropriate professionals before taking any health-related actions. The reader agrees that she/he is solely responsible for any actions she/he may take as a result of reading this book or any potion thereof.

Praise for Dr. Young and *American Health$care*

American Health Scare should be thoroughly read by persons who wish to understand how, why and where we are wasting our dwindling health care resources. Dr. Young examines the pieces of our health system thoroughly and provides a practical, reasoned physician's view of the economic challenges we face. He provides **excellent written arguments** against the spending status quo.

~ Christopher Gregory, DocOnomics.com

There are many things I appreciate about Dr. Young and his book, but chief among these is **his profound skill at untangling the many mysteries and conflicts within health care today**. Richard is an excellent physician, but what sets him apart in these pages is his ability to communicate. I'm not a doctor – and I don't play one on TV – but I have an array of docs overseeing my health. Through Richard's wisdom in this book, I now grasp many of the medical, ethical, legal, religious, and financial issues in medical care. Not only do I now feel more capable of being proactive with my health, **I thoroughly enjoyed reading this book** and highly recommend it to you.

~ Preston Gillham, Nonprofit Consultant, Leadership Mentor, and Author, www.PrestonGillham.com

Dr. Young brings **a needed voice of reason** to the cacophony of our healthcare "debate". He expresses the concern that "more healthcare" is not necessarily "better healthcare" and that one-size- fits-all solutions may fit no one.

A new models of care, based upon the patient's life-values is offered. Maybe a family vacation is better use of limited resources than selection of a trendy as-seen-on-TV wonder pill.

This is kind of science-based wisdom that we need to lead us through our most difficult decisions.

~ Charles Kurtzman, Past Governor, Rotary International

This book is written by **a great teacher** for regular folks who are bewildered by health care in the US and all the claims about what is needed to improve it. Its direct, blunt style is at once **engaging and understandable** by people who just want the whining to stop and better, affordable care to start.

~ Larry Green, MD, Professor of Family Medicine
Epperson-Zorn Chair for Innovation in Family Medicine, University of
Colorado Denver, Chair of the Board of Directors of the American
Board of Family Medicine, Member of the Institute of Medicine.

Table of Contents

Introduction   **1**

Part I: The Problem

Chapter 1: Don't Be Afraid of Change   **8**

Chapter 2: The Government Industrial
            Medical Coalition: GIMeC   **21**

Chapter 3: How GIMeC Thinks   **60**

Chapter 4: How GIMeC Thinks: Part 2   **89**

Chapter 5: The Enormous Cost of U.S. Healthcare   **107**

Part II: Heading Toward a Solution

Chapter 6: What Can We Learn From
            Other Countries?   **126**

Chapter 7: Why Aren't There More Family
            Physicians?   **157**

Chapter 8: The National Bigotry Against Family
            Medicine   **172**

Chapter 9: Now You Play Doctor – Order Tests   **209**

Chapter 10: Now You Play Doctor – Order
            Treatments   **222**

Chapter 11: An Ounce of Prevention Costs a
              Ton of Money   239

Chapter 12: Really Expensive Drugs and Devices   255

Chapter 13: Sugar Diabetes   265

Chapter 14: Keep the Government Out
              of My Medicare   277

Chapter 15: Get Your Motor Running   284

Chapter 16: A Few More Issues   293

Chapter 17: God and American Medicine   308

Part III: Solutions

Chapter 18: Solutions — Introduction   322

Chapter 19: Family Medicine Care   326

Chapter 20: Basic Healthcare   336

Chapter 21: Final Thoughts   347

Appendix   363

Acknowledgements

I have so many people to thank. In spite of their very busy schedules, Jonathan Nelson and Robert Earley graciously reviewed very early and very crude versions of this book. Their feedback encouraged me to press on.

Carol Proctor, Susan Linguist, Tawny Kilbourne, and Preston Gillham reviewed the next version, which wasn't refined much further. Each contributed their unique perspective, which enhanced the manuscript. I especially thank Tawny for his thorough editing of that manuscript and re-educating me on fundamentals of grammar.

The next wave of reviewers included Chuck Kurtzman, Terri Barton, Suzy Holloway, Judith Manriquez, and my dad, who was a great sport by letting me tell his story. Thanks Dad! During this phase I also began attending the weekly meetings of the DFW Writer's Workshop. Their detailed and constructive feedback was a crucial source for polishing my manuscript. I especially thank my carpool buddy, John Bartell.

The next wave included two more of my DFWWW colleagues, Virginia Traweek and Tracy Ward, who on their own volition volunteered to read the entire manuscript and give their thoughts. Two family physician colleagues, Maureen Swenson, MD and Doug Curran, MD provided great insight and encouragement. Other reviewers included Diane Searce and her husband Phil (who wrote a great book on WW II pilots called *Finish Forty and Home*), Chris Gregory of Doconomics, and my son David. I also thank Bridget Boland, whose professional book editing and general support made the final product that much better. I also attended a workshop at the Mayborn Nonfiction Writer's Conference. I thank my fellow workshop participants and our excellent moderator, Susannah Charlson.

I also acknowledge the excellent review of the Nataline Sarkisyan case presented by David Isch, PhD, who is a healthcare ethicist.

I thank Paul Black and Jay Johnson of Novel Instincts Publishing for their expert guidance that took my book to a higher level of quality.

Most importantly, I thank my wife for putting up with my late night and weekend writing and for all her love and support of my crazy dreams. I couldn't have done it without her.

To Dr. Margaret Scott Gaines, my technical writing professor at the University of Texas at Austin, who showed an engineer the real purpose and meaning of the English language.

To the children of America, who should be able to grow up unencumbered by the excesses of their parents and grandparents.

INTRODUCTION

I'm a family physician. I think American healthcare costs too much, and I think physicians are part of the problem.

I wrote this book because I'm worried about America's future. American businesses have become more efficient over the last 10 years, but their employees can't feel it. Workers are more productive, but the fruit of their labors is missing from their paychecks because it's being sucked into the healthcare system. As well, U.S. businesses face a competitive disadvantage because they pay so much more for healthcare than companies in other countries. I'm not talking just about China, either. I'm talking about developed countries such as Australia and Sweden.

I want a future that allows America to continue to make things and sell them to other countries. I want a future in which our children or grandchildren don't pay for the excesses of this generation, and unless we change course now, they'll drown in an ocean of federal government debt. America's healthcare system is a significant contributor to this debt, and new approaches must be implemented to prevent imminent disaster. During the health reform debates of 2009-2010, several commentators talked about bending the healthcare cost curve at some ill-defined point in the future. The cost curve doesn't need to be bent; it must be snapped off and reattached at a lower level. The root causes of expensive American healthcare have not been addressed. I will expose the core issues of the crisis that the special interests don't talk about.

Although I've practiced family medicine for 19 years, I'm actually more of a teacher. I work at America's largest family medicine residency, the John Peter Smith Hospital Family Medicine Residency Program in Fort Worth, Texas, where I take new doctors fresh out of medical school and teach them to be family physicians. My daily work environment is a tax-supported public hospital and clinic system. Almost all of my patients have low incomes, and many didn't graduate from high school. Of course, I also care for patients in the insured healthcare system; I've worked in the emergency rooms of several private hospitals and a few private clinics; and as a researcher, I've published papers in peer-reviewed medical journals.

From my experience inside the system, I have identified two fundamental issues that we must face to achieve significantly more affordable healthcare.

First, we must recognize that most of the major American cultural, political, philanthropic, and medical institutions think alike. They make rarely questioned assumptions about the role and purpose of healthcare within society, and these assumptions are often wrong and almost always lead to more expensive healthcare. Because of these unchallenged assumptions, special interest groups have received carte blanche to scare people needlessly. If you don't rush out and plunk down $200 for a "simple" test, you could die soon, and it will be your fault. If you don't undergo a third series of toxic chemotherapy cancer treatments – miserable every moment from the first dose to the last – you aren't a fighter. Or even worse, you have insulted God by not squeezing every possible second out of the life He has given you, even though overly aggressive treatment often kills people faster than comfort care.

Second, to achieve significantly less expensive healthcare, we must change the very way we think of the system. The most important change involves the relationship between doctors and patients. Should doctors order every possible test at every single visit, or should they be allowed to use judgment and be good stewards of precious medical resources? Should doctors insist on offering every conceivable experimental treatment, no matter how rare the chance of success, or are some treatments just too expensive to justify?

Many difficult truths must be exposed and debated to achieve a level of healthcare reform that will significantly lower costs. Because I address these difficult truths, I must say there are paragraphs in this book I didn't enjoy writing. I wish the world were simpler, but it's not. We can't solve America's healthcare cost crisis by ignoring difficult realities or believing in voodoo medical economics.

This book is divided into three sections. The first section defines the multitude of problems that must be fixed. I identify the major special interest groups, show how they all think alike, and demonstrate how that thinking harms average Americans. The groups include those typically demonized as the culprits for expensive healthcare, such as insurance companies, but they also include some you may not have realized were problems, such as disease advocacy groups. From this discussion, I arrive at four major assumptions that must be challenged to achieve significantly more affordable healthcare.

The next section explores a number of complicated issues that must be addressed: how physicians are paid, the care of patients with chronic diseases, the role of risk in decision making, and connections between religion and healthcare.

The final section lays out my proposed solutions. If you're happy with your current healthcare coverage and can afford it, I don't propose to take it from you. However, some people may want decent, reasonably affordable coverage. That option doesn't exist now, and I will show how it can.

I wish I could just list all of the changes necessary to create an affordable healthcare system. But if I did, the list would seem strange. There are too many common myths and misconceptions promoted by special interests that I must debunk for my proposed solutions to make sense. I highlight aspects of the overall solution at the end of each chapter to give you a sense of where I'm going, but I will consolidate the major points in my Solutions chapters at the end of the book.

Along this journey, I was guided by two underlying assumptions that aren't commonly mentioned in healthcare reform proposals. First, I assume you should control the distribution of your healthcare dollars. If you feel a system encouraging a lot of tests and experimental treatments is in your family's best interests, I support your right to make that choice. Just be ready when the bill comes. If you feel your family's overall health would be improved by moving to a better neighborhood, taking a vacation, not having the stress of living paycheck-to-paycheck, or sending your children to a better school, you should have that option as well. You shouldn't be coerced into putting all of your resources into the healthcare system to improve your family's health. I propose solutions that assume the healthcare industry isn't the only source of health.

Second, I assume your health insurance benefits at work really are part of your wages. You should control the distribution of those wages between take-home pay and insurance premiums your employer pays on your behalf. Similarly, America's elderly receive money from the federal government each year in the form of Social Security and Medicare benefits. They should have the same right to move money from healthcare to income as they see fit.

Ultimately, my proposed solutions are about choices. I fundamentally believe America is great because it respects the integrity and intelligence of her citizens and allows them to make the best decisions for their families. I want you to have choices that currently don't exist. Thank you for spending your valuable time to see the healthcare system from a different perspective. By working together, maybe we can bring a healthy dose of sanity and a sense of proportion to our dysfunctional healthcare system, and thereby save our children's future.

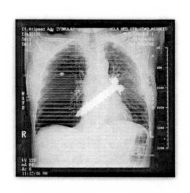

Part 1

The Problem

1 | Don't Be Afraid of Change

Curtis was a 41-year-old man in great physical shape. He went to the gym regularly, had an ideal body weight, had no significant chronic medical conditions, and had no family history of serious medical conditions.

He saw his family physician for a routine visit. The doctor listened to his heart and heard a soft heart murmur, which is the sound of blood rushing through the heart that may or may not be serious. It was nothing to worry about; the doctor was just informing his patient of all his findings, because the issue might come up in future physical exams.

Curtis wanted a second opinion, so he scheduled a visit with a cardiologist who ordered an exercise stress test. For this test, a patient is hooked up to an EKG machine and walks on a treadmill. The result was normal, but the cardiologist thought a sonogram of the heart, an echocardiogram, would be a good idea. That test also was normal. But to be extra sure there was absolutely nothing wrong, the cardiologist convinced Curtis to have a heart catheterization. At this point Curtis had a few doubts, but felt he would put his health at risk if he didn't follow the doctor's advice. The heart catheterization was also normal.

Curtis' insurance company was billed $28,000 for the cardiologist's office visits and tests. Was this journey an example of a doctor taking excellent care of his patient by being thorough, or an example of a healthcare system out of control? Reasonable people could argue either position. However, for those who believe the expensive tests were unnecessary, there is hope that someday they might have much more affordable healthcare.

SCARING THE PUBLIC

Why did Curtis agree to all the tests, even as his own doubts began to build? The trusted authority figure of the cardiologist was a huge factor. In spite of the patient empowerment movement, most patients still want their doctors to tell them what to do. They might politely listen to their doctor's discussion of the pros and cons of different options, but in the end they still say, "What would you do, doc?" or its variant, "What would you tell your mother to do?"

I wasn't in the room when the cardiologist talked to Curtis, and I don't have the cardiologist's version of the story. Nevertheless, I suspect there wasn't a lot of discussion. More likely, the cardiologist said, "I would like you to have a heart cath, just to be sure."

The root cause of why Curtis agreed to the full menu of heart tests goes even deeper. Healthcare special interest groups have scared the American public into embracing every expensive medical technology, promising a longer and better life as a result. Over the last four decades, Americans have been so bombarded by misinformation about the effectiveness of many common medical tests, procedures, and treatments that they believe they won't live another year unless they receive a litany of expensive interventions. Supported by the public's anxiety, a complex web of special interests – bureaucrats, physicians, hospitals, and drug companies, to name just a few – have created an uncoordinated and inefficient healthcare system that is technologically impressive, but completely unaffordable. Why do patients with no symptoms allow themselves to have needles stuck in their veins, X-ray plates squash their breasts, and fingers inserted into their rectums? It's more than concern – it's fear.

An example of a special interest group unnecessarily scaring the American public occurred when Dr. Lucy Marion, spokeswoman for the U.S. Preventive Services Task Force, discussed the 2009 recommendations for mammograms in women ages 40-49 on CNN. Instead of calling for mammograms for all women in that age range, the Task Force's report recommended only that women have discussions with their doctors about the risks and benefits of mammography.[1]

Dr. Sanjay Gupta barked at the petrified spokeswoman, "You're saying that some lives just aren't worth it."[2]

The great mammogram scare of 2009 revealed special interest groups at their worst. The media took a relatively benign report and twisted it into a major controversy. Breast doctors and radiologists claimed thousands of women would die if they didn't get mammograms. Strangely, insurance companies were silent. The fact is, they make money every time a claim is submitted because their contracts with their corporate customers commonly include a fee that is a percentage of each claim. More tests mean more income for the insurer. Senators called for hearings. Cancer researchers and special interest groups used the free air time to plead for more taxpayer money to invent new tests and treatments.

Few in the media reported that we've been down this road before. A consensus panel was convened by the National Institutes of Health in January 1997 to review all the clinical trials of mammograms.[3] The panel concluded the evidence didn't support a universal recommendation for or against mammograms in 40 to 49 year olds. The U.S. Senate passed a resolution condemning the panel and convened hearings. By March 1997, the panel caved to pressure and changed its mind, recommending mammograms beginning at age 40.

Few reported that the evidence to demonstrate that mammograms save lives in average-risk 40- to 49-year-old women is weak. No sound bite addressed the high cost of mammography. No network mentioned that almost all other developed countries[4] – including Britain,[5] Canada,[6] and Australia[7] – start routine mammograms at age 50.

One of the most self-interested beliefs of the current healthcare system is that good health must come from technology. No wonder television commercials talk about making healthcare human again (though in a brilliant marketing ploy, the hospital system or medical equipment manufacturer is really selling more technology). In today's system, a person with a disease doesn't have a name. She is just the bone cancer in Room 831 who needs a bone scan, CAT scan, PET scan, and radiation treatment. The truth is, health comes from many sources other than lasers, gamma knives, and mechanical ventilators.

Fifty years ago, people had lower expectations of the healthcare system. They didn't expect to get through life without scars, wrinkles, aches, or pains. A snapshot of a home 50 years ago could simultaneously include a general practitioner performing a minor procedure on the kitchen table, children taking some horrible-tasting syrup for a cough, and a family caring for a dying elderly relative. Physicians' tools were limited.

Families expected their doctors to try hard and to care, but not to restore critically ill patients to perfect health. Some of these values and expectations must be renewed to restore a sense of proportion to American healthcare. Today, patients are bounced from doctor to scanner to surgical center to lab and back to doctor. I'm not calling for a return to the medical practices of the 1950s, but in terms of expectations and treatment, we have to strike a middle ground between that era and the bloated mess of today. Our expensive healthcare system affects all of us, and the deficits created in our governments and our families will crush our children with debt if we don't change course now.[8]

National surveys have found that 90 percent of Americans believe our healthcare system needs a major overhaul (though the insured tend not to want their individual benefits changed much), but 36 percent feel our system is so dysfunctional it needs radical change.[9, 10] I hope to convince everyone to consider more fundamental changes to our existing system.

THE EFFECTS OF EXPENSIVE HEALTHCARE

Expensive healthcare has unintended harmful consequences. Hard work and improved productivity at the workplace often don't result in more personal income.[11, 12] An estimated 25 percent of workers are trapped in dead-end jobs, simply because those jobs come with health insurance coverage.[13] Ironically, Americans have worked themselves into poor health trying to maintain their health insurance benefits!

For example, examine the American automobile industry. Excessive healthcare costs played a significant role in GM and Chrysler filing for bankruptcy in 2009.[14] General Motors spent approximately $5.2 billion per year on healthcare in 2005, which translates to $1,500 more per vehicle than foreign manufacturers.[15] In 2006, Toyota in North America paid $280 per vehicle for healthcare for its current workers, and paid nothing for retiree healthcare.[16] GM paid $395 for healthcare for current workers and $950 for retirees. These additional healthcare costs mean GM must charge more. Its cars become less competitive. GM sells fewer cars. GM supports fewer jobs.

The sad irony of this situation is that expensive healthcare for the few remaining GM workers causes the health of the surrounding community to worsen. Job loss is a major source of stress associated with poorer health. Even a one percentage point increase in the unemployment rate is associated with an increase in suicides and heart attacks.[11] Stress is suspected as a contributing factor to a three-fold increase in the heart attack rate in New Orleans since Hurricane Katrina.[17] While these limited projections are hard to measure precisely, the overall conclusion that being underemployed or unemployed leads to poorer health is entirely plausible.

Over-priced healthcare also affects city, state, and federal budgets. As government at all levels is forced to pay more for the healthcare of government employees and government-sponsored health programs such as Medicaid, other programs suffer. A large number of middle-class families find it increasingly difficult to pay college tuition because state cutbacks to higher education have caused college expenses to rise faster than general inflation.[11] When more and more state spending is devoted to healthcare, less is available to support education, which in turn causes universities to increase their tuition and fees. Rising healthcare costs adversely affect the entire economy.

The pens doctors carry in their pockets possess incredible power and have been called the most expensive technology in healthcare. Physicians' orders can cause hundreds of thousands, even millions, of dollars to change hands. The doctor/patient relationship has expectations defined by decades of interactions between patients, lawyers, legislators, and physicians. Honestly, though, someone needs to ask the question: Should doctors have unfettered power to move money from one entity to another without the consent of the people who ultimately pay for the care?

HEALTHCARE COSTS AND KICKING TIRES

When most experts today talk about healthcare costs, they typically focus only on insurance issues: co-pays and deductibles, pharmacy benefits, and the number of uninsured. They rarely talk about meaningful issues beyond healthcare financing. This includes the much-debated healthcare reforms of 2010.

Imagine you were thinking about buying a new car and all you considered was the cost of insurance. Yes, it is important to know your monthly expense for car insurance, but this has little to do with the affordability of the car. What car to buy? A Kia or a Ferrari? That decision results in car payments of $200 or $2,000 per month. Whether your yearly car insurance deductible is $250 or $500 has much less impact on the total cost of owning a car. Similarly, in healthcare discussions too much time is spent arguing if a pharmacy co-pay should be $5 or $10, while almost no thought is devoted to discussing which drugs actually provide cost-effective benefits and should be widely available.

Even the most intelligent patients allow their physicians to perform controversial and expensive tests on them. President Obama received several expensive medical tests at his annual check up in 2010.[18] He had a PSA test, which at best is controversial, but really has been shown in clinical trials to be worthless.[19] He had a virtual CAT scan colonoscopy to check for colon cancer. Medicare determined in 2009 that there is inadequate evidence to conclude this test is appropriate for colorectal screening and doesn't cover it.[20] As for the timing of the test, Obama was screened for colon cancer two years before standard age recommendations in the U.S., and 12 years sooner than in Britain. He had a CAT scan of his heart, even though the American Heart Association states this test shouldn't be used to screen for coronary artery disease.[21]

American taxpayers spent somewhere in the range of $5,000 on unproven medical technology for Obama's exam. The President's health was no better after the tests than before. In fact, some would argue his health is now worse because he increased his future cancer risk from the unnecessary radiation exposure of the CAT scans.[22] This episode was a perfect example of what's wrong with American medicine: overuse of expensive technology by doctors and patients who assume it results in better health.

The President publicly stated that more prevention lowers costs.[14] Wrong. Prevention rarely save money! This myth, perpetuated by American medicine and most other special interest groups, is explained in Chapters Four and Eleven. Congress grasps the core issues no better.[23] Neither political party has addressed the fundamental causes of over-priced healthcare.

Fifteen years ago, I lived through the HMO era and watched greed distort the few good ideas in managed care. (For those too young to remember, the managed care companies abused the system with practices such as paying executives bonuses for denying expensive treatments and systematically denying legitimate claims to maintain cash flow, while at the same time paying their CEOs more than $100 million per year in salary and stock options.) I ultimately concluded that all the special interest groups in the healthcare industry think alike. They prosper from selling fear. I call this collection of special interests the Government-Industrial-Medical Coalition (GIMeC – pronounced "gimmick").

How expensive is American healthcare? During the healthcare reform debates of 2009-2010, many agreed healthcare costs were too high, and that the situation was worse than the previous major reform era of the early 1990s (Table).[24]

Measurement	Early 1990s	2009-2010
Healthcare spending as a percentage of GDP	12.3 percent (1990)	17.3 percent[25] (2009)
Per capita healthcare spending	$3,167 (1992)	$8,447 (2009)[26]
Number of uninsured	35.4 million (1991)	52.0 million (2010)[27]
Unemployment rate	7.5 percent (1992)	10.2 percent (2009)
Federal deficit in one year	$269 billion (1991)	$1.4 trillion (2009)[28]
Percentage of people who say the system needs to be completely rebuilt or needs fundamental changes	90 percent (1991)	90 percent (2007)

The U.S. spends more on healthcare than the entire economy of France,[29] and has spent almost twice as much per person than most other developed countries for many years (Figure).

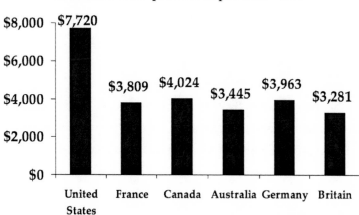

Health Care Costs per Person per Year – 2008

Based on data from the Organization of Economic Cooperation and Development, 2008.[30]

The political reality is national healthcare expenditures represent income to industry stakeholders, whose self-interests encourage more spending. Almost every previous effort to improve U.S. healthcare has resulted in more health insurance regulations or payment reform, but none have addressed the deeper, root causes. For the most part, the reforms passed in 2010 just expanded insurance coverage. The chief actuary for Medicare, Richard Foster, predicted that the 2010 changes will not even slow down the growth of government spending on health care, much less reduce costs.[31]

NECESSARY CHANGES

For America ever to have reasonably affordable healthcare, the relationship between doctors and patients must change. The current model – that all possible healthcare services be provided no matter how rare the benefit or expensive the service – is unsustainable. Until we accept this reality, healthcare costs will continue to rise faster than personal incomes, and sometime soon health insurance will be available only to the very wealthy. The great American healthcare irony – we spend the most but get the least – will only grow worse.

To achieve radical change in healthcare, two concepts must be managed that enormously impact the bottom line – risk and cost. The underlying reasons doctors make medical decisions must evolve. The values and expectations of both doctors and patients must transform.

In healthcare debates, worries about insurance coverage must be de-emphasized. The most important contributors to healthcare costs are the types and volumes of medical services provided. If a doctor orders $1,000 in tests or treatments, it doesn't matter if an insurance company, Medicare, Medicaid, or a person paying out of funds in a health savings account writes the check. Regardless of the source, $1,000 changed hands. If the tests are unnecessary, and the treatments are unproven, they shouldn't be ordered in the first place, and there is no cost to the healthcare system.

Too much care is provided by specialists who focus only on one body part, not the whole person. It is in everyone's best interest to have a healthcare system built on a solid foundation of family physicians, because we will not only be healthier, we will pay less.[32] For that to happen, America needs many more family physicians, and Medicare and insurance companies must actually encourage family physicians to provide the care patients expect.

Organized medicine in America – for example, the American Medical Association (AMA) – frequently promotes conventional medical interventions to improve patients' health. The AMA has no interest in engaging the country in a serious discussion about the way healthcare dollars are spent. Rather, it focuses on lobbying for insurance companies and government sources to cover any test or treatment that might possibly help a patient, and for doctors to be free to order these interventions without regard to cost. I say you don't need every possible test and treatment to be healthy.

Unfortunately, a complex system requires complex solutions. GIMeC promotes simplistic and erroneous ideas that serve only to maintain its own interests. Many in the healthcare field believe that one administrative change, such as medical malpractice reform or insurance industry reform, will fix everything. If only it were that easy.

A real solution to expensive American healthcare will be accomplished only when we finally achieve "health scare" reform. Over the last 40 years, GIMeC has thrived by scaring the American public into believing that anything less than the most aggressive healthcare possible is foolish and dangerous. When enough people overcome this fear and see overly aggressive healthcare for what it is – an enormously expensive undertaking for marginal gain – they will regain control of their resources, and affordable healthcare will finally exist. Curtis, in retrospect, now sees the fallacy of cardiac testing gone wild. He should be able to choose a health insurance plan that discourages these practices, thereby reducing how much he spends on healthcare so he can instead spend that money on other pursuits more likely to support health and happiness for himself and his family.

American healthcare is technologically impressive but completely unaffordable. It shouldn't be. We should have access to healthcare options that reflect a different set of values than those advocated by GIMeC. Significantly more affordable healthcare will require fundamental changes in the role and purpose of healthcare in America. Change is always difficult, but don't be afraid. Reasonable, compassionate healthcare can exist without bankrupting our children's future.

2 | THE GOVERNMENT-INDUSTRIAL-MEDICAL COALITION: GIMeC

It took me years to see that the primary reason American healthcare costs so much is that all the healthcare special interest groups think alike. Not only that, many of their beliefs are wrong, at least much of the time.

Throughout my journey in medicine, many times I felt like the little boy in "The Emperor's New Clothes." I would sit in a room of doctors at a medical conference listening to a speaker make a claim that felt good but reliable scientific evidence said was wrong, and all I saw was a bunch of heads nodding in agreement. I would watch the evening news and hear a spokesperson from a disease advocacy group make an exaggerated claim, then see the reporter smile and nod in agreement and never challenge the assertion. I'm here to tell you, these people are naked.

My journey has not been a smooth, linear experience. More typically, there have been periods of both calm and confusion, pierced by the occasional "Ah-Ha!" moment. After enough light bulbs went off, I started to identify some patterns.

TWO CELEBRITIES

The stories of two celebrities with serious health conditions fascinated me. The first was Mickey Mantle. He died relatively young of the complications of hepatitis, cirrhosis of the liver, and liver cancer.[1] These diseases afflicted him largely because he was an alcoholic infected with hepatitis C. He received a liver transplant before he died, but not without controversy. Some people thought he received the new liver suspiciously quickly, and he was discovered to have liver cancer soon after the transplant (which didn't save his life).

After he died, his family established a foundation to increase organ transplant awareness.[2] The foundation's primary purpose was not to reduce the behavior that caused his liver to fail in the first place – excessive alcohol consumption. Instead, the foundation's very existence seemed to imply you can drink all you want, and when your liver becomes a non-functional ball of scar tissue, you can order up a new one. A medical miracle awaits you, and someone else will pay for it. The doctors and hospitals will be paid handsomely for the high-tech procedures; the insurance companies will profit by taking a percentage of the claims. (To be fair, the foundation does have an alcohol abstinence pledge buried in its website, but the vast majority of the content is about organ transplantation.)

Another example was Christopher Reeve. He was a horse-jumping enthusiast good enough to try out for the Olympic equestrian team. At a competition, his horse suddenly balked at a rail. Mr. Reeve flew forward off the horse, landed on his head, broke his neck, severed his spinal cord, and became a quadriplegic.

Mr. Reeve's optimism after the injury was inspiring. He was convinced he would walk again and invited the world to follow the journey with him toward that goal. Sadly, he never came close to walking again. Along the way, he made many TV appearances and testified before Congress to advocate spinal cord injury research, specifically stem cell research.[3]

Similar to the Mickey Mantle situation, there was a lack of effort to advocate for fewer neck injuries in the first place. Why didn't he call for a ban on the sport of horse jumping so others wouldn't share his fate? If this was too drastic, why didn't he advocate limits on the height of the rails, or demand riders wear protective neck gear? In his vision of the future, people could jump horses all they want. When the occasional neck fracture and spinal cord injury happens, doctors will inject stem cells in your body, and you will be completely restored to your previous abilities. Mr. Reeve advocated for a high-tech solution that GIMeC loves to promote: a miracle in a vial.

The efforts of the Mantle and Reeve families to try to turn their painful experiences into hope for future generations is laudable and deserves our respect. Nevertheless, their work was guided by the prevailing culture of GIMeC, which produced unintended negative consequences.

THE IMPETUS TO WRITE

Watching the evening news in 2007, I was struck by three healthcare stories presented nearly back-to-back. One was a union threatening a strike over a company's proposal that they pay a larger share of their healthcare costs. Next was the story of a lab scientist who announced a discovery of a protein that has something to do with Alzheimer's. He gushed about how this could lead to new tests and cures, but of course those were years and years away. Finally, a politician proposed legislation that insurance companies be forced to cover an unproven medical screening test. (I knew it was unproven, but the health beat reporter didn't do her homework and inform the audience that it was unproven.)

None of the reporters or anchors gave any indication these three stories were connected. The high cost of healthcare was shown to harm businesses and their workers, but the next two stories touted the dubious future benefits of unproven, expensive technologies. I screamed something profound like, "Aaaaahhhhh," and decided I couldn't stand it anymore. I had to try to expose the GIMeC conspiracy and its faulty beliefs, or risk living in a country that would slowly test and treat itself into rampant unemployment and bankruptcy. I bought a cheap laptop on eBay and started writing.

THE MEDIA

I first concluded that the media loves to tell rat stories, which can only mean Americans love rat stories.[4] The image of a scientist in a white coat with caged rats and test tubes behind her looks scientific, and these images fit easily on a TV screen. The general script for such stories is invariably the same: "Scientists at Big Medical University announce the discovery of an abnormal protein that builds up in people with a certain disease." While a cure is always 10 to 15 years away, the scientists are encouraged by the results. The discovery of this abnormal protein could lead to the development of new drugs to treat the disease, but much more research, and a whole lot more dollars, are necessary. Recent examples include studies in mice potentially leading to new diet pills,[5] out-of-hospital treatments for heart attacks,[6] better treatments for Parkinson's disease,[7] and treatments to repair or replace damaged organs.[8] But once the rat story is told, the media rarely follows up to see if the early promises have resulted in a single proven treatment.

Interesting stories contain conflict and emotion, so the media uses our fear of disease and dying as a "hook" to snag our attention. Unfortunately, the result is a distorted picture of health in America and false hope for a disease-free future. Reporters constantly need new stories, and these rat and test tube stories are easy to tell.

A special favorite is the You-Could-Be-At-Risk story. The danger could be something in the water, something in the air, something you do that you should stop doing, something you don't do that you should. The lurking evil could be a side effect of a medicine or a complication of a procedure. The risk is something you are currently unaware of that the media claims you should know. If you are uninformed, your health is at risk, and you should be afraid.

For example, a 2000 story in *The New York Times* reported the association of elevated homocysteine, an amino acid naturally found in the blood, with an increased risk of heart attacks and strokes. It quoted a physician expert advising, "People should not have to wait five or more years for the research results before trying to lower their own homocysteine levels."[9] However, studies in 2004 and 2005 showed lowering homocysteine levels by taking vitamins did not affect stroke and heart attack rates.[10, 11] As an example of an intelligent person who acquiesced to the media hype and recommendations of his physicians, President Obama had his homocysteine level measured at his check up in 2010.[12]

A corollary of the You-Could-Be-At-Risk story is the Know-Your-Number story.[13] These stories typically invoke some disease lurking in the shadows that will jump out and bite you when you least expect it. The reporter interviews an expert who advises you to run to your doctor's office for a "simple blood test" so you will know your number. An example is a plea from a doctor in a magazines and newspapers that people should "insist on routine screening" to see if they are at risk for a disease,[14] even if there is no solid evidence such testing is beneficial.

Another favorite of the media is the Suffering-Victim-Versus-The-System story. The conflict in the story is a woman pitted against ignorance, the government, and the healthcare system. An example is the story of a 56-year old woman in Iowa who has a rare disease of the lungs, lymphangioleiomyomatosis (LAM).[15] It is ultimately fatal, although it's so rare there is no good research to predict how long she might live.

She went to 50 events with presidential hopefuls in 2008 and told them about her illness. She advocated for more healthcare dollars devoted to research, intervention, and prevention. She claimed LAM is frequently misdiagnosed or missed by doctors who don't have experience with this condition. She claimed 250,000 people have LAM and don't know it. We all empathize with the woman with the disease. We all want her to be cured and live a long and healthy life.

In this kind of story, the reporter rarely challenges the interviewee's point of view. The reporter needs her to appear sympathetic, not as someone grasping at straws. The victim claims the disease is frequently misdiagnosed and more common than doctors think, but factual data to back up the claim aren't available. When a reporter interviews an expert on a rare disease, he is commonly a basic scientist or other researcher who wants more funding. This inherent conflict of interest – the temptation of the researcher to exaggerate how frequent and bad the disease is – never seems to cross the reporter's mind.

Biases in healthcare stories have been observed by others.[16] Reporters admit that emotional stories are easier to sell and that they have a bias to tell their audience to take action. A review of eight stories on lung cancer CAT scan testing found six stories failed to adequately discuss the potential harms of such screening; four stories failed to discuss the costs of such screening, which range from $200 to $1,000 per scan; and five stories relied on a single source, the authors of the published study, and failed to present independent perspectives.[16]

For the media to accurately advance public health, many of the stories I mentioned should end with the reporter saying something such as, "A medical expert wants you to be concerned about a potential health risk. However, the expert couldn't produce scientifically valid proof that either early detection or aggressive treatment of this condition saves lives or improves health. Therefore, don't worry about it for now." It's a boring conclusion, but usually the truth.

THE LAWYERS

Doctors and many other Americans really can't stand lawyers. But for the moment, I'll fight the temptation to bash the lawyers too hard.

All doctors are human. We do make mistakes. It's one of the hells of our profession – knowing that any error or oversight could result in injury or, worse, death. I understand that a legal system must exist to allow people who had less-than-stellar care, and suffered injury because of it, to be compensated for their injuries.

But in our current system, people who suffer harm typically receive only half of the settlement amount.[17, 18] A portion of the other half covers court costs and expert witnesses. The bulk of it lines the lawyers' pockets. Our inefficient legal system directly contributes to bloated healthcare costs. Many other countries handle medical malpractice differently. Most importantly, when money is awarded, the victim benefits more than the lawyers.[17]

In Canada, the total cost of settlements, legal fees, and insurance comes to $4 per person each year; in the US it is $16.[19] Average payouts to American plaintiffs are $265,103, while payouts to Canadian plaintiffs are actually higher, averaging $309,417.[20] Yet malpractice suits are far more common in the US, with 350 percent more suits filed each year per person.[19]

One justification for drastically reducing the number of medical malpractice lawsuits is the belief that healthcare costs would plummet. This argument doesn't hold true. A radical overhaul of our legal tort system wouldn't significantly impact the cost of healthcare. It would have some effect, just not as big as people think. In fact, the total cost of all malpractice awards each year is only about 0.5 percent of all healthcare costs.[19]

A better reason for drastically reducing medical malpractice cases is the indirect expense of the claims – the habit of doctors unnecessarily ordering tests and procedures to protect themselves from lawsuits by practicing so-called "defensive medicine." A widely quoted estimate of the cost of defensive medicine in the U.S. states that it adds about 5 to 9 percent to overall healthcare costs.[21]

Defensive medicine contributes a little more to our excessive healthcare costs, but the issue is actually much more complicated.

Suppose a patient saw a doctor with the common symptoms of sinus pressure and nasal drainage. For most people, these symptoms are the result of a cold and will get better on their own with minimal or no treatment. But what if a doctor thought to herself, a tumor could be in my patient's sinuses, causing the symptoms. I better order a $1,500 MRI just to be sure there is no sinus tumor or other rare disease. Is the doctor practicing defensive medicine, or is she taking excellent care of her patient by being thorough? Reasonable people could argue either position. The plaintiff's lawyers expect the doctor to order the test.

Or imagine a person is discovered to have a brain tumor and immediately visits a lawyer. Together, they start the process of suing the doctor. The lawyers order all the medical records of the client and start backtracking through them to see if the client ever reported any symptom that might possibly have been a result of a brain tumor, like dizziness, tingling, or blurry vision. If the lawyers find even one of these symptoms in their client's medical records, they start their attack by accusing the doctor of failing to meet the standard of care. They deploy the shoulda-coulda-woulda attack: the doctor should have ordered an MRI at the first sign of dizziness and detected the tumor earlier, an operation could have happened sooner, so the patient would be alive and well today. The plaintiffs assume that early detection guarantees the injury (or death) would not have occurred or been as severe. The concept that ordering too many tests or too many treatments might actually harm people never enters the conversation.

When talking about tort reform, lawyers basically say, "The bad doctors are for changes in medical malpractice laws, but the good doctors aren't because they have nothing to worry about." Actually, most doctors are sued at some point in their careers, since there are an average of 161 claims per 100 physicians.[22] A fairer depiction of the malpractice landscape is that rare things happen rarely. If a doctor practices medicine long enough, her patients will experience weird and rare events. Here are a few examples: people contract meningitis without a fever or headache; people drive themselves to an ER with a broken neck from an accident that happened two days before; and people contract colon cancer with no changes in their bowel habits or blood in their stools.

The current legal standard for doctors is perfection. No disease is rare enough to be reasonably missed; no test or treatment is too rare or expensive to order. Is a doctor who frequently orders expensive tests to look for rare conditions a thorough physician, or one who practices defensive, expensive medicine? Who is more thorough: a doctor who spends enough time talking to her patient to learn that after his symptoms started he had a normal CAT scan and MRI at another facility, or a doctor who takes five seconds to check off those tests on an order sheet?

INSURANCE COMPANIES

Health insurance as it now functions is a relatively recent development in our nation's history. In 1940, only 10 percent of the U.S. population had some form of health insurance.[23] There was no prevention to speak of. Mammograms, vaccines, and colon cancer testing hadn't been invented. Healthcare accounted for about 4 percent of the overall economy, compared to 17.3 percemt in 2009.[24]

That all changed after World War II. As the economy adjusted to the millions of soldiers coming home from the war looking for education and jobs, a period of high inflation ensued. One of the remedies was the creation of wage and price controls. Employers needed workers for their factories. They couldn't attract them by offering higher wages, but they could sweeten the benefits pot. That gave birth to the American tradition of employer-sponsored health insurance.

The early part of my career coincided with the explosive growth, then shrinkage, of the managed care industry. That hugely mismanaged fiasco shaped a lot of my current beliefs.

One of the unfortunate consequences of the managed care era was the disappearance of non-profit health insurance companies in the U.S. At the beginning of the managed care era, most insurance companies were non-profits.[25] As insurance companies gobbled each other up to gain larger and larger market share, the for-profit companies bought up the non-profits. The non-profits did not have the ability to raise enough capital to keep up, especially after a federal government program to help the non-profit HMOs was eliminated. They could not borrow enough money from banks nor could they create and sell shares of stock. As a result, for-profit plans now dominate the health insurance market in most states.

The for-profit health insurance industry is much less efficient than the non-profit industry. Journalist Maggie Mahar and healthcare analyst Niko Karvounis of the Century

Foundation reported that in the late 1970s nonprofit HMOs spent about 94 percent of premiums on members' medical treatments; by the late 1990s, for-profit HMOs spent less than 70 percent of their earnings on patients.[26] The Commonwealth Fund estimated in 2009 that the cost to our economy of the administration and net cost of private health insurance, which includes profit in investor-owned plans, was approximately $150 billion.[27]

Many members of GIMeC promote a fear of "socialized medicine," though other countries have much lower administrative costs than the U.S. In 1999, for instance, the costs for health insurance administration were $752 per person higher in the U.S. than Canada,[28] with similar differences compared to European nations.[29] It is true some European nations have national health plans run by the government, such as Britain and Sweden, but others, such as the Netherlands and Switzerland, are managed by private health insurance companies. An important difference with the U.S. is that these European companies are not permitted to make a profit. They still compete for patients, since larger customer bases mean larger salaries for the administrators of the plans. But even so, their cost of healthcare administration is more on the order of 2 to 5 cents of every dollar paid in premiums.[30]

Let's face facts. For-profit insurance companies exist to make money for their shareholders. That's it. They're not in business to donate to charities or give away merchandise unless it ultimately improves their bottom line. Corporations are considered to be persons in our legal system. They can sue and be sued. But a very important distinction between a legal corporate person and a human person is the corporation does not have a soul.

Non-profit organizations usually have a soul, or at least a conscience. Their boards make decisions based on the mission of the organization, not the bottom line. However, many of them may be quick to remind us of their day-to-day survival reality: no money, no mission. They still have to pay their bills to achieve their goals.

I realize non-profits act like for-profit companies sometimes. But at least in a non-profit organization, there are community members on its board who can question the organization's motivations and actions. This may not always happen, but it's reasonable to believe that non-profits are more likely to make decisions based on a larger sense of right and wrong.

Also in contrast to for-profit insurance companies, the federal government is more efficient with administrative overhead than most people probably realize. One study estimated Medicare administrative costs were 3 percent of its total budget, Medicaid 6.7 percent, and private health insurance plans 12.8 percent.[28] A non-profit HMO like Kaiser Permanente claims administrative costs of just 4 percent.

One reason for the low administrative costs of Medicare is a lack of advertising and marketing expenses. Medicare requires many fewer employees to process its claims than do private insurance companies. The administrative apparatus of Medicare houses one employee per 10,000 beneficiaries; whereas most large private insurers hire 15 or more employees per 10,000 beneficiaries.[28]

A fair estimate for the administrative costs of the entire healthcare system, including costs to doctors and hospitals, is about 25 percent,[25, 31, 32] which is still a lot of money spent to push paper. But since the collapse of managed care, administrative costs have skyrocketed. The Commonwealth Fund calculated administrative costs for private health insurance rose much higher than workers' earnings from 2000 to 2007: 109 percent for administrative costs vs. 24 percent for workers' earnings.[33]

Of all the GIMeC constituents, however, the insurance companies are the least wed to some of the GIMeC beliefs. Some insurers understand that primary care delivers exceptional value (though they don't understand why). They understand hospital care is more expensive than outpatient care. So why aren't they leading any big reform efforts? I can think of at least three reasons.

First, insurance companies were seriously burned by the managed care fiasco. The venom spewed by the American public towards HMOs in that era was well deserved. Some companies paid executives bonuses to deny expensive claims and dump patients with expensive conditions. We shouldn't be surprised that happened. The insurance companies' trade-off was actually very simple. Several hundreds of thousands of dollars of care could be spent on a patient, or that money could pass to shareholders. This tension never disappears in for-profit plans. Today's insurance executives are in no mood to lead cost-containment efforts. They've thrived since the collapse of the managed care era without the added headaches of cutting costs.

Second, the insurance industry charges some large employers' health plans per claim. When a company hires an insurance company to manage healthcare benefits for its employees, the insurance company may set its payment rate as a percentage of each bill submitted. The corporation may be charged $100 for a doctor's visit, which means the insurance company collects about $12. If you see five different doctors two times a year instead of seeing one family physician four times a year, the insurance company makes more money.

Third, I don't think many people realize how beholden the insurance companies are to the big employers in America. The process of insurance is nothing more than a bunch of people – all the employees at a company, for example – throwing their money into a big pot and agreeing to the following: There are a thousand of us standing around this pot of money. Three of us will have a heart attack, two will get cancer, five will sprain an ankle, and so on. At the beginning of the year we don't know which one of us will experience an expensive health event, but we pledge to each other that whoever becomes sick or injured, the others will soften the financial blow and help pay for most of the costs.

At many large companies, the decision of which health plans to offer starts with hiring a benefits broker/consultant who charges 4 percent to 11 percent of the premium dollar for advice.[30] The consultant recommends co-pay amounts, the services covered under a "wellness" benefit, and so on. Next, the company bids out the package to insurance companies in the local markets to administer the plan. The result of this process is your personal insurance package is dictated much more by your employer than the insurance company. Therefore, major reform of employer-funded health insurance is more likely to happen when the large corporations that pay for most of their employees' healthcare, not the insurance company middlemen, say enough is enough.

THE GOVERNMENT

Many Americans believe the government is largely responsible for our dysfunctional healthcare system. I believe the government's role is complicated. In some ways, Medicare and even Medicaid are very efficient. On the other hand, as I will discuss later, my time as a medical student at a Veterans Affairs hospital was awful. My days were filled waiting on lazy, dysfunctional file room clerks, admitting patients to the hospital without good reason, and watching honest, altruistic new employees have the spirit sucked out of them. I will discuss the two largest government healthcare programs, Medicare and Medicaid, throughout the book. In the meantime, let's consider two other federal agencies that influence the entire healthcare system and deserve comment.

THE NATIONAL INSTITUTES OF HEALTH (NIH)

The NIH is the largest single funder of biomedical research in the U.S., contributing roughly the same amount of research money as all U.S. drug companies combined.[34] The NIH funds research in basic science, such as learning how normal cells become cancerous and unraveling the human genome, and also funds clinical trials of experimental drugs and medical devices.

The fundamental problem with the NIH is that it historically funds research in miracles, not efficiency. It funds research to discover new treatments for diseases, but rarely funds research comparing new discoveries with established treatments. It funds research on specific diseases affecting a single part of the body, but rarely funds research on the best approach to diagnose and treat common, yet complex, symptoms such as low back pain or fatigue. NIH invests in new tests, but neglects to determine the best use of these tests, especially compared to established tests. It pursues its mission with little regard for the ultimate cost to the healthcare system. A new federal research initiative in comparative effectiveness research will help determine the best tests and treatments for some conditions, but its overall budget is a small fraction of the NIH budget,[35] and many are concerned that oversight of this new initiative is overly influenced by the medical industry.[36]

What's more, research on the cost-effectiveness of healthcare options is explicitly forbidden! When I worked at a research facility for a chemical company prior to medical school, the chemists calculated the costs of raw materials and estimated a possible sales price of the potential product before they launched any major research project. If a new chemical manufacturing process would require one dollar of raw materials to make 50 cents of product, the proposal was doomed to failure.

Medical researchers have no comparable reality check. They don't have to estimate a reasonable product price before they begin their research. Experience shows the American market will tolerate almost any price for a new drug. The eventual price consumers will have to pay has no influence on medical research priorities. To be fair to these medical researchers, American society seems reluctant to set a maximum price on any particular drug. At what point should we say, "Enough is enough"?

Thus, we have a healthcare system that does some miraculous things, but is extremely inefficient and expensive. A federal agency separate from the NIH that has some role in researching questions of healthcare system efficiency, the Agency for Healthcare Research and Quality (AHRQ), has barely 1 percent of the budget of the NIH. Even worse, most of AHRQ's budget is spent on activities such as periodic national health surveys and bioterrorism preparedness, not medical efficiency research.[37] To look at this issue another way, federal and foundation support for research on efficiency and value in healthcare amounts to less than 0.1 percent of total health expenditures.[34] Imagine a business that only spent 1/1000th of its budget to become more efficient. It wouldn't be very competitive or last very long.

Many members of Congress have enhanced their political legacies by supporting more taxpayer funding for the NIH. The NIH showed its appreciation by naming seven buildings on its campus in Bethesda, Maryland, after former key members of the Senate or House appropriations committees.[38] In fairness to the NIH and Congress, they pursue what the American people want: miraculous tests and cures. Unfortunately, we are arriving at the point where we can't afford more miracles. I have never seen any of the NIH scientists express even a hint of remorse for the economic harm caused by their ultra-expensive inventions. They find the miracles and accept the accolades; paying for the miracles is someone else's problem.

THE FOOD AND DRUG ADMINISTRATION (FDA)

The FDA contributes to inefficient healthcare in two ways. First, it doesn't insist that new drugs be compared to existing drugs before approving them. Second, it has lenient standards for approving new medical devices. The FDA has a complex relationship with companies in the medical industry. It regulates them, but also depends on them for data.

THE PHARMACEUTICAL INDUSTRY

Drug companies deliver some amazing drugs. That's their job. They invent new drugs and sell them for a profit, and there's nothing inherently wrong with that. New drugs make the quality of our lives better and help us live longer, an estimated 4.7 month increase from 1980 to 2000.[39]

Drug companies also are hugely profitable. In one recent year, they accounted for only 2 percent of the Fortune 500 companies, but 52 percent of the total profit.[40] Pharmaceutical firms have shown higher net returns for their shareholders than other Fortune 500 companies for the last two decades.[41] Drug companies spend $19-$20 billion per year on advertising and marketing,[42] which is 63 times more than the total budget for AHRQ, and also more than the drug companies themselves spend on research and development.[29]

Spurred by successful marketing efforts, drugs have been the fastest rising segment of healthcare costs in the U.S. over the last 10 years. Prescription drug spending in the U.S. increased from $12 billion to $200 billion between 1980 and 2005, which translates to an average annual increase of 11.9 percent per year over 25 years,[23] a much higher rate of inflation than any other major segment of healthcare.

When criticized, the pharmaceutical industry justifies its profitability by claiming it is a high-risk business. What they don't say is how often their new drugs are actually innovative, high-risk products. If a company invents a new drug that works differently than any other, this drug is said to represent a "new class" of drugs, which is risky to develop. Other companies quickly line up to invent drugs similar to the innovative drug, which doctors call "me-too" drugs. When the me-too drugs reach the market, they are rarely cheaper than the first drug, usually selling for about the same price. They are commonly marketed as having some better property than the first drug: less nausea, less acne, better sexual performance, etc. To receive FDA approval for a me-too drug, the company only has to show that the me-too drug works better than a placebo.[41] The FDA does not require the drug company to sponsor studies comparing the me-too drug with the original drug in head-to-head clinical trials. Just 22 percent of the drugs approved by the FDA represent major advances; the other 78 percent are me-too drugs.[37] In addition, much of the basic scientific research that drug companies rely upon is funded by the NIH. Barely 15 percent of the original studies that support drug patents are funded by the drug companies that then apply for those patents.[41] With such high percentages of me-too drugs and government funding for research, the drug companies' claim that they are in a high-risk business lacks credibility.

THE MEDICAL DEVICE COMPANIES

The first cousin to the drug industry is the medical device industry, which makes things such as pacemakers and artificial hips. Many of the dynamics of the drug industry are duplicated in the device industry – with one important distinction.

Federal oversight of new drugs began in 1938, but regulation of devices did not begin until 1976.[43] The latter date is important because the device companies had a loophole written into the FDA regulations stating they simply have to show a new device has "substantial equivalence" to an older device.[43] If there is a chain of new devices preceding 1976, a company may never have to prove the device was truly effective in the first place, and sometimes previous problems are overlooked.

This chain of approvals can lead to sad cases. In 2001, Lana Keeton, a 54-year-old woman with urinary incontinence, had surgery with a new FDA-approved mesh to restore the bladder to its proper position.[43] The mesh eroded through her bladder wall, and the woman required procedures during the next eight years to remove pieces of the mesh. She also had recurring urinary infections and pain. This particular mesh was approved using the previous-device approval process, though it turned out an earlier version of the mesh had been recalled as "adulterated and misbranded."[43] The mesh is now off the market, and dozens of lawsuits are in progress.

The second problem with device approval is the amount of proof required. The FDA bar is set lower for devices than drugs. For instance, a company manufacturing surgical plates and screws for back surgery just has to show the devices stabilize the back after disk surgery, not that the devices reduce low back pain for many years. Likewise, a company making a device that zaps painful nerves has to show the device temporarily knocks out nerve function without damaging too much surrounding tissue; long-term effectiveness is never questioned. A review of cardiovascular devices by researchers at the University of California at San Francisco concluded that approval by the FDA is often based on weak studies prone to bias.[44] Sadly, this seems the rule, not the exception.

DOCTORS

OK, I'll admit it. The cup on my desk is full of pens with the names of drugs on them. I received them as freebies from representatives of drug companies, a practice now forbidden. My supply should last for at least another year. I'd like to think the brief sales pitches that accompanied these pens didn't corrupt my medical decisions, but maybe I'm just deluding myself.

But the truth is, I missed out on the golden era of drug and device company excesses. In medical school, I heard stories of physicians flown with their families to ski and beach resorts for four-day weekends. In return, the doctors would have to listen to a half-day sales pitch disguised as medical education. Just when I was about to graduate from medical school, the drug companies and doctors agreed to reign in some of these abuses. Further restrictions were announced in 2009, which is when the ban on pens came into effect.

Although they are loathe to admit it, doctors are people, too, and can be influenced by attractive salespeople who are still allowed to bring food to their offices. Some doctors' offices schedule complete meals provided by the drug companies for the doctors and their entire staffs most days of the week. The pharmaceutical industry spent more than $7 billion a year on direct marketing to doctors in 2005 – about $10,000 per doctor[45] – and employed approximately 90,000 salespeople – one for every five doctors (recent layoffs may have reduced this number somewhat).[41] Drug companies also influence patients directly. They spend more than $4 billion a year in direct advertising to the public (Viagra commercials, for example).[45] For every dollar the drug industry spends on direct advertising to the public, it increases revenue by four dollars.[46]

Drug companies also influence doctors in other ways. They pay for doctors to write diagnostic and treatment guidelines.[47] They give money to disease advocacy groups and discuss their products with these associations' members, who then commonly advocate that these drugs must be made available to everyone who might possibly benefit, no matter how preliminary the scientific proof of the drug's effectiveness. At one of these disease association meetings, the President of the American Medical Association, Nancy Nielson, MD, PhD, described the discussion with some of these disease advocates as, "the most anti-science one I had been in for a long time."[47]

Drug companies grow angry when doctors don't support their view of the world. Documents released in Vioxx litigation found that employees of Merck, one of the largest pharmaceutical companies, discussed a "list of 'problem' physicians that [they] must, at a minimum, neutralize."[48] This list included more than 30 U.S. physicians who were described as "important from a business perspective in terms of influence and/or prescribing" and "not as supportive of Merck and/or Vioxx as we would like."[48] Merck tried to neutralize these doctors with offers of money for research, education, and funding for medical schools.

There are ways to minimize the effect of drug companies on physicians' practices, but it isn't free. The state of

Pennsylvania spends about $1 million a year on its pharmaceutical "unsales" force – 11 consultants, including some former drug company sales people, assigned to the 28 counties with the highest concentrations of seniors enrolled in discount drug programs.[49] This unsales force visits doctors in hospitals and clinics and tries to convince them that less-expensive drugs are just as effective as the expensive drugs. For example, the cost of a 20 mg daily dose of cholesterol drugs can range from 13 cents for generics to $4.53 for the more expensive brand names.[49] The program saved Pennsylvania $572,000 per year on heartburn medicines alone.[49]

MEDICAL SCHOOLS

While we're on the subject of doctors, it would be a good time to talk about the place that produces them. Medical schools train the next generation of doctors, produce much of the medical research in the U.S., serve as important economic engines for their communities, and are home to most of the American winners of the Nobel Prize in medicine. One estimate of the economic impact of medical schools and their affiliated teaching hospitals was $512 billion in 2008.[50]

Many physicians who are professors at a typical medical school lead triple lives. They teach medical students, care for some patients, and conduct research funded by outside organizations such as drug companies, the federal government, and foundations. Of the three activities, research commonly dominates the medical professors' thoughts and careers. Research sucks millions of outside dollars into the school, whether the source is private foundations, generous donors, or government agencies. Some medical schools have different tracks for their professors. They might have a teaching track or a clinical care track, but the big promotions and all the publicity belong to the researchers. Medical schools are extremely dependent on outside revenue streams. Among the top 20 research medical schools, upwards of one-third of their revenue comes from outside research donations and contracts.[51]

The researchers (and their bosses, the medical school administrators) are the ones who promise the miracles – the cure "we're oh-so-close to." The researchers attract the huge donations – the $50 million buildings bearing the name of a wealthy couple. The researchers are admired by medical students and held up by the institution as the ideal physicians – the physician-scientists who ease suffering and save lives with their discoveries.

But these same researchers are not burdened by issues of cost-effectiveness when they submit their grants requests to invent a new drug. They do not have to estimate how much the drug they're trying to invent will ultimately cost. All they have to do is convince someone with access to bags and bags of money that they can find a cure for a horrible disease.

The problem with medical schools is a lack of balance. The predominant culture says every doctor should be this combination of basic scientist and clinician. The truth is, most practicing physicians don't need the amount of basic science the medical schools want to teach in order to provide top-quality care. If medical students had unlimited brainpower and time, all that basic science would be justified. Unfortunately, when medical schools push a large basic science curriculum, they must sacrifice time that could have been spent teaching the practical aspects of caring for patients.

By practical aspects, I'm not referring to bedside manners. Many medical schools teach students how to draw a picture of a cholesterol molecule, but say nothing about the basic guidelines of when to order cholesterol tests or what cholesterol level justifies treatment. Which would you prefer that your doctor knew? I find that medical students today can tell you where a chromosome was damaged to cause lung cancer, but they can't interpret a chest X-ray. They can tell you what happens on a microscopic level to cause an electrical signal to fire through the heart, but they can't interpret an EKG. Medical schools seem focused on training the next generation of laboratory researchers, not a cadre of broad-minded physicians who can actually care for patients.

Medical schools are funded by fear. The more medical schools can scare people into believing a long list of dreaded diseases is lurking in the shadows, held at bay only by the intrepid researcher handicapped by his lack of funding, the more dollars pour in from donors and state and federal governments.

AMERICAN MEDICAL ASSOCIATION

After young doctors graduate from all their training, some join the American Medical Association (AMA), though the majority don't. (Full disclosure: I have been a member of the AMA for two decades.) The same core beliefs exist within the AMA as at the medical schools, so those points will not be repeated. Suffice it to say that between the AMA's newsletters and its other mailings received during my career, every disease known to man has had an advocate pronounce that primary care physicians should screen for it so that it can be caught early. Oh and by the way, with more research dollars we could cure the disease, and *we're this close* to finding a cure.

The AMA appropriately represents universal physician interests on many issues, particularly those such as reducing the impact of medical malpractice lawsuits, making sure Medicare and Medicaid have adequate funding, and fighting unreasonable policies of the insurance companies.

On the other hand, the AMA has been mostly silent, until very recently, on the power of generalist physicians' care. The AMA is primarily an organization of "ologists" – specialists in one field or another. A strong generalist physician base is a threat to the AMA's status quo. The AMA certainly hasn't led any discussions about a more limited role for the healthcare system in society. "More is better" is simply assumed.

HOSPITALS

To achieve a more affordable healthcare system in the future, hospitals must be part of the solution because they are the single largest contributor to healthcare costs, accounting for roughly one-third of all costs.[52]

In the managed care era, one of the interesting horse races was between the hospitals and the managed care companies. Who would become dominant? Who would ultimately define the prices charged for a day in the hospital? In many markets, hospitals consolidated to the point that they commanded enough market share to gain the upper hand in setting prices. If a managed care company walked out of a negotiation because the company thought the prices demanded were too high, the remaining hospitals lacked the capacity to care for all the managed care members. The hospitals won.

Hospitals achieved the upper hand because politicians and influential citizens often viewed them as local resources with long histories of community involvement. Managed care companies were seen as menacing national behemoths that couldn't care less if cherished local institutions survived or not.

As a result of this consolidation, hospitals now hold a powerful position to dictate charges for all their services. Medicare regulations put a damper on hospitals' ability to charge whatever they want, but not much. Consequently, bed costs per day in American hospitals run about three times as much as most European hospitals: $1,850 per day vs. $653 per day in 1999.[53]

When I walk into the lobby of many private hospitals, I see expensive leather chairs and couches, shiny surfaces, and hand-painted portraits of local leaders on the walls. Many hospitals are appointed like expensive hotels. Someone has to pay for these amenities.

I do have some sympathy for hospitals because the federal government forces them to absorb many unfunded mandates. The government may require hospitals to track some new drug side effect or emerging infection, for example, and report what they are doing to minimize the potential dangers. Hospitals commonly have to hire a new nurse to oversee such projects – more measurements require more personnel to collect data and write reports. And, of course, the results are filtered through a series of administrators and meetings, all of which take an enormous amount of time and human resources. The hospital absorbs these expenses from its general revenues. Do the Feds then calculate an estimated cost of these mandates and raise the allowable hospital fees to meet the requirements? No.

The Feds typically pay the hospitals nothing. PricewaterhouseCoopers estimated in 2001 that 15 percent of healthcare inflation was caused by unfunded government mandates and regulations.[54]

Hospitals also must cover the costs of treating uninsured patients who show up at the ER door. Sometimes, treatments can run into the hundreds of thousands or even millions of dollars, because hospitals are required to cover legitimate medical needs no matter what they cost. One potential advantage of a national healthcare plan would be to decrease some of the ridiculous markups hospitals currently charge in the name of covering unfunded mandates and uninsured patients.

Hospital charges are often like Pentagon charges. Hospitals would charge $600 for a toilet seat if they could get away with it. The charges hospitals generated for their services in 2004 were three times the Medicare-allowable cost, which means they were more than three times what it actually cost them to deliver the care.[55]

One of the greatest injustices of the American healthcare system is that these inflated charges are billed to the uninsured working poor in America. For some of these people, they absolutely cannot pay these exorbitant bills, and the hospital ends up eating the cost of care. However, many conscientious Americans spend years trying to pay their debts, and some are simply unable. *Newsweek* told the story of Julie Basem, a 20-year-old uninsured dancer living in New York who injured her knee and sought care.[56] About $40,000 later, her only way out of the jam was to declare bankruptcy.

Our current situation isn't entirely the hospitals' fault. The lion's share of the blame falls on Medicare, whose complex rules (which I don't pretend to fully understand) encourage hospitals to increase their charges as much as possible. Some of the Medicare reimbursement formulas are based on charges, not actual costs.

What's worse, Medicare doesn't just expect hospitals to report their unpaid charges. Medicare forces them to aggressively pursue their uninsured customers. For one federal uncompensated care program, the hospital has to prove to the bureaucrats that it tried *at least four times* to collect the full amount charged to uninsured patients who were admitted. Medicare doesn't allow hospitals to initially charge uninsured Americans on a more reasonable sliding scale.

NON-PROFIT DISEASE ADVOCACY GROUPS

Finally, I've come to the sad conclusion that well-meaning disease advocacy groups also contribute to the exorbitant cost of American healthcare. I'm talking about organizations such as the Susan G Komen Foundation for the Cure, the American Cancer Society, the American Heart Association, etc.

One problem I have with them is that they wrongly have convinced the public that catching a disease in its early stages will – without a doubt – lessen its impact on an individual's life. I'll explain why this is often untrue in Chapter 4.

My main problem with these groups, however, is that they are extremely single-minded, and none of them seriously considers the impact that increased spending on "their" disease has on the greater healthcare system. They rarely, if ever, compare the resources required for their advocated positions to other possible uses of those resources. You will never hear one of these groups issue a statement such as, "We could use a much more expensive technology on thousands of people, which will allow us to detect a few more cases of (fill in the blank) than the tests we use today. But overall, the impact would be small, and since there's no proof that this expensive new technology would actually save lives, we should stick with the old technology." These groups assume the newer the technology, the better. The costs are someone else's problem.

To give just one example, the use of cholesterol medicines in young people has been rising rapidly. The number of people 20 to 44 years old taking cholesterol medicines jumped 68 percent in a six-year period, so roughly 4.2 million Americans in this age group now take cholesterol medicines.[57]

"This is good news, that more people in this age range are taking these medicines," claims Dr. Daniel W. Jones, president of the American Heart Association.[57] But at best, this undertaking will cost a lot of money over a lot of years and save very few lives. (I'll expand on this point in the next chapter.)

To give credit where it's due, the American Cancer Society recently had the courage and honesty to question some of its past beliefs, although news accounts stated the Society made changes on its website "quietly."[58] The Cancer Society now recognizes screening for breast, prostate, and certain other cancers come with a real risk of overtreating many small cancers while missing cancers that are deadly.

I have a dream. Actually, a twisted daydream. I want to take the representatives of every disease advocacy group (and their ologist supporters) and lock them in a room. My instructions would be: "You can come out of the room when you all agree on one disease that someone could contract and ultimately die from without labeling it a 'tragedy.' This chosen disease must not be fought with fundraisers, 5K races, t-shirts, colored ribbons, or more research to find a cure. You are not allowed to cop out and choose 'old age.' You must agree on a specific disease before you can leave." I seriously doubt anyone would ever come out of that room.

GIMeC AND THE ROLE OF HOPE

How has the GIMeC belief system become so integrated into American healthcare? By telling us all what we want to hear, GIMeC has subverted the important role of hope in the way Americans deal with injuries, illness, and death. Hope is important for any person or society, but it is especially crucial to the American psyche. Americans are optimistic by nature. Americans love to celebrate individuals who succeed, including those who overcome life-threatening diseases.

How many times have you watched a story on the news about a person with cancer? The reporter typically states the person is a fighter, determined to defeat the dreaded disease. The story inspires us and gives all of us hope that one day, if we are faced with a similar diagnosis, we will fight and be cured.

What's wrong with this picture? GIMeC has warped our perspective into believing the only source of hope resides in CAT scans, laser surgeries, and chemotherapies. GIMeC doesn't accept other sources of hope, such as the possibility a person might be better off going through the last phase of his or her life not controlled by doctors' visits and toxic treatment regimens.

Many people don't desire as much aggressive medical care as they're given. For many years, researchers at Dartmouth have studied variation in medical care across the country. They conclude patients generally prefer less intense care than is ordered by doctors, even after families and caregivers make extensive efforts to inform those doctors of the wishes of the seriously ill patients.[59]

A team of researchers in Southern California tried to create care environments friendlier to patients' wishes. They developed a program in five hospitals to improve the care of patients at the end of their lives, but the researchers were unable to affect how often the patients' wishes were achieved.[60] Among the patients who preferred to die at home, the majority (55 percent) actually died in the hospital. At the same time, less than half (46 percent) of those who preferred to die in the hospital actually did. The local healthcare systems forced patients to conform to its excess hospital capacity. The beliefs of GIMeC trumped the patients' wishes.

When should a patient with a severe illness, such as a recurrence of cancer, stop expecting a cure? It's a very difficult question to answer. If and when a person accepts that she will die from this cancer, how can there be hope?

Hope persists, but it must be based on different expectations. Patients who accept that they have entered the final phase of their lives hope for successful closure. They hope for good relationships with their families, including mending old grievances. They hope for good days in spite of the disease. They hope for one more Christmas with their grandchildren. They hope for a gentle death. They hope for life after death. Hope not only can exist without technology, it does.

GIMeC

Now that I have discussed all the major co-conspirators of GIMeC, let's group them by category for future reference:

Government

- o *Medicare*
- o *Medicaid*
- o *NIH*
- o *FDA*

Industries

- o *Legal industry*
- o *Insurance companies*
- o *Pharmaceutical industry*
- o *Medical device industry*
- o *Media*

Medical Establishment

- o *Medical schools*
- o *Doctors and their professional organizations (the AMA and related groups)*
- o *Hospitals*
- o *Disease advocacy groups*

THE GIMeC ASSUMPTIONS

In this chapter, I alluded to the core beliefs that GIMeC almost never challenges. Let's call them the POEM assumptions:

- Prevention saves money
- Ologist (specialist) care is best
- Early detection cures everything
- More treatments equal better care

PART OF THE SOLUTION

Each of the members of GIMeC must change for a more efficient and caring American healthcare system. Some of these changes could happen quickly – as in, right now – but others will require serious reworking of our medical culture and governmental regulations. Medicare and Medicaid are behemoths that require major overhauls. Since it is premature, at this point in our journey, to discuss some of my proposed changes to these programs, I will add pieces to that puzzle throughout the book.

NIH

We can't afford every medicine the research industry, including the NIH, has created. Inventing more drugs costing $5,000 per dose will only make healthcare more expensive.

A much larger share of federal research dollars must be diverted to research on healthcare efficiency, rather than spending almost every penny on discovering miracles. The new federal research initiative called "comparative effectiveness research" will help, as will a small new NIH research program in health economics,[61] but the balance of funding for miracles compared to efficiency remains seriously out of touch with the real needs of the healthcare system. Doctors who want to practice medicine ethically but efficiently have little high-quality research to guide them.

FDA

The FDA should insist that all new drugs be compared to the existing treatment for a particular disease or symptom before the drug is approved. The FDA also should insist that medical devices meet the same standard of proof as drugs. The FDA is already moving in that direction in a few areas, but it is taking baby steps on what will be a long journey. Also, as a nation we need to recognize that regulatory efforts to reduce risks, such as some drug side effects, become exceedingly expensive as the risk becomes rarer. There has to be *some* level of risk that we just accept as part of life.

THE LEGAL INDUSTRY

The tort system must allow more of the damages awarded in medical malpractice cases to go to the victim. Lawyers and juries have to accept that rare events occur rarely, and it is extraordinarily expensive and unrealistic to try to prevent every possible rare event that might potentially occur.

THE INSURANCE INDUSTRY

For those of you with private employer-sponsored health insurance, you and your employer are the key to a more affordable healthcare system. Major reform of the healthcare finance and delivery system can start with the large corporations that actually pay for much of U.S. healthcare. Start a conversation with your company's benefits managers and tell them you would like to consider radically different approaches to healthcare.

THE PHARMACEUTICAL AND MEDICAL DEVICE INDUSTRIES

The next time you don't feel 100 percent, ask yourself: "Do I really need a pill, or would a little time and patience allow my symptoms to run their course?" Resist the urge to run to your doctor's office after you see a pharmaceutical ad on TV. If something mentioned on a TV ad didn't really bother you before, why should it now?

Also, encourage your company's health plan to tell drug and medical device companies demanding exorbitant prices for their new products: "No. We won't buy your product because it costs too much."

THE MEDIA

Be a discriminating consumer of claims of medical companies or doctors with something to sell. Because so many news stories are based on the assumption that early detection of disease makes all the difference in the world, be slow to rush out and pay for a screening test you've never heard of. I will expand on this point when I talk about the limits of early detection.

MEDICAL SCHOOLS

More family physicians must be on the faculty of medical schools and teach more of the courses. The curriculum should lessen the emphasis on basic sciences and return to teaching more practical patient care. Most importantly, federal and state governments must create a funding environment that ensures the long-term success of family medicine professors and departments. My family physician educator colleagues and I receive money from Medicare to offset the cost of running a training program. Because these educational dollars are based on dollars charged to Medicare, the ologists and their multi-thousand dollar procedures have a huge advantage over doctors receiving just $50 per patient visit.

Attracting outside research dollars will always be important to medical school faculty members. Therefore, the NIH should establish a new research institute, the National Institute of Family Medicine. Its mission will be to answer the clinical knowledge needs of family physicians in practice. Examples include research to find the most efficient methods to investigate and treat vague or mild symptoms, to compare treatments for common symptoms and diseases, to explore the intersection of mental and physical health, to study complex healthcare systems and make them more efficient, and to maximize the delivery of healthcare to rural America.

AMERICAN MEDICAL ASSOCIATION

The AMA must change the structure of its House of Delegates to insure a 50/50 mix of generalists and ologists (and no, OB/Gyns aren't generalists). It must acknowledge that doctors are a large reason healthcare is so expensive. Medical malpractice pressures explain some of the expense, but that's only a small part of the story. The AMA must develop a new understanding of medical ethics that balances the needs of individuals with the needs of the community.

HOSPITALS

Hospitals should be challenged on their charges. If you serve on the board of a hospital, question requests to spend large amounts of money on amenities that are attractive but don't directly contribute to patient care. Medicare must change its rules so hospitals can set sliding scales fees that are reasonable for uninsured patients, most of whom make average to below average wages.

DISEASE ADVOCACY GROUPS

Disease advocacy groups must be willing to balance the needs of their causes with the needs of the greater healthcare system. They must be more humble and slower to recommend that physicians order numerous tests and treatments without definitive proof of effectiveness.

3 | HOW GIMeC THINKS

ONE NIGHT IN THE ER

As many family physicians do, I worked in emergency rooms for 11 years, including a full-time position at a Level 2 trauma center for two of those years. As soon as I finished my intern year and acquired the necessary licenses and certificates, I signed on as a moonlighter with a company that held ER physician contracts in many hospitals. My first jobs were 48- to 60-hour shifts covering a rural ER over an entire weekend. Small town hospitals hired people like me to give their local family physicians a break over the weekend so they would be less likely to burn out and leave town.

These shifts were great on many levels. The locals appreciated me being there and "giving Doc Billings a break." The local ambulance systems knew these small ERs didn't have the capacity to handle major traumas or burns, so I never saw those patients. Everything else was fair game, though. As for the medical capacity of the entire county that weekend, I was it. It was an ideal environment for a young physician to gain confidence that he could handle anything that walked through the door. For the most part, few clinical situations entered the rural ER that I hadn't already learned to handle in my large urban family medicine residency. Help for the more unusual cases was only a phone call away.

Usually, my biggest challenge over the weekend was to avoid being overfed. My first few weekends, a sweet elderly woman who cooked meals for the patients and nursing staff would ask me what I wanted to eat, then bring it to my call room a few minutes later. I didn't want to be rude, so I kept saying "yes ma'am" as she asked if I wanted another type of vegetable, then "my famous biscuits," followed by "the best chocolate pie you ever had." The portions were obscene. Several nights of limited sleep caused by the sting of acid reflux convinced me that I somehow had to politely decline her offerings. We eventually reached a happy medium.

Over time, I inched up the ER food chain and transferred to larger volume ERs that paid more per hour. At that stage of my career, one weekend a month I left my family medicine job and worked Friday night in an ER, slept Saturday, covered the ER again Saturday night, then showed up for work back at my family medicine job on Monday morning. I might drag a little on those Mondays, but it wasn't too bad. I was still relatively young.

Covering the graveyard shift of an urban emergency room in 2001, my first patient one night was a 70-year-old woman whose chief complaint was chest pain, according to the intake nurse. The patient told a completely different story.

Whenever I start a conversation with a patient, I always begin with an open-ended statement like, "Hello Mrs. Jones. I'm Dr. Young. What can I do for you this evening?" Or, "What brings you to the ER?" I want my patient to feel completely free to set the agenda. Maybe later in the visit I'll steer the conversation to something I need to cover, but at the beginning, it's her show.

That night, Mrs. Jones (a pseudonym) said, "I feel fine. Can I go home?"

I waited a few moments. "Why did you come here in the first place?"

"I just wasn't feeling myself earlier. I was tired and had a little trouble breathing, but I'm fine now."

At this point I felt I needed to be more direct. "What about your chest pain?"

"I don't have any chest pain."

"What about earlier?"

"I never had chest pain."

The conversation went on like this for another five minutes. She'd had heart surgery five years earlier. People with blocked coronary arteries can experience shortness of breath without chest pain, especially elderly women, but it's unusual. I asked her about the symptoms that led to the bypass to see if any commonality existed between that event and her current feeling. But she'd had classic-sounding anginal pain five years prior, which led to the bypass, and she'd felt nothing like that the day I saw her. I asked her half a dozen other chest-pain related questions, and she steadfastly denied any of those feelings that day or even during the previous few months.

I asked her to wait a moment so I could talk to the nurse who wrote "chest pain" in her note. As I feared, the day nurse's shift had ended, and she already had driven away.

I finished my exam of Mrs. Jones. Everything was perfectly normal for a 70-year-old woman: a few wrinkles and sun-damaged skin, some arthritic joints, but clear lungs, good pulses, normal vital signs, and only a very soft heart murmur. I convinced her to stick around a little longer to let me get an

EKG. It was technically abnormal, but looked exactly like one recorded on her a year earlier. Faced with this woman who said she had no symptoms and wanted to go home, I filled out my paperwork and discharged her with the usual list of warnings – come back immediately if the symptoms return, etc. She climbed in her car and drove herself home.

Our forms had a lot of preprinted information on them. To document that a person had no chest pain, I drew a straight line through that preprinted phrase. I remember thinking at the time that I should write out more on a separate piece of paper to document how many ways I attempted to find out whether she had chest pain. However, the early evening is the busy time for an ER, and other patients were stirring, poking their heads out of curtains and asking whoever would make eye contact, "How much longer before the doctor sees me?" ER doctors, driven by patient satisfaction report cards, also are pressured by hospital administrators to see patients quickly. I concluded that I had appropriately documented Mrs. Jones had no chest pain and moved on to other patients, a decision I would regret later.

The punch line to this story isn't that she walked out of the ER and died that night of a heart attack. In fact, over the following week she saw her primary physicians twice and called their office two other times. They made a few chronic medication adjustments and reassured her that nothing was seriously wrong with her.

A week after I saw her, she walked into a different ER in another part of town with a packed suitcase. Her chief complaint was that she just didn't feel well and had come to "check myself into the hospital." Mrs. Jones' vital signs were essentially normal. The ER docs at that facility started a typical work-up of tests and hung a bag of IV fluid, probably as much out of habit as any other specific reason.

While this work-up was underway, Mrs. Jones told the ER doctor she was nauseated. The ER doctor ordered a commonly used drug called Compazine to relieve her symptom. I probably would have done the same if I had been there. The nurse gave the medicine through Mrs. Jones' IV port. About five minutes later Mrs. Jones crashed. She became unresponsive, and her blood pressure dropped from normal to barely detectable. The ER team inserted a plastic tube in her windpipe, hooked her up to a breathing machine, ran in more IV fluids, started another IV medicine to force her blood pressure back up, and alerted the ICU doctor on call. The resuscitation efforts were successful. She made it to the ICU with improved vital signs.

Why did Mrs. Jones crash? It turned out she had a heart condition called mitral valve prolapse. Once in a great while, Compazine can cause a sudden drop of blood pressure in patients with this condition.

I had never heard of this rare side effect prior to this case. I don't blame the ER doctors for giving her Compazine. I had given the same medicine to hundreds of patients with no hint of that bad reaction. It's completely unreasonable for anyone – patients, lawyers, reporters, quality inspectors – to expect doctors to memorize every rare side effect of the thousands of drugs approved for use. (Electronic health records won't really help, either. But more on that later.)

In the ICU it was determined that Mrs. Jones had too much fluid in her chest caused by an exacerbation of her pre-existing heart failure. She didn't mention she had this condition when I saw her, but that wouldn't have changed anything I did.

It's impossible to know how much of the fluid in her chest had been building up over the few weeks prior to her second ER visit, how much had built quickly from the sudden stress on her heart caused by her reaction to Compazine, or how much was the result of the IV fluid pumped into her veins during her time in the ER. The chest X-ray demonstrating the excess fluid wasn't shot until after she made it to the ICU.

Mrs. Jones came off the breathing machine in two days and remained hospitalized for a week. She was discharged to a skilled nursing facility for rehabilitation, which is common when elderly patients become deconditioned after being bed-bound in a hospital for a week, especially if part of that stay included being paralyzed by medication in an ICU. Three weeks later she went home.

Throughout all this, she never had a heart attack. A few weeks later she told her primary doctor that she felt mostly back to normal, although she was a little weaker overall. About a month after that she was readmitted to a hospital with heart failure and again was moved to a rehabilitation facility. This time, she couldn't really regain her strength, had discussions with her healthcare team, and decided to sign an Advance Directive stating she didn't want any future resuscitation efforts. She enrolled in a hospice program and some two months later died from heart failure.

THE SUMMONS

Six months after Mrs. Jones died, a stranger appeared at my front door and handed me a folded document of a few pages. I was being sued for medical malpractice.

Mrs. Jones had a son who was upset at her death and the care she received over this entire period. She apparently lived alone, and her son was an only child. His father was either long gone or dead. The details of what happened after I saw her came from her medical records, which I received as part of my legal defense.

The summons is weighted down by all the expected legal verbiage, but in essence the plaintiff's major claim was that I should have admitted her to the hospital and called a cardiologist to evaluate her. If I'd done so, according to the claim, she certainly would still be alive today.

Don't feel too sorry for me just yet. The ER is widely recognized as a high liability environment because of cases such as this. If nothing else, statistically a small number of patients seen in an ER will die within a short time of leaving. It doesn't take a genius attorney to construct an accusation that the ER physician could possibly have done something to prevent the death. Everyone who accepts the role of ER physician knows this is one of the downsides of the job.

This case is a useful launching pad to discuss the underlying beliefs of GIMeC that lead to these kinds of lawsuits. Remember the four POEM assumptions of GIMeC from Chapter 2? These four assumptions are the most important factors driving our unaffordable healthcare system. Three of the four were prominent in this case.

ASSUMPTION #1 – OLOGIST CARE IS BEST
WHAT EXACTLY IS AN OLOGIST?

Doctors are commonly described as being one of two types: specialists or primary care physicians.

Any person, doctors included, wants to be thought of as special. Unfortunately, that root word, "special," carries implications of the relative value of doctors and the best approaches to healthcare systems.

But let's level the rhetorical playing field and look at physicians in a slightly different way. Some doctors take care of the whole person; those are the generalists. Some doctors take care of only part of a person, or perform only certain procedures. Most of their titles end in the suffix -ologist: cardiologist, dermatologist, urologist, etc. (For the purpose of this book, let's lump all the surgical fields into this category, as well.) Ologist physicians dominate America's healthcare system.

An ologist might take care only of your bones, your skin, or your liver. Ologists might cut off only pieces of you and sew you back together. Some ologists might limit their cutting to just a few body parts. Some ologists do nothing but knock you out so you don't feel anything when another ologist cuts you open. Yet another ologist will look at the piece of you that was sliced off under a microscope to help make a diagnosis. Ologists do many amazing things. Many Americans know an ologist saved their lives or made a significant impact on their quality of life, such as easing pain or restoring sight. Healthcare systems will always need ologists. The more important questions are: how many ologists are really needed, and how exactly should they be used?

Tests have been conducted to compare the relative knowledge of ologists about their favorite body part to generalists. As expected, the ologists scored better.[1] Other studies measured disease-specific performance on things such as whether an ologist's or generalist's patients are taking a certain drug for a certain disease. The ologists tended to do better in those measures, too, but not by much.[1] However, when the view is at 50,000 feet and the measure is the overall health of a population, having more ologists just doesn't help.[2]

THE "MISTER POTATO HEAD™" APPROACH TO HEALTHCARE

Ologists believe in the Mister Potato Head™ approach to healthcare, which assumes each major body part is separate from all the other body parts. In this model of healthcare delivery, if you have a heart problem you go to the heart doctor. If you have a nose problem you go to the nose doctor, and so on. This approach assumes the body parts are not interdependent.

There are at least two problems to this approach. First, the body parts *are* dependent on one another. Second, a multi-ologist healthcare system is not what the majority of Americans want.

Two independent research firms conducted a national study of Americans about their thoughts on an ideal health care system from about 2002 to 2003.[3] The people interviewed said they wanted a doctor who knew them as a person, knew their medical history, and provided the majority of their care. If they need something unusual, surgery to remove a gallbladder for example, they wanted a doctor who did a lot of those procedures to take care of that particular need, but afterward they wanted to return to their personal physician for the majority of their care. They didn't want to bounce from doctor to doctor if one physician could meet their needs.

How many times have you or someone you have known asked an ologist about a health concern not directly related to that ologist's favorite body part? For instance, if you mentioned headaches to your cardiologist, how likely is it that he or she would ask about your symptoms, examine your head, and prescribe an effective treatment for the headaches?

Ologists are quick to hold up their hand and say, "That's not my field (or even, "That's not my problem"). You need to see another doctor." At this point, the ologist commonly will support his body-part brethren and advise the patient to see another ologist, not her family physician.

A classic example of how Mister Potato Head™ healthcare can prove harmful is a patient hospitalized with both heart failure and kidney failure. Usually, a heart does better when it has to pump less body fluid (blood); a kidney does better with more fluid. I have personally observed, on more than one occasion, a conflict between ologists caring for a patient with both diseases. The heart doctors write orders to decrease or stop IV fluid; the kidney doctors write orders to increase it. The two ologists rarely convene to discuss the treatment trade-offs and compromise. Rather, the unwitting patient receives the amount of IV fluid ordered by the doctor who saw the patient last. Patients such as this need generalists to make the difficult decision of balancing the needs of the heart and the kidney to arrive at the best solution for the whole person.

A MAN WITH CHEST PAIN

To illustrate how ologists can waste healthcare resources through their love of technology, consider another case of a man with chest pain. Ed was about 63 when his chest started hurting, and the pain progressively worsened with exercise over the span of a few weeks. Ed was still employed, active, and had no medical problems to speak of. His pain got to the point that it would begin with relatively little exertion, so he went to see his family physician. The family physician ran an EKG and saw no immediate problems, but recognizing these symptoms as a bad thing, he referred Ed to a cardiologist, who appropriately ordered a series of tests that showed Ed had significant cholesterol blockage in one of the arteries supplying blood directly to the heart muscle.

So far, this is an example of the appropriate use of an ologist. The family physician did not have the keys to the heart lab at the hospital, but that's where Ed needed to be. This ologist added value, because the right test was done at the right time without inefficiency or duplication of services.

The ologist was able to maneuver a small balloon into the blocked artery, blow up the balloon, significantly push back the blockage, and thereby improve the flow of blood through the artery. Ed had an uneventful recovery and was pain free when he went home.

Ed's care now became unusual in that he did exactly what he should have. He changed his diet, lost weight, restarted his abandoned exercise program, and took his cholesterol medicine consistently.

Ed saw a different cardiologist for follow-up care, who to his credit wasn't enamored with the typical, high-dollar cardiologist toys: heart catheterizations, balloon procedures, stent placements, etc. This doctor viewed himself as more of a preventive cardiologist and enjoyed discussing new theories on diets and the like. Ed kept seeing his family physician, but left all of the cardiovascular monitoring up to the cardiologist, including decisions about cholesterol drugs.

The family physician now couldn't do much for Ed because his well-controlled cholesterol blockage was his only significant medical issue. Ed made it clear by his actions he wanted to keep seeing his cardiologist, even though he was having no further heart symptoms. Ed also felt the family physician was rushed, whereas the cardiologist spent more time talking to him. (I'll talk more about why this happens later, in the chapter on how physicians are paid.)

The cardiologist provided appropriate care, but he would order extra blood work, such as cholesterol tests, not supported by top-quality research. Some of the cholesterol panels cost more than a thousand dollars just for blood work. He would periodically order other tests costing several thousand dollars each, such as cardiac scans also not recommended by standard medical guidelines.

All these extra tests were for a man who had no chest pain, who could walk on a treadmill for an hour at the maximal heart rate for his age, who lost enough weight to return to the weight he was in his forties, and who kept detailed logs of his cholesterol levels, liver tests, and medicine doses for years on an Excel spreadsheet. To put it another way, his insurance company initially, then Medicare later on, wasted gobs of money on unnecessary tests.

When the cardiologist ordered nonstandard tests, he was taking money away first from the other employees where the man worked – they all contributed some of their wages into the insurance pool paying for the tests – and next from the American taxpayers when Medicare took over payment of his medical bills. I'm sure the cardiologist meant well and believed he provided top-quality medical care to his patient. But did he really have the right to force so much money to change hands without the consent of the people actually paying for the care, when the justification for ordering these tests was so flimsy – he just felt like it?

A better approach would have been to ask Ed how much exercise he could do without chest pain. That conversation would have supplied enough information to tell a reasonable physician the man's heart was just fine. As expected, the many thousands of dollars invested in testing Ed showed what was clear before the tests were ordered: his heart was working properly.

Now 16 years later, Ed is 79 and still walking on the treadmill for an hour several days a week. He is still thin. He is still taking his medications as he should. He still hasn't had a bit of chest pain. His ability to put his heart under stress with exercise and his complete lack of symptoms were a more powerful predictor of his longevity than any battery of expensive tests could be. He's in great health partly from the system, but more importantly because he began to make smart choices and take care of himself. And Ed – he's my father.

Parents, they never listen.

GENERALISTS

A generalist physician will take care of any part of your body, including mental health concerns. The most complete generalist, the family physician, can care for any person who walks into his office or hospital unit. The patient could be either sex, any age, and have any symptom or disease.

A common misconception about family physicians vis a vis the ologists is that only the best medical students become ologists. For the most part, ologists are trained completely separate from family physicians. The best family medicine training is in hospitals and clinics where the family physician trainees are not bullied by legions of ologists. Many ologists do not have the skill set patients expect in their personal doctors. One skill is the ability to establish long-term relationships with patients. Another is the talent to explain complex medical realities in common English, which is important for a doctor to humanize the healthcare experience for patients.[3] Family physicians occasionally have office visits spent translating something an ologist told the patient or family in medical Latin.

Some ologists simply prefer clear-cut diseases and treatments. Surgeons in particular are more comfortable diagnosing a single problem, doing the surgery to fix it, then ending the relationship with the patient as soon as recovery from surgery seems assured.

On the other extreme, some ologists advise their patients to continue seeing them just to follow a condition, even if there is nothing to do if the condition changes. It is the culture of many medical fields to practice this form of recreational data collection. For example, a person might have a rare condition for which there is no treatment. Ologists commonly tell those patients to be retested every year, just to "follow up" on the disease. If there is no proven treatment even if the disease worsens, what's the point of the yearly office visit and tests?

Many ologists are uncomfortable with uncertainty and feel they must order every test possible to be a good doctor. Family physicians are more comfortable with uncertainty than all other physicians, which means they don't feel pressed to order every test in existence to care for you.[3] Patients commonly tell their family physicians about symptoms that are ill-defined and evolve over time.[4] Many of the issues patients discuss with ologists are different from those they discuss with their family physicians. Therefore, family physicians use different problem-solving approaches than the ologists.[5] Faced with the same patient concerns as ologists, however, family physicians order fewer tests and procedures, yet provide the same or higher-quality care.[5]

Frankly, some ologists have control issues. Many are uncomfortable working with healthcare teams. They can be inflexible and insist that a diagnostic or treatment approach be carried out their way, or they will decline to participate in a patient's care. These ologists are less comfortable working with other healthcare providers, such as nurses, physical therapists, and counselors, and often will do so only to the extent they can control the other providers' actions.

National surveys and interviews concluded family physicians are more comfortable with complex patients than all other physicians[1] and handle more complexity per hour than cardiologists and psychiatrists.[6] Family doctors are more comfortable making the best of imperfect situations, which could arise from multiple chronic diseases in the same patient, co-existing mental health issues, family issues, or financial issues. Family physicians are more likely than other physicians to consider the added complexity of financial burdens on their patients when they make medical decisions.[7]

Ologists will sometimes protect their business turf even if it is inconvenient for their patients. A family physician colleague is convinced that OB/Gyns tell their new mothers to take their babies to pediatricians, because if a new mother takes her baby to a family physician, one day the family physician might mention, "I could take care of your well-woman exams, your contraceptive needs, and your baby at the same office visit." Convenient care at that level would drive business away from the OB/Gyns.

BACK TO MRS. JONES

When I teach my family medicine residents, the question of when to refer a patient is a commonly discussed. Humility is a cornerstone of family medicine. If a patient's condition can be narrowed down to a single body part, some other doctor knows more about it than me, and in most cases can perform procedures I shouldn't. On the other hand, in medicine as in life, too many cooks spoil the broth. My bottom-line exhortation to my residents is to ask another physician to get involved only if that physician will likely add value to the patient's health. The family physician asking for help must have a specific question he wants answered by the ologist, otherwise the only thing that changes is an increase in the chance of a medical error.

In Mrs. Jones's case, there was absolutely no reason to call a cardiologist to traipse down to the hospital on a Friday night. His presence would have added no value to her life. There was nothing for him to detect.

So why did the plaintiff's lawyer believe this particular shoulda-woulda-coulda attack could be successful? Mainly, lawyers are convinced that it's worth it to roll the dice in front of a jury in hopes of the multi-million dollar payout. They believe that some juries can be convinced that somehow, some way, a cardiologist could have miraculously saved the patient.

ASSUMPTION #2 – EARLY DETECTION CURES EVERYTHING

Mrs. Jones's lawyers claimed that if I had ordered a bunch of tests, I surely would have caught some abnormality, and had that been addressed the day I saw her, she would have still been alive five months later. Almost without exception, GIMeC members extol the virtues of early detection without ever questioning this assumption. Frankly, many efforts to improve health by finding disease at an early stage simply aren't effective.

THE TALE OF TWO SEEDS

It is true that people whose cancers are detected at a small size are more likely to be cured than those whose cancers are detected at a larger size. From this, many people conclude that early detection is extremely important to prevent deaths from cancer. Unfortunately, reality isn't so simple.

To illustrate this point, imagine you have several prize rose bushes, and two birds simultaneously drop two different seeds at the base of two different bushes. One seed is a fast-growing vine; the other a slow-growing shrub, like a holly. If left alone, both invading plants will overwhelm the rose bushes. The vine will ultimately kill the rose bush by enveloping it. The holly will kill the rose bush by growing larger than the bush and covering it up. Each can damage or kill the rose bush if not removed before it reaches a critical size.

Now imagine you were away from your garden for many weeks. While you were gone, both seeds germinated at about the same time and started growing. When you return home, you go outside to inspect your prize flowers and see the vine growing halfway into one of the rose bushes. The holly by another rose bush is less than a foot tall. The vine is impossible to remove without damaging the rose bush because it grew so fast and is intertwined in the branches. The holly is much easier to remove. It barely reaches the lower branches. The damage caused by the invading plants was determined by the speed and nature of their growth, not when they were detected relative to when they started.

The same reality exists in cancer detection. People assume a small cancer is more curable because it's caught early. A more accurate understanding is a less aggressive cancer not only grows slower, but is less likely to invade the surrounding tissue or break apart and spread throughout the body (metastasize). The small cancer's slow growth and lack of aggressiveness is the reason it's detected at an earlier size, and also why treatment is more successful. The timing of detection actually has little to do with a positive outcome.

THE TALE OF TWO BLOOD TESTS

For a slightly different take on this issue, imagine two women with the same cancerous tumor in January, but neither knew it. Each had no symptoms. One woman had a screening blood test showing a protein produced by the cancer leaked into her blood and was at a level of 10, which was above normal. Further tests revealed the tumor, and treatment was begun. In spite of appropriate medical care, she died in September.

The second woman noticed symptoms in May. Her doctor recognized the symptoms could mean cancer. Tests were performed; the tumor was discovered; and treatment was started. The level of the same protein in this woman's blood was

100 when the symptoms started because the tumor had grown since January. She died in September.

On the surface, it might look like the first woman benefited from early detection. She lived eight months from the time the cancer was detected by the blood test – January to September. The symptom-detection woman lived just four months from the time the cancer was detected – May to September. The simplistic observation was misleading. Early detection didn't affect survival.

These two realities – hidden diseases detected at a small size are often small because they grow slowly, and early awareness of a hidden disease creates a false impression that survival time is longer – explain why early detection doesn't improve health nearly as often as most assume.

CARDIOVASCULAR SCREENING TESTS

An entire industry has sprung up to test symptom-free people for all sorts of blood vessel diseases. The companies run ads in major newspapers and make their services convenient by putting their equipment in mobile vans. The charge for a package that includes testing for blocked arteries in the neck, abdomen, and legs might cost around $200. Promoters of this technology claim, "People are realizing that proactive healthcare is much better than reactive."[8]

Some evidence exists that screening for an abdominal aortic aneurysm, a weakening of the major artery carrying blood from your heart to your lower body, cuts the death rate from aneurysms in half, although there does not seem to be an increase in the overall life expectancy of those screened.[9] The test is only effective in men ages 65-74 who have smoked, and isn't at all effective in women. The other blood vessel tests offered by these companies have no proof they lead to better health for patients without symptoms.

What really saddens me about this service is that some people without insurance buy these tests in the false belief that they will prolong their lives. They could have spent $200 on other things to make their lives better, but the fear instilled by these ads causes people to spend money on unproven tests.

PROSTATE CANCER

For years, urologists and cancer doctors promoted PSA screening for the early detection of prostate cancer. The PSA test stands for Prostate-Specific Antigen. It is a protein the prostate gland makes that gets into the bloodstream. All normal men have small amounts of PSA in their blood.

Two large clinical trials on the procedure were recently published, one in the U.S. and one in Europe.[10, 11] The U.S. study found absolutely no difference in total deaths or prostate cancer deaths between the men who were in the PSA testing group and those who were in the "usual care" group. The European study found a slight difference in prostate cancer deaths in the men who received routine PSA testing (20 percent fewer), but no reduction in the overall death rate. In other words, approximately as many men died from the complications of prostate cancer treatments as were saved by early detection. Another review of six clinical trials of prostate cancer screening concluded the evidence was overwhelming that no method of detection saves lives.[12] Why doesn't the PSA test work?

The first reality is no medical test is perfect or 100 percent accurate. Every test has the potential to be wrong in two ways. The test could say you have a disease when you really don't, or that you don't have a disease when you really do. The PSA test is imperfect in both directions.

Other conditions cause PSA levels to be high. The prostate gland can be irritated or enlarged, which causes it to release more PSA, which increases the level of it in the blood. But the most common reason for the PSA level to rise without cancer is a condition in older men called benign prostatic hypertrophy (BPH), which restricts the flow of urine through the prostate gland. A typical BPH symptom is when older men wake up several times at night to go to the bathroom. These men frequently have increased levels of PSA but no dangerous cancer in their prostate gland.

On the other hand, it's also true that prostate cancer becomes more common as men get older. Many men in their 60s and older have prostate cancer. Two-thirds of men in their 70s and more than four-fifths of men in their 80s have prostate cancer – not pre-cancer, actual cancer.[13]

As much as the media and the prostate cancer advocacy groups imply that there is an epidemic of men dying of prostate cancer in America, prostate cancer causes less than 5 percent of all deaths, even at the ages with the highest incidence of prostate cancer. Most older men have a mild form of prostate cancer. It is usually not very aggressive and most men actually die with prostate cancer in their body, *not* because of it. They die of other diseases such as heart attacks, strokes, and other forms of cancer.

The PSA-pushing ologists find it hard to accept the proof that routine PSA testing doesn't save lives. Even under the most optimistic assumptions, the number of lives potentially saved is minute. If we only considered the results of the most optimistic study, they imply routine PSA testing increases life expectancy by only 2.6 days.[14] Aggressive PSA testing and treatment will cause many men to suffer the side effects of the prostate cancer treatment – such as incontinence and impotence – and the costs will be extraordinary. Yet, the PSA pushers will continue to scare Americans into submitting to tests costing billions of dollars a year, many of these costs in procedure fees for the ologists.

I propose the PSA test be renamed – the Procedure Stimulating Antigen.

OTHER CANCERS

To demonstrate once again that the value of prevention is overstated, let's consider other cancers. Although GIMeC clearly has convinced the American people that early detection is crucial for all cancer care, there actually are only three cancers for which nearly all doctors agree that it saves lives: breast, cervical, and colon (and now possibly lung). For other cancers, a range of speculation exists regarding how effective early detection might be.

A recent national study found 87 percent of adults believe routine cancer screening is almost always a good idea, and 74 percent say finding cancer early saves lives.[15] Two-thirds said they would want to be tested for cancer, even if nothing could be done, and 56 percent said they would want to be tested for pseudo-disease: cancers growing so slowly they would never cause problems during a person's lifetime even if untreated. Clearly, the GIMeC assumptions have penetrated the American psyche.

Here is a partial list of cancers for which there is no proof early detection saves lives in typical American populations

Bladder cancer

Blood cancers
Acute lymphoblastic leukemia
Acute myeloid leukemia
Hodgkin's lymphoma
Multiple myeloma
Non-Hodgkin's lymphoma
Other lymphoma types

Bone cancers
Bone marrow cancers
Osteosarcomas

Brain cancers
Astrocytoma
Gliomas
Medulloblastoma
Other brain cancer types

Esophageal cancer

Eye cancers

Female cancers
Endometrial cancer
Ovarian cancer
Uterine cancer (non-cervix)
Vaginal cancer
Vulvar cancer

Gallbladder cancer

Head and neck cancers

Kidney cancers

Laryngeal cancer

Lip and oral cancers

Liver cancer

Male cancers
Penile cancer
Testicular cancer

Muscle cancers
Sarcomas

Other cancers
AIDS-related cancers
Carcinoid tumors
Mesothelioma

Pancreatic cancers

Pituitary gland cancers

Prostate cancer

Skin cancers
Basal cell cancer
Melanoma
Squamous cell cancer

Stomach cancer

Thyroid cancer

Even in a disease where early detection is proven, the amount of benefit is likely smaller than most people believe. Breast cancer is an example. How much do mammograms affect a woman's life expectancy? Many people might guess it increases the life expectancy by a significant amount, maybe even years. Mammograms actually increase the life expectancy of a 50-year-old average-risk woman by six to twelve days.[16, 17]

Evidence for this reality comes from the original clinical trials of mammograms. In those studies, women who received regular mammogram screening still could have widespread breast cancer when detected by the mammogram. Mammograms *reduce* the risk of dying of breast cancer, but they don't *eliminate* the risk.

Many breast cancers were cured before the invention of mammograms. If a woman feels a lump and further tests determine the lump is cancer, it is still surgically removed, with chemotherapy or radiation treatments usually given after the surgery. Fifty percent of all breast cancers are cured by treatment after symptoms develop, so early detection doesn't make a difference in women with non-aggressive tumors.[16]

On the other side of the spectrum, just because a cancer is first detected by a mammogram doesn't mean it's curable. About 35 percent of women in the studies whose cancer was first detected by a mammogram eventually died of breast cancer.[16] Therefore, early detection doesn't make a difference in women with aggressive tumors, either.

The breast cancer death rate in even the most optimistic mammogram studies was only reduced by about 30 percent.[18] Since half of all cancers in those studies were cured without mammography, the ultimate outcome of whether or not women who developed breast cancer actually died of breast cancer was a 15 percent difference. In other words, of all the women who are diagnosed with breast cancer because a mammogram found the lump, only 15 percent will survive the cancer because the mammogram detected the cancer early, and that may be an optimistic assumption.[16] The other 85 percent of women with breast cancer will ultimately live or die regardless of whether they received a mammogram.

For that matter, most women never have breast cancer. The American Cancer Society exaggerates the impact of breast cancer. The organization's latest figure is one in eight women will get breast cancer.[19] For starters, this number is an estimate, not something directly measured. It is calculated assuming a certain rate of new breast cancer cases per year, no matter how old the woman.

Just because a calculation estimates a person will develop a cancer does not mean the cancer will have any impact on that person's life. In other words, if we looked really hard, we could find a number of breast cancers in 90-year-old women with Alzheimer's dementia living in a nursing home. These women usually have high blood pressure and other chronic diseases such as diabetes, heart disease, and a history of strokes. The breast cancer may be there, but it won't ultimately cause her death. This reality is something the Cancer Society doesn't tell you. An estimate of the number of women whose lives are even threatened by breast cancer is more like six percent, or one in 16.[16]

I'm not telling any woman to refuse mammography. Mammograms probably extend lives, just not as often as the breast cancer ologists and disease advocates lead you to believe.

PART OF THE SOLUTION

To fix the healthcare system, I ask you to consider the following proposals:

The relationship between ologists and generalists should be thought of as a yin and yang reality. One must balance the other to achieve the perfect whole. The physician workforce must be balanced, not favored towards the ologists as is currently the case. The unique values and strengths of the two physician camps must be respected and supported.

Ologists add the most value to your health when their input into your care is focused and brief. Long-term patient care, the handling of complex situations, the management of symptoms and diseases not fitting into neat categories, and cost-effective care, are best provided by family physicians. Take a moment to examine your values about the best use of doctors. If you give yourself a small cut from a moment of carelessness with a kitchen knife, do you assume the best care is provided by a plastic surgeon? Or do you assume it's a waste of the healthcare system's money to pay higher fees to a plastic surgeon than a family physician, since your scar will look the same? (Yes, I admit my bias that I assume the results would be the same. I can't find any clinical trials that have studied the issue.)

If you have a cardiologist who wants to see you every three months to draw your blood and review your blood pressure and cholesterol medicines, do you assume you're receiving top notch care from an expert in cardiovascular disease? Or do you question if it's really necessary for you to make so many trips each year, since a family physician could manage these problems and most of the other concerns you may have?

Having said this, I recognize all doctors are human and therefore imperfect. As one friend told me, doctors are not interchangeable. Second and third opinions are valuable in some cases. It is difficult for any doctor to diagnose and treat rare conditions. Some doctors are comfortable doing unusual procedures, others aren't. Any system seeking balance between the attitudes and cultures of generalists and ologists must maintain some flexibility.

For a final example, imagine you were concerned you had thyroid disease. Your overall energy level was low, you learned about your symptoms on the internet, and you concluded your symptoms could be the result of a weak thyroid gland. A family physician can diagnose and treat this condition for the rest of your life. Consulting an endocrinologist for this symptom adds no value or health to your life.

But what if the tests the family physician orders come back with bizarre results that don't fit a classic pattern? Now the expertise of the endocrinologist might be valuable. But all this requires is one or two visits to the endocrinologist to sort it all out. The endocrinologist can suggest a diagnosis and treatment plan. The family physician can take it from there. You shouldn't be condemned to see two doctors for the rest of your life for your underactive thyroid gland when you only need one doctor, your family physician.

The next time you listen to or read a news report on health, listen closely to what the expert or reporter says. If the story only concludes that some people are at increased risk for a disease because the result of a blood test is high (a KNOW-

YOUR-NUMBER story), there is probably no action for you to take. If the story concludes that taking a pill will lower the number on the blood test, there is still probably no action for you to take. A blood test result that becomes lower doesn't necessarily translate into better health. If the story concludes that if you have a certain risk factor AND a test will find that risk factor AND there is a treatment for the risk factor AND the treatment will not only improve a blood test number but will decrease the rate of serious health conditions such as heart attacks, strokes, and death -- now go see your family physician. You can relax. Very few news stories sound like this.

The next time you hear of someone who is diagnosed with cancer and who seems fine after the initial diagnosis and treatment, these words will likely be spoken, "It's a good thing it was caught early." Unfortunately, this statement is usually inaccurate.

It's understandable why so many people say this. All of the special interest groups of GIMeC have pounded this idea into the American psyche for decades. This phrase implies we control our future. We won't die of cancer, because if it's caught early it won't get us.

The truth is the person with the newly-discovered cancer has no control over the type of cancer she has. The next time you hear of someone who seems to be cancer free after treatment, consider a more humble response. Take the timing of the discovery of the cancer and the illusion of control out of your statement and say something like, "She's lucky. The cancer was not very aggressive."

There must be some agreement between patients and their doctors about the time when medical journeys reach the humility point. Doctors and patients must accept that hope can persist even though no more tests or experimental treatments are offered. Begin thinking about what a humility point might look like to you for some of the common diseases, such as heart disease, cancers, strokes, and Alzheimer's disease.

For people who are comfortable with these thoughts, I will propose they be allowed to separate themselves from the rest of the insured population and pay lower healthcare costs as a result. I will provide more specifics in the Solutions chapters.

4 | How GIMeC Thnks – Part 2

ASSUMPTION #3 – MORE TREATMENTS EQUAL BETTER CARE

The GIMeC assumptions could be summarized in the phrase "more is better." In Mrs. Jones' case, this assumption marched along in lock step with the assumption that early detection would have made a difference. If I was expected to find something early it would have done no good to just watch it. The assumption by the plaintiff was that I or another doctor could have treated the hidden abnormality, thus allowing her to feel better and live longer.

To further explain my decision making that night, one of the small influences on why I decided to let her go home was that the year 2001 was about the time the Institute of Medicine (IOM) made the big stink about 45,000 to 90,000 people dying each year from mistakes made in hospitals. I think those numbers exaggerate the problem, but I fully agreed with the spirit of the IOM report that bad things can happen to people in a hospital that wouldn't happen at home (like tripping over an IV line and breaking a hip). Therefore people should only be admitted to a hospital if the potential benefit clearly outweighs the risk.

To be clear, this issue played a minor role in my final decision to discharge her from the ER. However, several lines of research show in healthcare, sometimes less is more.

THE DARTMOUTH STUDIES

Researchers at Dartmouth University examined the relationship between medical resources used and the resulting health outcomes in a population of people nearing the end of their lives.[1] In other words, they tested the POEM assumption that more medical interventions result in better health.

They compared costs and outcomes in patients in two California regions, Los Angeles and Sacramento. They measured how many people lived, how often they were in the hospital, and how much was done to them.

In Los Angeles, the patients used 61% more hospital beds, 128% more intensive care unit (ICU) beds, and 89% more physician labor in the management of chronically ill patients during the last two years of life compared to Sacramento. In spite of this intense use of medical resources, the quality of care for patients with heart attacks, heart failure, and pneumonia was worse in Los Angeles. Patients didn't enjoy this aggressive care either. Patients rated 57% of Los Angeles hospitals as below average, compared to 13% of Sacramento hospitals.

What are the cost implications of the overly aggressive care in Los Angeles? If the Los Angeles hospitals had functioned at the same level as the Sacramento hospitals over the five years of the study measuring these differences, the savings to the Medicare system would have been approximately $1.7 billion.

Why is there so much variation in the aggressiveness of care? One reason is there is no high-quality research to inform the medical community about which patients really benefit from expensive healthcare facilities such as ICUs compared to other hospital units. GIMeC just assumes ICUs are best. There are no clinical guidelines for doctors to follow, because there is no research on which to base the guidelines. There is essentially no research on which patients to admit to the hospital, when to schedule a revisit after an illness, when to refer a patient to a home health agency or hospice service, or when a referral to an ologist actually helps the patient. The NIH funds research to discover new things, not how to use our existing resources most efficiently.

BRAIN ANEURYSMS

A brain aneurysm is a weakness in the wall of one of the arteries supplying blood to the brain. Aneurysms usually form where one artery splits into two smaller branches. The weakness manifests itself as a bulging of the artery wall, which becomes thin and can burst. The worst case scenario is if the aneurysm suddenly ruptures, a significant amount of blood can be pumped outside the artery into the closed space where the brain is trapped within the skull. The pressure on the brain rapidly increases from this growing pool of blood. The excess pressure then causes the person to have a stroke or die. The whole process can cause death in a matter of minutes.

There is some genetic predisposition for brain aneurysms. Close relatives of a person with a brain aneurysm are more likely to have aneurysms themselves. Researchers wanted to know if early detection of aneurysms improved patients' health. The researchers started their journey with people who had ruptured brain aneurysms.[2] They invited the parents, children, and siblings of these patients to enroll in a study to see if aggressive testing and treatment would prevent stroke or death. These relatives did not know if they had brain aneurysms when they agreed to participate. 625 of these relatives had MRIs and 25 (4%) were found to have aneurysms themselves.

Some people might wonder why this experiment was conducted in the first place. Of course, detecting an aneurysm early and fixing it is better for a person who has one. The problem with the assumption is it underestimates the harm caused by fixing the problem. All procedures have risks, and the risks of operating on brain aneurysms are very similar to the disease itself. The surgery can cause strokes and death.

Of the 25 people who were found to have aneurysms, 18 elected to have surgery to repair them. Of those, 11 were left with worse physical function and one was disabled. The authors estimated on average, aneurysm surgery increased life expectancy by 2.5 years for these 18 subjects (or by 0.9 month per person originally tested), at the expense of 19 years of decreased function per person. They concluded screening people at increased risk for brain aneurysms was not warranted.

Many people with no family history of aneurysms or no symptoms have aneurysms. In a different study, MRIs of the head were performed on 2,000 middle-age and elderly adults with no symptoms of brain disease.[3] They found asymptomatic small strokes in 7.2% of these study subjects, aneurysms in 1.8%, and benign brain tumors in 1.6%. The point is, many people have asymptomatic abnormalities that will be discovered if enough tests are done. There is usually no proof that finding the abnormalities early will actually improve health, though GIMeC assumes this to be the case.

THE MEDICAL OUTCOMES STUDIES

In the late 1980s and early 1990s, a series of studies called the Medical Outcomes Studies were completed. Their purpose was to measure differences in medical resources used and health outcomes in patients with common conditions who saw different kinds of doctors. They wanted to know if ologist care led to better health compared to primary care, and how the doctors differed in practice styles. The researchers studied patients with high blood pressure and diabetes and compared their outcomes based on whether they saw ologists who consider themselves experts in high blood pressure (cardiologists) or diabetes (endocrinologists), general internists, or family physicians.

For high blood pressure, patients of cardiologists had more office visits, more prescriptions, more lab tests per physician visit, and were more likely to be hospitalized.[4] There was no difference between the three physician types for average blood pressure, complications, or physical function.

For diabetes, patients of endocrinologists were found to have higher hospitalization rates, more office visits, more prescription drugs, and more lab tests per physician visit than family physicians.[4] There was no difference between the three physicians for average sugar levels, physical functioning, and diabetic complications.[5] (disclosure: the only outcome better with endocrinologists was fewer foot ulcers. Since the publication of this study, the major primary care organizations have provided a lot of education about foot care to their doctor members. National healthcare quality organizations added the expectation that all doctors check their diabetic patients' feet on a regular basis. I would be amazed if there is still a difference in foot ulcers between the different doctor types now.)

OTHER STUDIES OF HEALTH OUTCOMES
AND MEDICAL SPENDING

A separate study of patients with new episodes of low back pain compared outcomes between care provided by family physicians, chiropractors, and orthopedists.[5] Patients of chiropractors had many more office visits compared to the other doctors. Patients of family physicians were much less likely to receive X-rays than the other two doctors. Patients of orthopedists were more likely to receive MRIs or CAT scans and be hospitalized than patients of the other doctors. Pain scores and measures of physical function were the same between the patients of the three types of doctors. Costs were higher for patients of chiropractors and orthopedists than those of family physicians.

Other studies measured how often expensive procedures are performed in different regions of the country. For example, studies have concluded a large proportion of expensive high-tech procedures such as coronary artery bypass surgery[6] and carotid artery surgery[7] are performed for inappropriate reasons, such as patients who didn't have enough arterial blockage to justify the risk of the procedure. The response from the ologists and organized medicine when presented with those findings was to discredit the results.[8]

THE HUMILITY POINT

One of the contributors to our culture of more is better is our nations' difficulty in asking a fundamental question: when is it OK to let go?

This issue commonly arises in cancer care. How many rounds of radiation or chemotherapy must a patient go through before she and her doctors decide enough is enough? When is it reasonable for a patient to humbly accept that her life will end and the cause of her death will be a cancer spread throughout her body?

This dilemma crops up in diseases other than cancer and is probably more common than you think. If a doctor cares for a person with chronic back pain who has tried all of the therapies with at least some proof of effectiveness but still reports significant daily pain, now what is the doctor supposed to do? Should he order experimental and unproven treatments, no matter how expensive the treatment or questionable the effectiveness? When should his efforts to comfort her shift from attempting to eliminate the pain to just taking the edge off it and encouraging her to stay functional in spite of it?

What about a patient who says she is tired all the time? Several rounds of testing yielded normal results. How many more tests should the doctor re-order on the rare chance that one of the tests will now show an abnormality that wasn't there before? How many treatments should the doctor offer to try to improve the symptom even though there is no clear cause and no previous treatment worked well?

What about a patient who has inoperable heart disease who keeps showing up to the emergency room because of chest pain? The emergency room doctors order expensive tests and hospitalizations. But other than making his medications stronger, hoping the side effects won't make his overall quality of life worse, no other treatments will open up the narrowed coronary arteries (though the pain can still be treated). At what point does the patient decide to stop going to the emergency room for chest pain?

One of the conventional axioms of medicine that must remain in the minds of American doctors, no matter what direction our healthcare system travels, is to cure when possible, relieve sometimes, but comfort always. It has been my experience that most Americans will have a difficult healthcare journey at some point in their lives. They will have a nagging symptom, feeling, or disease with no easy answers. They will try a variety of tests and treatments that give some relief, but remains incomplete.

The humility point is the moment a person says to herself that she has had enough of the healthcare industry and now accepts a new reality to her life. This could be a relatively benign, but annoying, symptom such as when she realizes she can't play tennis like she used to because her feet hurt too much. The humility point could be much more profound, such as the moment she accepts she has dementia and can't drive anymore.

MORE TREATMENTS – SUMMARY

I have given a few examples showing that aggressive care doesn't always mean better care. In the fee-for-service world of doctor and hospital payments, ologists and some healthcare facilities have incentives to order more tests and provide more treatments. I'm not accusing the ologists and healthcare facilities of blatant greed, though I do believe the amount of money they make to provide some treatments affects their insight. Ologists performing expensive procedures truly believe the procedures are in the best interest of their patients and always worth the cost.

GIMeC wants you to believe more is necessarily better, but a line of evidence in the medical literature finds the opposite. Aggressive expensive medical care is commonly helpful, but patients and physicians shouldn't assume more tests, procedures, and treatments lead to better health. One thing is certain: aggressive medical care is much more expensive than the alternative.

ASSUMPTION #4 – PREVENTION SAVES MONEY

Like most Americans, for years I assumed that prevention was the golden ticket to maximizing personal health for me and creating more affordable healthcare for everyone. Buzzwords like regular check ups, disease screening, and early detection just felt right, and I heard no medical or business leaders say anything to contradict these beliefs. I even remember in my engineering days before I went to medical school telling my young engineer friends that I signed up for the new HMO insurance plan, because I believed in prevention.

However, as I learned more about healthcare economics than my standard medical education provided, I was exposed to research that came to different conclusions than the feel-good insurance company brochures. I learned that many common medical preventive services not only don't save money, they cost a fortune.

I will attempt to explain why this version of reality is true. But first, let me make clear a few caveats. By "prevention" I mean doing things such as X-rays, blood tests, or other non-invasive tests to people who have no symptoms related to the disease in question. Finding prostate cancer in a man with no urinary problems that started with a PSA blood test is an example of prevention. Diagnosing prostate cancer in a man who tells his doctor he has difficulty urinating isn't.

I believe that preventing future disease by making healthy lifestyle choices creates many additional years of high-quality life and probably saves money if the individual makes these choices without requiring a lot of expensive programs. Compare a person who eats the equivalent of a smallish chicken breast sandwich, a piece of fruit, and a glass of water each meal versus a person who eats the equivalent of a triple-decker cheeseburger, super-sized fries, and a milkshake every meal. I believe the first person spends less on food, has a longer disease-free life, and spends less on healthcare.

I will also present a simplified example of medical cost-effectiveness analyses here. This science is very complex and the highest quality cost-effectiveness studies require input from many scientific disciplines. My example will deal with life-and-death issues. More formal cost-effectiveness analyses include quality-of-life considerations. Many appropriate medical tests and treatments don't increase life expectancy but increase patients' well-being by improving discomforts such as difficulty breathing, painful joints, and depression. A discussion of how these legitimate treatment goals are incorporated into cost-effectiveness studies is beyond the scope of this book.

With these understandings out of the way, I will start my explanation that prevention doesn't save money with a bit of family history.

MAMU ECONOMICS

Mamu was the name we called my grandmother. As in so many families, her nickname was coined when one of the first grandchildren, me, attempted to say the word "grandmother." My grandfather came out better in the naming process. He was called Granddaddy. Mamu used to drive Granddaddy crazy in many ways. One was when she earnestly tried to save money. She and my grandfather were children of the Great Depression and despite the financial success they enjoyed in their later adult lives, they never forgot the hardships of those earlier years.

Mamu was a big-time coupon clipper. She got excited when she found a coupon for 50 cents off a can of green beans. It didn't matter to her that the store offering the great deal wasn't the neighborhood grocery store, but was miles away.

She would take her coupon, get in her car, and drive off for the distant store. She would typically spend 50 cents in gas, four dollars in wear-and-tear on her car, and would buy something else for three dollars she had not thought of buying when she left the house, but caught her eye at the store. She would then come home proud of the time and effort she spent being a frugal home manager.

In the end, she spent $7.50 to save 50 cents. She meant well. My grandfather learned long ago that it was pointless to try to convince her she hadn't saved the money she thought. When Mamu made up her mind, trying to change it was useless.

Unfortunately, most preventive services in healthcare don't save money either. Thirty years of medical economic studies demonstrate a consistent pattern. In health care the saying, "An ounce of prevention is worth a pound of cure" should be replaced with "An ounce of prevention costs a ton of money."[9] In medical prevention, later savings rarely make up for the initial costs of tests and treatments.

A few preventive services in healthcare actually save lives, health, and money. Childhood immunizations are one example. One dollar of childhood immunizations is estimated to save about ten dollars in economic costs later.[10] Prenatal care also probably saves money in the long run. It takes lots of doctors' visits and tests to equal the cost of one premature infant's prolonged stay in the intensive care unit, which can easily be over a half million dollars. Prenatal care is estimated to save about three dollars for every dollar spent.[11]

Other interventions impact health, prevent disease, and save money, but have nothing to do with the healthcare industry. A group called The Trust for America's Health estimates an investment of $10 per person per year in proven community-based programs to increase physical activity, improve nutrition, and prevent smoking could save the country $16 billion annually within five years of implementation.[12] This is a return of $5.60 for every $1 invested.

Very little else in healthcare works so well or saves money in the long run.

A SIMPLE COST-EFFECTIVENESS EXAMPLE

Let's spend some time understanding the reality in a little more detail that an ounce of prevention costs a ton of money. Pretend the political will developed in Texas to completely eliminate deaths from tetanus, which is in theory a completely preventable disease. If every adult got a tetanus shot every 10 years, they would all be immune and the disease would be unable to do much damage.

If a statewide campaign was launched to find all the adults who are not up to date with their tetanus shots, roughly 10 million adult Texans would need one. Pretend they magically showed up to be vaccinated with no advertising campaign. We won't include the costs of a campaign to raise awareness to get people up to date with their vaccinations. (A more formal cost-effectiveness analysis might include such costs, because they would be legitimate costs required to get the job done.) Assume a tetanus shot costs only $5 and has to be given every 10 years to maintain its effectiveness.

As for the savings generated by this effort, assume tetanus illnesses would cause a person to be hospitalized, but not lead to death, and would be prevented at a cost of $100,000 per hospitalization (my estimate).

So this is how the program would stack up:

Costs: 10,000,000 people vaccinated times $5 per shot = $50,000,000
Savings: 5 hospitalizations per year times $100,000 = $5,000,000 savings over 10 years
Lives saved: One life saved per year over 10 years = 10 lives

Therefore, the net cost of the program would be $45,000,000 ($50 million minus $5 million) to save 10 lives. Only one Texan dies of tetanus in an average year. So this works out to $4,500,000 to extend a life. Ten years later the shots have to be given again, because a tetanus shot is not a one-time intervention. This is a difficult reality to consider. A more rigorous published cost-effectiveness analysis of tetanus vaccines found the cost to extend a year of life to be much higher, at more than $1,000,000 per *year* of life.[13]

Common medical interventions have widely different cost-effectiveness values. The older childhood immunizations save money,[10] the newer vaccines don't.[14-16] Few medical interventions save money or are even cost neutral.

EPILOGUE TO THE MRS. JONES CASE

Also happening at the time I saw Mrs. Jones, the woman in the ER who told me she didn't have chest pain, was an environment of runaway lawsuits in Texas. This was just before tort reform passed, which did a great job calming down the toxic atmosphere and encouraged doctors in high-risk fields to come back to the state. The malpractice insurance company hired by the ER company I worked for went bankrupt. This caused my case to be kicked to a state-mandated backup insurance fund, which only had a total payout limit of $300,000. The other gem was the rules of this fund prohibited it from paying pre-judgment interest, which is set by statute at 10% per year guaranteed.

The practical threat to me was that if a jury felt Mrs. Jones was seriously wronged and awarded her $1,000,000, and the jury believed the GIMeC assumptions that I was at fault from not doing more and tagged me with 50% of the total damages ($500,000 total), I would be burned two ways. First I'd be out the $200,000 difference between my portion of the damages and the fund limits. Second, because the resolution of this case took four years, I'd be out another $200,000 from the pre-judgment interest the fund was prohibited from paying ($500,000 times 10% times four years).

Another dynamic of this case is that I was burned by the embarrassment of osteopathic medicine: the one-year D.O. It turned out Mrs. Jones' primary doctors had no more training than osteopathic school and one year of internship. They called themselves family physicians (and one even said he was also an allergist) with no training or board certification in those fields. This phenomenon is part of the tradition of osteopathy, though to its credit this tradition is fading away.

In the discovery process, it turned out that on the morning of the day I saw her Mrs. Jones saw one of these doctors and complained of chest pain. They told her to go to the ER immediately, but she arrived about 10 hours later. I'll never know why she so vehemently denied having chest pain at any point that day when I talked to her. These doctors completely washed their hands of the responsibility to care for her symptoms when they saw her. They did not get an EKG, call a colleague to see her through an appropriate work up, or arrange to care for her in any hospital. They only told her to go to an ER to "get a complete cardiac work up." Anything that happened afterwards was the fault of the ER doctor. Clearly their definition of "emergency" was different from mine.

I had the following discussion with the lawyer assigned to represent me by the state fund. I pointed out that the whole early-detection-would-have-saved-her argument was especially weak in her case, because she had been diagnosed with heart failure four years prior to me seeing her. The average life expectancy for a 70-year-old woman after a new diagnosis of heart failure is about three years.[17] She had already lived longer than expected.

The lawyer responded, "If we tell the jury that, it will come across as doctors making excuses. All they'll hear is two groups of doctors arguing -- you said she was fine, the other doctors said the ER should have ordered a lot of tests. They won't understand the technical information and they'll probably end up awarding money and blaming everyone." This is what some lawyers really think of juries, at least in technical cases. I also pointed out that the plaintiff's expert witnesses completely missed the fact Mrs. Jones received Compazine, which explains why she went into shock in the next ER a week later. My attorney didn't seem to care about that. In her mind the dynamic of the case was that the defendant doctors were arguing with each other, which meant there had to be a settlement.

The case went to mediation and my choices were to invest tens of thousands of dollars of my own money to fight this at the risk of losing $400,000 just to assuage my pride, or sucking it up and getting on with my life. I sucked it up. I agreed to a settlement of $150,000. Now you can feel a little sorry for me.

Let me say here that I hope this confessional has given you some insight on what it's like to be sued for medical malpractice. The original pain is bad, but in a way it gets worse because it never goes away. There is no forgiveness in medical malpractice. There is no "after a few years we'll forget about it and move on." For the rest of my career any time I have dealings with any type of medical insurance company, hospital, or other medical facility, I'll have to dredge up this experience from my darkest memory files and relive this case. The people reading my story usually don't react much. They probably assume I was wronged to some degree, but that I could have done something better.

The dollar amount of lawsuits is not why doctors get emotional when talking about the toll of the constant threat of lawsuits that hangs over our heads. The pain is in the lifelong cut we are forced to keep reopening.[18]

PART OF THE SOLUTION

Don't fall for the worksite wellness plans springing up all over corporate America. This advice may sound foolish to many people, but hear me out.

I am totally convinced that many academics in the organizational aspects of healthcare and business people simply do not understand the basic cost-effectiveness realities I covered in this chapter. I have observed this ignorance to include hospital administrators, healthcare economists, masters of hospital administration, insurance executives, chief financial officers, administrative physicians, and others. I have seen it in prestigious journals such as *Health Affairs*. They have drunk the POEM Kool-Aid™ and don't even think to question the assumptions.

It's beyond the scope of this book to cover the topic exhaustively, but I find the worksite wellness research literature to be very weak. In a nutshell, I don't think any single study, much less the body of literature, accounts for costs and outcomes enough to explain what is really happening. There are too many other changes happening at the same time as the wellness plans, the accounting in the research is too often sloppy, and there is almost no information on health outcomes.

A typical worksite wellness plan has employees filling out a risk assessment, being weighed, having blood drawn, and maybe having a few other tests. The healthcare plan or physician then takes this information to see if the employee is at increased risk for some bad disease down the road. The "high-risk" person is encouraged to see a doctor, and maybe eat better and exercise more to lose weight.

The weight loss part is fine, but the medical cost-effectiveness literature makes if very clear that labeling people as having a chronic disease, doing more tests, writing prescriptions, and insisting these new chronic disease patients now start seeing their doctors for regular check ups does not save money. Certainly not in the short run, but not in the long run either. In other words, the worksite wellness plans are spending upfront money (risk assessments) to cause even more money to be spent (clinic visits, tests, and treatments), with no substantial payback later to make up for the initial costs.

To the degree there is any financial merit to worksite wellness, using the risk assessment process as a roundabout way to get employees to begin a relationship with a family physician might yield some early cost savings, especially if the employee is one of these people who goes to an urgent care center or ER for most of his care.

I'll explain some of these concepts a little more in the chapter "Sugar Diabetes."

5 | The Enormous Cost of Healthcare

CURRENT HEALTH COSTS & OUTCOMES

If you feel you pay an outrageous amount of money for healthcare, you're not alone. Cost is the number one concern among Americans about healthcare, greater than worries about quality of care or safety. Almost half of Americans polled in 2009 worried they could not afford healthcare in the future.[1] Americans aren't so worried about getting the wrong drug from a pharmacy or having the wrong arm amputated during surgery. They're worried about how to pay for it all.

The purpose of this chapter is to straighten out our facts before we move forward. Many numbers in this chapter are depressing, but they are unavoidable if we want to confront reality and create meaningful solutions to our healthcare mess.

IMPACT OF HEALTHCARE COSTS ON FAMILIES

The high cost of healthcare traps Americans in lousy jobs. In an online survey of 26,419 Americans by the AFL-CIO, 48 percent say they or a relative are unhappily stuck with a job just for the healthcare benefits.[2] Even though 77 percent of respondents have health insurance for their households, one-third skips recommended medical care because the deductibles are too expensive.

Half of all people who filed for bankruptcy in 2001 cited medical bills as the primary cause, which means 1.9 to 2.2

million people were bankrupted by the healthcare system. [3] Among those who filed for bankruptcy, out-of-pocket medical costs averaged $11,854 since the start of the illness, although the majority (75.7 percent) had insurance at the onset. A national survey in 2007 found 62 percent of bankruptcies were heavily influenced by medical debt.[4] Every 30 seconds in the U.S., someone files for bankruptcy in the aftermath of a serious health problem. (Disclosure: Critics of the study generating these estimates claim the study exaggerated the problem.)[5-7]

Even having health insurance doesn't protect some families. A 15 year old named Brittney was diagnosed with ovarian cancer and underwent extensive treatment.[8] She seemed to be in the clear, but then the cancer was found in her spinal cord. The insurance company would not pay for further treatment. The family had a $3 million dollar policy, but its annual limit was $75,000. The recommended back surgery cost over $300,000. The family held fundraisers and bake sales. After several months, Brittney qualified for Medicaid, but the family still owed for the previous medical care. Brittney died at age 16, leaving behind both her family and a mountain of debt.

Of all people who filed for bankruptcy during the two years before the filing, four in 10 lost their telephone service, two in 10 went without food, and four in 10 did not fill a prescription.[3] In contrast, only 7 to 14 percent of bankruptcies are attributable to health misfortune in Canada.[5] In other developed nations, such as Britain, medical bankruptcy is almost unknown.[4]

CURRENT HEALTHCARE COSTS FOR FAMILIES

A typical family of four's average annual medical spending – health insurance premiums plus out-of-pocket expenses – reached $18,074 in 2010.[9] From 1996 to 2006, the employee's average contribution for an annual health insurance premium has increased from $1,800 to $3,330[10] for family coverage. Little cost difference exists between insurance products; HMOs and other insurance models are not significantly different. Health insurance as a job benefit provided by employers declined from 80 percent in 1980 to 60 percent in 2007, especially in lower wage jobs.[11]

HEALTHCARE INFLATION

Over the last several decades, healthcare inflation has far outpaced general inflation. The amount of your family's money devoted to healthcare has grown more than any other expense. Healthcare now costs American families more than food or housing.[12] (See Figure)

Components of U.S. Personal Consumption Spending 1970-2000

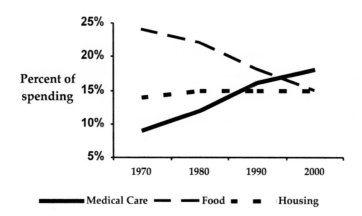

THE COST OF PRIVATE HEALTH INSURANCE

The inflation rate for healthcare insurance has been relentless since managed care started to collapse in about 2000. Over the last 10 years, the general inflation rate has averaged about 3 percent; the inflation rate for health insurance premiums has averaged about 9 percent (See Figure).[13]

Annual Inflation for Health Insurance Premiums, Wages, and Overall Inflation, 1988-2007

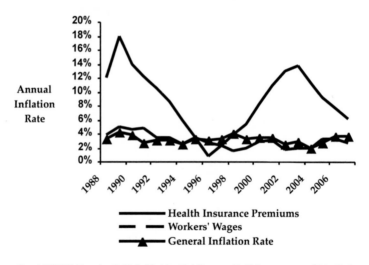

This divergence in the inflation rates means health insurance premiums increased 114 percent from 1999 to 2007, while workers' earnings rose just 27 percent.[14] This difference is why many American workers have noticed their health insurance premiums sky-rocket since 2000. However, the percentage of the total cost of health insurance that workers must pay has actually remained fairly stable: about 16 percent of premiums for single coverage and 28 percent for family coverage.[14] In other words, the total amount of money you're expected to pay in deductibles and co-pays is much more now than 10 years ago, but your employer, who pays for the majority of your healthcare costs, has felt the same pain.

THE OVERALL U.S. SITUATION: PAST, PRESENT, AND FUTURE

The U.S. only spent 5.2 percent of the total economy (Gross Domestic Product, or GDP) on healthcare in 1960[15] and 8 percent in 1975.[16] It spent 17.3 percent of the GDP on health care in 2009, or $2.6 trillion.

Health spending is expected to become 20 percent of GDP by 2015.[16] The Congressional Budget Office estimates that if major changes don't occur, healthcare will become 49 percent of the GDP by 2082.[17] Let that sink in. Half of our total economy will be spent on healthcare if we don't make significant changes!

Over the last 40 years, Medicare and Medicaid spending has averaged 2.5 percent higher growth per person than the overall economy.[16] In 2007, the Congressional Budget Office calculated federal spending on Medicare and Medicaid was 4.6 percent of GDP and Social Security was 4.2 percent, or 8.8 percent of the GDP combined.[16] By 2050, Medicare and Medicaid spending *alone* will more than double to about 20 percent of the GDP, roughly the same share of the economy the entire federal budget accounts for currently.[17]

U.S. HEALTHCARE COSTS COMPARED TO OTHER COUNTRIES

Rich countries spend more on healthcare than poor countries. In rich countries, more resources are spent on tests and treatments, marginally effective therapies, and convenient times and places for high-tech healthcare to be provided. U.S. healthcare is 42 percent more expensive than predicted based on wealth trends compared to the rest of the developed world.[18]

Health Expenditures and GDP per Person

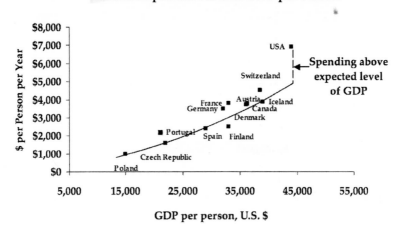

MYTH BUSTING: THINGS THAT DON'T CONTRIBUTE MUCH TO HEALTHCARE COSTS

The media makes assumptions about the cost of healthcare that are, at best, exaggerated. Other GIMeC members also perpetuate a few myths about the causes of high healthcare costs. These myths are as follows:

1. THE AGING POPULATION

Estimates of the contribution of the aging population to the cost of healthcare from 1940 to 1990 concluded barely 2 percent of the increased cost was caused by an aging population.[14] This reality is not predicted to change much over the next several decades. In other words, the tremendous impact that retiring baby boomers will have on overall healthcare costs will be determined more by how many there are, not simply the fact that they're growing older.

2. WE SPEND TOO MUCH AT THE END OF LIFE

Each year, 5 to 6 percent of Medicare beneficiaries die, and in so doing consume 27 to 30 percent of Medicare payments (not 30 percent of a person's healthcare costs over an entire lifetime).[19] However, just one-fifth of people in the top 5 percent of Medicare spending in a given year die by the end of the year.[20]

More hospice care will not save us from high healthcare costs. Home hospice saves between 31 and 64 percent of medical care costs in the last month of life for terminally ill patients.[19] Nevertheless, the longer a patient receives hospice care, the smaller the savings. During the last six months of life, average medical costs for patients receiving hospice care at home are 27 percent less than for conventional care, and the savings with hospital-based hospice care are less than 15 percent.[21] Savings decrease further, to 0 to 10 percent over 12 months of hospice care. Put differently, if a person under hospice care dies about a year after enrolling in hospice, there are essentially no cost savings compared to other approaches. The cost of a year of daily home nurse visits and treatments becomes equivalent to a few admissions to the hospital.

Most enrollees in hospice care do not survive one year, so there is at least some potential for cost savings if everyone enrolled in hospices in their final days. It turns out, though, that the savings don't amount to much. If each of the 2.17 million Americans who die each year completed an advance directive, chose hospice care, and refused aggressive in-hospital interventions at the end of life, total health expenditures would be about 3.3 percent less, and Medicare costs would be about 6.1 percent less.[21]

3. IMPROVING SAFETY AND QUALITY

A complete discussion of the quality improvement movement in healthcare is beyond the scope of this book. However, some critics believe that if we spent more money on healthcare safety, massive savings would result. An estimate of savings from improved safety and quality in hospitals was $25 billion nationwide, or about 1 percent of total healthcare costs.[22]

THINGS THAT MODERATELY CONTRIBUTE TO HIGHER HEALTHCARE COSTS

1. DEFENSIVE MEDICINE

Defensive medicine is the practice of ordering rarely beneficial tests and treatments to avoid being sued. At most, it may account for 5 to 9 percent of health expenditures.[23] Should all defensive medicine disappear tomorrow, the U.S. would still significantly outspend the rest of the world on healthcare. Another estimate from 2010 is that defensive medicine contributed $55.8 billion in 2008, which is about 2 percent of all healthcare costs.[24]

The issue of defensive medicine is extremely complex and hinges on two concepts: risk and cost. I will explain the root causes of defensive medicine in the chapters on ordering tests and treatments.

2. FRAUD AND ABUSE

When politicians are pressured to explain how they will balance a budget without raising taxes or cutting services, a typical dodgy response is waste, fraud, and abuse will be reduced. There is evidence this might be a legitimate concern in healthcare. One estimate is $75 to $250 billion of healthcare billing each year may be fraudulent.[25] This documented surge in suspected fraud is one of the downsides of electronic claims processing, which makes it easier for sophisticated criminals to quickly set up and dismantle phony patients and companies.

well-stated

FORCES THAT MARKEDLY CONTRIBUTE TO HIGHER HEALTHCARE COSTS

Other forces GIMeC rarely talks about have a large impact on healthcare costs.

1. UNEXPLAINED VARIATION IN CARE

Average Medicare spending per enrollee in 2006 was $15,909 in Miami and $5,293 in Honolulu.[26] The difference was not explained by differences in prices, socioeconomic status, or degree of illness. Rather, it was related solely to the quantity of services provided and the high supply of ologists in Miami.[23, 26] Another review estimated more than half the variation in healthcare spending across the U.S. is caused by differences in the aggressiveness of medical services provided.[27]

The rate of operations depends on non-medical factors. The number of surgical and orthopedic procedures in a region is highly associated with the supply of surgeons and orthopedists.[23] A study of Medicare beneficiaries found 15 percent of heart bypass surgeries were justified by the doctors for marginally appropriate reasons and 10 percent were deemed inappropriate; 54 percent of angioplasties (where the coronary artery is widened with a balloon) had marginally appropriate reasons and 14 percent were inappropriate.[20] The rate of diagnostic heart catheterizations varies across the country and is most associated with the fear of lawsuits for not performing the procedure.[28]

In some regions, cancer patients may receive inappropriately aggressive treatment. More than 20 percent of patients with cancer receive chemotherapy in the last three months of life. This percentage is similar for patients whose cancer responds to chemotherapy and those whose cancer doesn't respond to treatment at all.[20]

When compared to other contributors of healthcare expenditures, regional variation in healthcare delivery is the largest factor by far in high-cost regions.[29]

2. SUPPLY OF HOSPITAL BEDS

Multiple studies have documented the relationship between the number of hospital beds per person in a region and the overall cost of healthcare in that region.[27] The phenomenon even has a pithy saying: "a bed built is a bed filled," which has been named Roemer's law.

Residents who live in areas with a greater supply of hospital beds are up to 30 percent more likely to be hospitalized than those in areas with fewer beds.[23] Availability of beds also drives the practice of admitting patients to the hospital with less severe illnesses (commonly described as admitting a person to the hospital as a precaution), staying in the hospital longer,

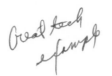

having the patient seen by more ologists during the hospital stay, and ordering more CAT scans and MRIs.

3. SUPPLY OF OLOGISTS

The more ologists there are in a region, the higher the healthcare spending.[30, 31] I will discuss this issue further in the chapters on international comparisons and family medicine.

4. GROWTH OF TECHNOLOGY

Medical inflation is commonly driven by the quantity of services provided. Laparoscopic gallbladder surgery is a technique developed in the last 20 years in which surgeons poke about three small holes in the abdominal wall and remove the gallbladder by using long, thin instruments. The patient does not receive a big incision and resulting scar. Experts thought the overall costs for treating gallstones would come down since patients receiving laparoscopic surgery recover quicker and spend less time in the hospital.[32] As predicted, the cost of gallbladder surgery fell 25 percent per procedure, but the rate of gallbladder surgery increased 60 percent. The total cost for gallbladder care actually increased after the introduction of laparoscopic surgery.

New technologies are prone to overuse and thereby generate excessive costs. Some of the explanation for this is the enormous investment by hospitals in expensive technology that is directly tied to their economic stability. For instance, a hospital may make a business decision to buy more cardiac equipment so it can advertise itself as a center of excellence for cardiac care. The hospital then must entice patients to come to its facilities because it has to pay for its investment in equipment and personnel. More patients with marginal indications for heart procedures visit the cardiac center, and many expensive procedures are performed.

5. CHRONIC DISEASES

By far the biggest driver of healthcare costs is chronic diseases, especially in the Medicare population. Between 78 to 83 percent of Medicare beneficiaries have at least one chronic disease; around 32 percent have four or more.[33, 34] Medicare beneficiaries with at least one chronic disease are responsible for almost 99 percent of program spending.[33, 34] The cost of chronic diseases is such an important issue, I will discuss this issue in depth later.

INTERVENTIONS THAT WON'T MAKE A BIG IMPACT ON HEALTHCARE COSTS

A few solutions were attempted over the last 10 to 20 years to rein in healthcare cost inflation. These interventions were commonly dreamed up by insurance companies or other well-meaning entrepreneurs. None made a big impact.

1. DISEASE MANAGEMENT PROGRAMS

A boondoggle that insurance companies and employers were sucked into during the last 10 years was disease management programs. The idea sounded reasonable: Enroll patients with chronic diseases likely to have high annual healthcare costs and make extra efforts to keep their chronic diseases in control and the patients out of the hospital.

Unfortunately, the disease management approach was flawed from the beginning. Companies separate from the patients' personal physicians were hired by the insurance companies to run the programs. Not surprisingly, many disease management companies are owned by insurance companies themselves. Large employers were willing to pay some of these disease management companies more than $100 per month per patient just to have some nurse from another state call the patient to check on him. Oddly enough, however, they weren't willing to spend a fraction of that to allow a patient's personal physician to spend a little extra time with her patient.[35]

The disease management nurses often had little interaction with the doctors' offices, other than to send them a mountain of paperwork that accomplished little other than create extra work for doctors and nurses.[36] The reports rarely contained any useful information, and many times the offices would have to take time to correct misinformation recorded by these companies.

A study of four disease management programs – coronary heart disease, heart failure, diabetes, and asthma – at Kaiser Permanente from 1996 to 2002 found the programs were associated with some improvement in the quality of care, but no cost savings.[36] Whatever savings were generated by fewer hospitalizations and ER visits were more than matched by the fees charged by the disease management companies.

Disease management for patients with heart failure discharged from the hospital was found not cost-effective for most patients.[20] The programs that successfully reduced costs were limited to high-risk patients, were initiated in the hospital or shortly thereafter, and included post-discharge, face-to-face encounters with nurse care managers rather than mere telephone contact. Another review confirmed these findings and found disease management saved money only when it enrolled patients with severe chronic diseases.[37]

A review of disease management programs for diabetes concluded, "[e]ven for the most optimistic picture . . . the net effect on diabetes-related costs would be an increase of about 25 percent."[38] The Congressional Budget Office concluded that "there is insufficient evidence that disease management programs can generally reduce overall health spending."[39]

The disease management fiasco serves to remind us that the insurance companies, and some of the health insurance consultants hired by large employers, just don't get it. Even in 2010, UnitedHealth announced plans to pay pharmacists to teach people with diabetes how to better manage their disease.[40] One of its senior executives demonstrated an ignorance of all of the cost-effective studies for diabetes prevention by exclaiming, "This will absolutely pay for itself." The GIMeC mentality led employers subsequently to waste billions of dollars and simultaneously undermine primary care.

2. ENCOURAGING PATIENTS TO SHOP AROUND FOR THEIR HEALTHCARE

Making patients responsible for the costs of their care may reduce expenditures for patients who are mostly healthy. However, no convincing evidence exists that cost-sharing reduces expenditures for the high healthcare users. People with bad asthma, for example, will go to the ER and sometimes be admitted to the hospital, no matter how excellent the outpatient care.

About 50 percent of a typical insured population is responsible for just 3 percent of healthcare expenditures.[21]

Forcing this half of the population to shop around for their healthcare will have minimal impact on total healthcare costs. On the other extreme, if you're having a heart attack, it's not the time to crack open the Yellow Pages and shop around for the best deal on doctors and hospitals.

Employees have been voting with their feet on this issue. So-called Consumer-Directed Health Plans – the very high-deductible health insurance plans – are offered by a growing number of employers, but enrollment in these products constituted just 5 percent of total enrollment in employer-sponsored plans in 2007.[41]

3. ELIMINATING MEDICAL ERRORS

Medical errors receive a lot of attention from the media and Congress. Unexpected complications, often resulting from medical errors, may catapult hospitalized patients from the low-cost to the high-cost category. One study estimated the cost of preventable errors was $5 to $10 billion per year, while another study pegged it at $17 billion annually.[20] Even if we assumed the high estimate, the cost of medical errors is less than 1 percent of total healthcare costs per year.

4. IMPROVED CHRONIC DISEASE CARE
UNDER CURRENT GUIDELINES

Excellent chronic disease care soon after diagnosis will not impact the cost of care over a person's lifetime. One study looked at patients in good health at age 70 years and compared them to those in poor health at 70 years of age.[20] People in good health lived longer, thereby incurring more years of medical expenses; those in poor health had more expenses per year but for fewer years. Total expenses until death were equal, suggesting improved chronic care before 70 years of age neither increases nor reduces health expenses over the lifetime of the patient.

I don't suggest that doctors abandon patients with chronic diseases. Nevertheless, several of the existing chronic disease guidelines written by the ologist medical societies make recommendations that have little evidence to support them and are extraordinarily expensive. I will give specific examples later.

RATIONING CARE

Americans must get over our national brain freeze whenever someone mentions rationing care. Healthcare in America is already rationed. We ration it by insurance status, social status, and income. For a politician to state he or she won't support any proposal that rations care just means he or she is clueless about current realities.

A study of injuries in Wisconsin found the outcomes of people who were injured in severe automobile accidents varied by insurance status.[42] Those with no health insurance received 20 percent less care and had a death rate 37 percent higher than those with health insurance. Even when corrected for other factors, this relationship held up. Another study of trauma patients estimated the uninsured were 80 percent more likely to die, even after adjusting for other factors such as co-morbid conditions.[43] Uninsured patients admitted to the hospital were more likely to die of a heart attack and stroke than privately insured patients.[44]

Other estimates of excess deaths resulting from a lack of health insurance range from 20,000 to 45,000 annually.[42, 45] These estimates are calculated from differences in mortality rates between insured and uninsured populations. Another study found the uninsured were more likely to donate organs for transplantation than those with private insurance, yet the uninsured were much less likely to receive organs for transplantation.[46]

Rationing affects quality of life, as well. People with migraine headaches who are uninsured or on Medicaid receive lower quality care than the insured.[47] These patients tend to seek care in ERs, where they are much less likely to receive standard acute and preventive treatments than in physicians' offices.

The literature on health disparities by income, insurance status, and race is burgeoning. It is beyond the scope of this book to review it. Suffice it to say that healthcare in America, just as in every other developed country, is already rationed. The more important questions are: how is that care rationed, and how fair and transparent are the approaches to rationing?

WHAT HAPPENS IF WE DON'T DO SOMETHING ABOUT HEALTHCARE COSTS?

If we're not willing to make significant changes in the way healthcare is delivered, the economic consequences will be staggering. For families trying to pay their portion of employer-sponsored health insurance premiums, the Kaiser Family Foundation estimated that typical health insurance premiums will continue to grow about 10 percent per year. At that rate, the average premium in 2013 will be $21,000, or 37 percent of the average American household income of about $57,000. How much of that cost will America's employers pay on their employees' behalf in the future?

And if we assume healthcare inflation and general inflation rates stay about the same for several decades, the annual cost of health insurance premiums will equal the average annual household income by the year 2033 (See Figure).[48-50]

Projected Annual Family Health Insurance Premium Costs and Average Household Income

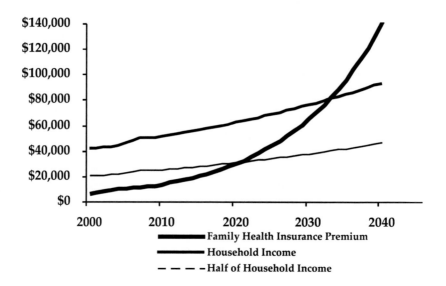

PART OF THE SOLUTION

Faced with this reality, don't panic if I or anyone else talks about limiting or rationing healthcare. Have the courage to confront the truth with both eyes open. Be willing to consider radical approaches to reduce the cost of healthcare in the U.S.

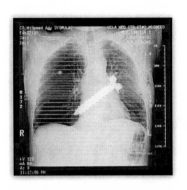

Part 2
Heading Toward a Solution

6 | What Can We Learn From Other Countries?

Other developed countries have better health at a lower cost than the U.S. for many reasons. It is beyond the scope of this book to cover the topic exhaustively; however, America could learn from the successes and failures of other healthcare systems.

Typical discussions comparing healthcare approaches among countries deal with insurance and payment mechanisms – whether a country has "socialized medicine" or not – which is ultimately a superficial and meaningless exercise. The real driving forces of efficiency in different systems are the attitudes and beliefs of not only doctors and hospitals, but more importantly the citizens who use the systems being compared.

To illustrate how many Americans react to reports of people with serious medical conditions, I'll begin with a story to remind us of common expectations of our system, followed by examples of how Europeans view and deliver healthcare differently, then show how their attitudes result in much more affordable healthcare systems.

THE CASE OF NATILINE SARKISYAN

The case of Nataline Sarkisyan received a lot of attention in 2007. A 17-year-old girl from California, Nataline was diagnosed with leukemia (a form of blood cancer) at age 14. After two years of chemotherapy, the cancer seemed to be cured but later returned. She received a bone marrow transplant from a brother, but soon afterward developed liver failure and required life support. Her doctors recommended a liver transplant. She was given a 65 percent chance of living six months after the transplant with no assurance the cancer would be cured.

The initial response from her family's insurance company, Cigna, was "[T]he procedure in question, given the patient's particular circumstances, would not have been an effective or appropriate treatment."[1] The Cigna plan "does not cover unproven and experimental treatment." Furthermore, Cigna contended, "[c]overage decisions are based on the best scientific and clinical evidence available, often utilizing external experts." Nataline's physicians appealed the decision, so Cigna had her case reviewed by external cancer and liver doctors.[2] Cigna continued to decline to pay for the transplant.

The family had hired a local plaintiff's attorney, Mark Geragos. Under media and legal pressure, Cigna HealthCare decided "to make an exception in this rare and unusual case and … provide coverage should she proceed with the requested liver transplant."[1] Cigna called Mr. Geragos' law office immediately after it decided to pay for the transplant. Mr. Garagos tried to reach the family, but couldn't. One hour later at the hospital, unaware that Cigna agreed to cover the transplant, the family decided to discontinue life support, and Nataline died.[3]

Soon after Nataline's death, Mr. Geragos held a news conference to announce that he planned to sue Cigna[4] and ask the district attorney to press murder or manslaughter charges against the insurance company. He claimed the insurer "maliciously killed her" because it did not want to bear the cost of the transplant and subsequent care.[5] "They took my daughter away from me," said Nataline's father at a news conference.

But was the liver transplant really medically appropriate, especially given the chronic shortage of organs available for transplant in the U.S.? Other transplant doctors were interviewed and said that, in general, they will not accept a patient without a 50% chance of living five years.[10] The operation UCLA wanted to perform was an extremely high-risk transplant. Although not commenting specifically on Nataline's case, Dr. Stuart Knechtle, who heads the liver transplant program at the University of Wisconsin at Madison, stated that transplantation is not an option for leukemia patients because the immunosuppressant drugs tend to increase the risk and growth of any tumors.[6] In his opinion, the procedure would have been futile.

This was an American response. What would have happened in other parts of the world?

Two recent cases give us a glimpse of how other developed countries react to sensational stories of young people with severe disease. Jade Goody was a reality TV star in Britain, appearing for several seasons on its version of *Big Brother*. She died in 2009 at age 27 of cervical cancer, which is mostly prevented with Pap smears on some regular basis. While this story was evolving, advocates called for the English National Health Service to lower the age at which cervical cancer screening starts from 25 to 20. The Advisory Committee on Cervical Screening voted unanimously that the screening age should not be lowered, saying, "Mild abnormalities are very common in the cervix of young women, which would often regress over time. This means women would have a lot of unnecessary investigation and treatment. Treatment can damage the cervix and increases the risk of premature births."[7] There are approximately 50 cases of cervical cancer in England each year in women under 25.

The next example is from Canada. Baby Joseph was 13 months old and was dying from a severe degenerative incurable brain disease in 2011.[8] It was so advanced he was in a vegetative state. At this point, he was blind and deaf and was missing all five brain stem reflexes considered necessary for life – gag, cough, eye movement, pupil and cornea responses. As his condition worsened, his doctors wanted to remove the mechanical ventilator and let him die in the hospital, believing his poor quality of life created unnecessary suffering. But the family would not give consent. The hospital took the family to court, which ruled that the family could not appeal the decision by Ontario's Consent and Capacity Board to have the child's breathing tube removed and initiate a do-not-resuscitate order and palliative care at home.[8,9]

The baby's parents wanted the same treatment for Joseph as their daughter received before she died at 18 months – a tracheostomy (a plastic breathing tube inserted directly into his neck – a more permanent device) and mechanical ventilation, which they hoped would allow them to take him home to die a peaceful death. Joseph's doctors argued that a tracheostomy may prolong the baby's life, but in this case it was futile and would likely cause much discomfort. The Board ordered that the breathing tube be removed a few days later to give the family time to say goodbye and make final arrangements. The doctors and medical center had planned to take Joseph home so he wouldn't die in the hospital.[9]

The parents accepted an offer from a U.S. right-to-life group, Priests for Life, to fly him to St. Louis to receive a tracheostomy.[9] Supporters were told it might cost up to $150,000 to pay for his stay in the pediatric intensive care unit. The tracheostomy tube was placed in his neck, and sometime after that he returned to his home in Canada. He died there when he was 20 months old.

There may be exceptions, but no European country, or Japan, or Australia, or Canada would have offered a liver transplant to Nataline. Her doctors would have informed the family that her liver was failing, there was nothing they could do to cure it, and they would switch their focus to providing excellent comfort care.

And informed of the bad news, a European family very likely wouldn't have alerted the media or hired a plaintiff's lawyer. They would have appropriately grieved for the death of a girl who was robbed of so many years of life, then moved on without adding years of legal fighting and media attention.

PROBLEMS WITH THE BRITISH HEALTHCARE SYSTEM

A young soccer coach in England injured his arm in his early 20s, and he saw his local general practitioner. She ordered an MRI, but because of the waiting list and the lack of a life-threatening emergency, the appointment was three weeks later. It showed that a biceps tendon was completely torn in half.

This injury is actually not quite as bad as it sounds. A bicep has two tendons on the upper half of the muscle, so a person can function with one torn tendon. A little strength is lost, but the arm still works normally. After the British doctors saw the MRI, they said there was nothing left to do. If he had been in the U.S., he probably would have gotten an MRI within a day and seen an orthopedic surgeon, who would have performed surgery to reattach the tendon.

As for the coach, his arm still works with a slight loss of strength not noticeable in daily life. When he flexes his arm to make his muscle bulge, his bicep looks like he has a small golf ball implanted under his skin. He calls it his party trick.

No national healthcare system is ideal. A significant source of discontent for British and Canadian patients has been long waits for medical services. Billions of pounds were committed to upgrade the British National Health Service (NHS) since 2000 to reduce waiting times.[10, 11] The latest figures show that not only have the long waits improved, but average times are down to two to four weeks to receive ologist care and related services.[12, 13] However, this improved convenience has come at a large cost, with little to no improvement in many national health measures.[11]

DIALYSIS IN BRITAIN

Whenever people talk negatively about healthcare in Britain, a common criticism is that Britain rations care. A common American misconception is that no one in Britain over the age of 65 receives dialysis, the treatment required when a patient's kidneys fail.

Dialysis was severely limited in Britain as late as the early 1980s, but not now.[14] Thirty years ago, it was uncommon for a British citizen to receive dialysis over the age of 55.[15] Today, many elderly whose kidneys fail are started on dialysis and continue receiving dialysis for years.[15, 16]

On the other hand, the rate of dialysis in Britain is on the low end of the range of European countries and about one-third to one-half the rate of the U.S.[14, 17] The U.S. has the highest dialysis rate in the developed world.[14] In Britain, regional variation exists in dialysis rates. Although not entirely explained by age, ethnic, or other factors,[16, 18] the variation is attributable in part to differences in funding levels.[18] The press in Britain still runs stories of kidney units turning away adult patients or offering inadequate treatment.[17]

Kidney failure is not less common in Britain than the rest of the developed world, but a British citizen is usually sicker when dialysis is started. It is rare for a person's kidneys to suddenly and catastrophically stop working completely. Most of the time, the deterioration of kidney function is a gradual process that is monitored by doctors on the basis of symptoms, blood tests, and urine tests. The moment a kidney doctor recommends starting dialysis is usually subjective and not based on a hard and fixed indicator.

When I asked some British physicians about dialysis in their country in 2007, I received e-mail responses that ranged from near indignity to an acknowledgement that sometimes dialysis is not offered to patients. The indignant physicians said dialysis was widely available all across the country and was commonly provided to elderly patients with co-existing chronic diseases. Other British doctors responded in ways that illustrated the subtlety and complexity of this issue. They talked of elderly patients whose kidneys slowly failed, were frail, and had many co-existing health issues that had reduced their quality of life. Those patients weren't always offered dialysis.

Should a demented patient with widespread cancer whose kidneys are failing be offered dialysis just because the family demands it? Taking costs out of the discussion, I say there is no right answer. Dialysis is not futile care. Without dialysis, the patient usually dies sooner than if dialysis is provided. In this example, on the other hand, dialysis does no more than keep a person with a low quality of life alive a little longer. Dialysis does not make a demented brain work significantly better or cure a cancer.

Kidney doctors in Britain are more reluctant than doctors in the U.S. to start dialysis in a person with poor quality of life. A study of kidney doctors in Britain, Canada, and America found American kidney doctors were less likely to comply with requests to terminate dialysis and more likely to provide dialysis for incompetent patients they initially refused to dialyze if asked to do so by the family.[19] No difference in dialysis recommendations was shown if the patient or family expressed no preference for dialysis. These results suggest cultural differences exist between Britain and the U.S. in both doctors and patients.

In almost all cases, to withhold dialysis is to ration healthcare. In countries that place limits on healthcare services, they develop a language and an ethical framework to live with this reality. When asked several decades ago why it was legitimate to deny dialysis to people over the age of fifty, a British kidney doctor responded that everyone who had completed five decades of life was "a bit crumbly."[15] More recently, British kidney doctors were reported to spread out dialysis sessions to less-than-ideal intervals in order to accommodate more patients, or to try to talk ill-feeling patients out of dialysis.[17]

British general practitioners also consider quality of life as a major factor in deciding who should be offered dialysis. One British general practitioner, Dr. Helen Stokes-Lampard, described her decision process as follows:

> *"For patients in whom quality of life was very poor anyhow or who had a terminal prognosis prior to renal failure, then not offering dialysis would be regarded as appropriate and ethical as we are not in the habit of providing invasive, futile treatment that will not improve quality of life and are not evidence based . . . . This might be couched in sensitive terms of 'little to be gained and a lot of hassle for you' or 'your body is very tired/worn out and each organ in turn is slowing down' or 'nature is taking it course' however we would never lie or conceal the option from a patient or their relatives."* (personal communication)

The relationship between doctors and patients who live in a healthcare system with an annual fixed budget is different from the current relationship in the U.S. British doctors have to balance the needs of their personal patients with the needs of all other patients.

ANOTHER COMPARISON OF THE U.S. AND BRITISH SYSTEMS

I read a story in *The New York Times*[20] that nicely illustrated the strengths and weaknesses of the British and

American healthcare systems. The author is a woman who had kidney infections while living in both countries.

British experience:

"*Getting sick in New York City decimated my bank account. In London, I didn't pay a penny. I should note, however, that a full 9 percent of my gross pay goes towards the equivalent of a health tax (For comparison's sake, according to the Commonwealth Fund, about half of working-age Americans spent five percent or more of their income on out-of-pocket medical costs and premiums in 2007.)*[21]

The system's problems, real and perceived, are such that the best jobs in this country offer private insurance [separate from the NHS]. A few of my friends have paid thousands of dollars extra to get private care when they gave birth. For this private care you get your own room instead of sharing a ward with other new mothers and their babies, and extra care from doctors and the nurses.

When I got sick [with a kidney infection] I wasn't afraid to call the doctor because of money. I was run through myriad tests and attended to by a fleet of nurses and doctors. I am now fully better. I can and do make appointments at my neighborhood doctor's office a five-minute walk from my house, without ever having to worry about being bankrupted."

U.S. experience:

"*The [kidney doctor] immediately put me at ease with his twinkly eyes and a hand on my shoulder. After an ultrasound, the doctor sent me home, armed with prescriptions for painkillers and a potent antibiotic. It was good to be at home instead of a hospital, but I was knocked out and slept much of the time. I soaked the sheets as I sweat through my fever.*

I saw the doctor two times during my convalescence and he called my home several times to check on me. After several ultrasounds, he determined there was no permanent damage to my kidneys. (Author's comment: I don't know the details of her case beyond what was written in the article, but these extra ultrasounds are a perfect example of American technological waste.)

After I recovered, I was hit with another shock: my insurance company refused to pay the roughly $4,000 I owed. Unable to pay the bill, I felt guilty for years that the doctors who had cared for me had been left holding the bag. With my family's help, I finally was able to pay what I owed, but by that point my finances were a mess and my credit record had taken a hit."

DIFFERENCES IN HOW DOCTORS THINK

Many common symptoms and diseases are treated differently by doctors in the U.S. compared to the rest of the developed world. In North America, France, and Finland, for example, guidelines for treating a sore throat include testing and treating patients with a positive Strep test with antibiotics.[22] The medical guidelines in at least four other European countries conclude that acute sore throats resolve without treatment, therefore testing and antibiotics are not recommended.[22] Also in Europe, antibiotics are infrequently prescribed for children with ear infections,[23] though anesthetic ear drops are prescribed.

Cancer treatments vary between countries. I once asked a doctor from New Zealand how they would treat a patient with essentially incurable cancer. In the U.S., the person would undergo chemotherapy, radiation, and other aggressive treatments. The doctor said in New Zealand, they would give the patient a bottle of morphine and a fishing pole. However, the New Zealand doctors wouldn't abandon the patient. They would continue to do everything they could to maximize his quality of life and keep symptoms such as pain and difficulty breathing under control.

In the U.S., many people are conditioned to seek the magic cure, no matter how unlikely. They search the Internet and look at every possible experimental treatment offered. They make pilgrimages to places like M.D. Anderson and Sloan-Kettering to see if they qualify for experimental drugs.

One study rigorously examined the effectiveness of experimental cancer treatments. It reviewed the success of experimental radiation treatments compared to placebo treatments. [24] In each of these clinical trials, half the patients received the actual radiation, the others did not; but neither the patients nor the treating doctors knew which patients received radiation until the end of the clinical trial. The people who received radiation lived no longer on average than those who received placebo treatments.

Most of these clinical trials turned out to be pretty harmless (or perhaps useless). The radiation treatment didn't help anything, but it didn't hurt much either. A few of the treatments worked – patients who received the radiation lived a little longer than those who received placebo treatments. However, an equal number of the experimental radiation treatments killed more people than placebo treatments. Patients who travel to big-name cancer centers seeking experimental therapies should realize that their chances of survival are not improved. They are equally likely to receive an experimental treatment that helps their chances as they are a treatment that hurts. Other studies of the effectiveness of experimental treatments find either a slightly increased chance of benefit for patients who received the experimental treatment[25, 26] or no difference – the harms equaled the benefit.[27]

Guidelines exist in all developed countries to help doctors make the best decisions for their patients. But doctors aren't robots. Variations in care exist even between doctors of the same country, although more substantial differences exist between the U.S. and the rest of the developed world. The guidelines in each country reflect the values of the physicians and broader culture of each country.

An example of differences between national guidelines is the care of high blood pressure. In Britain, there is now a series of chronic disease targets that general practitioners are expected to meet for their patients. The payment target to receive a quality-of-care bonus for blood pressure is 150/90 or less.[28] Some British commentators observed most heart attacks and strokes occur in people over the age of 55, and proposed 55 as a reasonable age to begin prescribing drugs for high blood pressure.[29]

The British Hypertension Society released guidelines in 2004, and stated most people should not take drugs unless their pressure is greater than or equal to 160/100.[30] It believes patients with certain co-existing diseases, such as diabetes, should have lower blood pressure goals. People also should be treated to lower blood pressure if the 10-year risk of cardiovascular disease is greater than 20 percent, but not for people with less risk.

In contrast, U.S. guidelines advise to screen and treat everyone with a blood pressure of 140/90 or greater starting at any age, and to lower the pressure even further in people with diabetes and kidney disease.[31]

The British guidelines implicitly include considerations of cost-effectiveness and were written to achieve the most bang for the healthcare buck from a societal point of view. It is extraordinarily expensive to treat otherwise healthy young people for mild elevations of blood pressure, as our American guidelines suggest.

NICE

Other guidelines are written by a government agency in Britain called the National Institute for Health & Clinical Excellence, which is known by the acronym, NICE. Created in 1999, its mission is to keep up with developments in medicine and make recommendations to the NHS about which tests and treatments should be provided.[32] A significant difference between the mission of NICE and any American healthcare agency is NICE is specifically mandated to consider the cost of healthcare in its decisions. Even if a treatment is effective, it won't be recommended if it costs too much.

NICE was in the news in Britain in 2006 over its decisions on drugs for Alzheimer's disease. NICE reviewed medical studies, analyzed costs, and decided in May 2006 to limit the availability of drugs for Alzheimer's patients.[33] NICE approved the use of a few drugs only for patients with mild Alzheimer's disease. Other Alzheimer's drugs available in the U.S. are not provided by the British NHS. American doctors generally have no limits on the types of Alzheimer's drugs they can prescribe.

In atypical British fashion, people got mad and sued the government. The plaintiffs came from several walks of life, including pharmaceutical companies and members of The Alzheimers' Society. They not only contested the specifics of this decision, but contested the legality of the existence of NICE in the first place.

The Royal Courts of Justice upheld the decision of NICE to disapprove the use of Alzheimers' drugs, and moreover ruled that the agency's existence was legal and that it had the authority to make those decisions.[34] A later appeals court ruling provided a small victory for the plaintiffs when it ruled that a NICE evaluation procedure was unfair.[35] NICE did not provide the drug company with a "fully executable" version of the cost-effectiveness model it used to conclude the Alzheimers' drugs did not meet cost-effectiveness targets for mild or severe disease. The court ruled the plaintiffs must have access to the information to formulate an appeal to NICE.

The legal and media hoopla elevated NICE from an unknown agency to one with unfavorable coverage in the British press.[36] Since then, courts ruled in favor of other NICE decisions,[37] but criticized some NICE processes for lacking transparency.[38] NICE received public support from government officials, who promised that when it determined certain treatments were appropriate, local health systems would provide those services quickly.[39] NICE is currently debating when to allow extremely expensive cancer drugs for patients with rare forms of cancer,[25, 26] and when to allow patients to cover some or all of the cost of expensive drugs themselves.[27, 28]

While the British people debate which healthcare services should be provided under a fixed annual NHS budget, four points must be emphasized. 1) The British explicitly acknowledge that healthcare resources are limited. 2) They have developed an objective process to guide those difficult decisions. 3) The British public is part of the conversation. 4) NICE decisions can be appealed.

NICE's chief executive, Andrew Dillon, recently responded to criticism from British cancer doctors who wanted very expensive drugs approved for renal (kidney) cancer.

> *"For Professor Sikora and his colleagues to maintain the credibility of their argument, they need to explain which patients – with other diseases – should forgo cost effective care in order to meet the needs of those with renal cancer. There is a finite pot of money for the NHS. If one group of patients is provided with cost ineffective care, other groups – lacking powerful lobbyists – will be denied cost effective care for miserable conditions like schizophrenia, Crohn's disease, or cystic fibrosis. NICE seeks to look after all patients who seek their care from the NHS."*[40]

PREVENTING HEART DISEASE BY LOWERING CHOLESTEROL

Guidelines also differ for testing and treating cholesterol. Statins are by far the most common class of drugs used worldwide to lower cholesterol. Commercials for statins such as Lipitor and Crestor are a staple of televised sporting events (and no, these aren't the drugs that give men erections).

The NICE guidelines say statins should be given only to adults who have a 20 percent or greater 10-year risk of developing the disease.[41] American guidelines say everybody should be tested at age 20, and testing should continue periodically for the rest of a person's life.[42] The 20 percent or greater criterion in the British guidelines means that many young and middle-aged Americans wouldn't have a high enough cardiovascular disease risk to qualify for cholesterol testing. Cholesterol is only a moderate predictor of heart attack risk over a 10-year period. Other factors, such as age and the presence of diabetes, can be more important predictors.

Another subtle implication of the British guideline is that women and men are treated differently with respect to age and cholesterol levels. For instance, a 50-year-old man with high blood pressure and diabetes who has a bad cholesterol (LDL) level of more than 160 would qualify to start taking statins, but a 50-year-old woman wouldn't. Women have a lower heart attack risk than men across the board, so it takes more co-existing risk factors for them to reach the 20 percent level.

Another not-so-subtle implication of the British guideline is it defines an age at which it is no longer appropriate to take statins: 75 years. At that point, all cholesterol testing and statin use may cease.

One of the justifications for this age limit is the association between cholesterol level and heart attack risk weakens as people age, and pretty much disappears by the time people get into their 70s (though there is evidence that treating high cholesterol with statins continues to extend lives in high-risk patients in this age group). Another reason for the age criteria is concern for cost-effectiveness. A 75 year old is not likely to live as long as a 45 year old, therefore some treatments become less cost-effective in the elderly compared to middle-aged people. Cost-effectiveness evaluations consider the value of each year of future life to be equal.

British guidelines specifically state the drug "with a low acquisition cost" should be used, and once treatment has started no future LDL cholesterol monitoring is necessary. American guidelines do not ask physicians to prescribe the low-cost drug. Once treatment has begun, a complicated set of LDL targets defines success.

As for drug side effects, statins can injure muscles and the liver. The British guidelines say checking for muscle damage in a patient with no symptoms isn't necessary. If a British patient develops muscle pain, his doctor can order the test to investigate the symptom. For liver damage, they recommend only three blood measures: just before starting treatment, six months later, and 12 months later. American guidelines state routine testing for muscle and liver damage should occur before starting the drug, every month for a few months, and periodically thereafter with no end point. Most drug side effects will happen within a year of starting a drug, and only rarely happen more than a year later.

The British spend much less for cholesterol treatment for several reasons: 1) Their drugs are cheaper per pill because the NHS is willing to forego purchasing a drug if it feels the drug company charges too much. 2) They treat fewer people because they define high cholesterol differently.[43] 3) Monitoring costs for side effects of medication are lower because they don't insist on a lifetime of blood tests. 4) The money they spend is better utilized because it targets high-risk people who gain the most by being treated.

What would happen if an American doctor tried to practice cost-effectively in the British style? He likely would be sued out of medical practice forever. A young woman who was denied cholesterol testing and treatment but later developed angina or had a heart attack could sue because it "could have been prevented if only detected earlier." Besides, American guidelines advise screening for cholesterol should start at age 20. Once a person takes a statin, she could develop nausea and vomiting, and her skin turn a little yellow (signs that her liver might be injured) before she had been on the statin six months. This would also be a rare occurrence, but another instance where she could sue the doctor for the pain and suffering it caused her, even if there was no permanent damage. Even more rare, she could develop permanent liver failure and live with either a damaged liver – and probably require more medicine for that – or be placed on a liver transplant list. Even more grounds for a good old American lawsuit.

How do different nations' guidelines affect the usage of medication? Researchers looked at the impact of various international cholesterol testing and treatment guidelines on a generic Western population – not the actual populations, whose usage also may differ because of lifestyle differences.[34] New Zealand's guidelines were the most efficient, recommending treatment to the fewest number of people (12.9% of adults vs. 17.9% for Australia and British guidelines). U.S. guidelines recommended treating the highest number of people (24.5% of the population) with almost no decrease in the estimated number of deaths. The main reason the American guidelines are so inefficient is they overly focus on aggressively testing and treating young people.

In fact, the best way to treat cholesterol disease would be to start a statin two to five years before a heart attack, because statins significantly reduce heart attack risk within two years of starting the drug.[32, 33] Of course, it is impossible to know in advance who will have a heart attack and when it will happen. For someone to have taken a cholesterol drug for 20 years before their heart attack means the first 15 or so years taking the statin was wasted.

HEALTH COMPARISONS BETWEEN DEVELOPED COUNTRIES

How does aggressive U.S. healthcare impact the health of Americans? The U.S. has the worst life expectancy of all the developed countries. It ranked 29th in the world as of 2007 and was tied with Poland and Slovenia.[44] A comparison of a few of the major developed countries is below. Infant mortality is also higher than most other developed nations.[44]

Figure 1 – Life expectancy at birth 2007

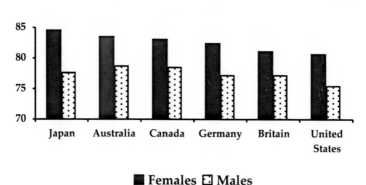

■ Females ▣ Males

Figure 2 – Infant Mortality

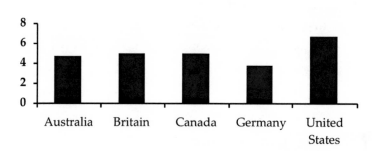

To be fair, some researchers believe the U.S. infant mortality rate looks worse than it is because other countries measure infant mortality differently.[45-47] Also, let's recognize that it's hard to compare health between countries. Reasonable people could argue the measures of life expectancy and infant mortality are too broad and crude to be meaningful. For example, if the Japanese live so long because of their inherent genetic composition and because they eat mostly fish their entire life, can we conclude the Japanese healthcare system is better?

In spite of our seemingly poor health, we don't get a break on the cost of healthcare. The U.S. has outspent the rest of the world on healthcare for decades.[48]

Figure 3 – Average spending on healthcare per capita

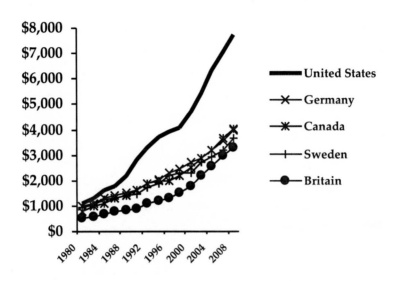

Reprinted by permission from the Commonwealth Fund

Wealthier Americans can't overcome the ill effects of inefficient healthcare. A study published in 2009 compared the overall health of Americans to Europeans on measures of six chronic diseases and functional levels.[49] American adults are less healthy than Europeans at all wealth levels.

WHY IS THE U.S. HEALTHCARE SYSTEM SO EXPENSIVE?

Differences in the basic components of a healthcare system don't explain the discrepancy in costs between the U.S. and Europe. The U.S. healthcare system doesn't differ substantially from Europe by the number of practicing doctors or nurses per capita, the number of acute hospital beds per capita, or the average number of days a patient stays in a hospital.[44] However, the cost of one acute inpatient hospital day in the U.S. is double that of Canada and three times that of most European countries.[50] There are two primary reasons for this cost differential: inpatients in U.S. receive more intensive tests and treatments per day than other nations and identical tests and treatments cost more in the U.S. than in Europe.

TECHNOLOGY AND AGGRESSIVE CARE

A key difference between U.S. and European healthcare is American doctors and patients are much more likely to assume newer technology results in better health. An international survey found people in the U.S. and Canada have greater knowledge and expectations of new medical discoveries than people in Western European nations.[51] These expectations influence the actions and decisions of physicians.

The U.S. healthcare system more aggressively detects and treats patients with mildly symptomatic or asymptomatic disease than in Europe. For example, seven out of 10,000 children were prescribed psychiatric drugs in 2005 in Britain, mostly for attention deficit disorders; in the U.S. it was 45 per 10,000 children, or nearly seven times as many.[52] Also, high blood pressure is treated more aggressively in the U.S. than Western Europe.[53]

The U.S. has about twice the number of MRI scanners per capita compared to other developed nations, except Japan.[44] It has three times more cardiac surgery units and heart catheterization labs than most other developed nations, except Germany.[44] As you might expect with so much more capacity to do procedures, angioplasty (the balloons that open up blockages in the coronary arteries) rates are twice as high in the U.S. than most other countries.[44]

Cardiac procedures by country

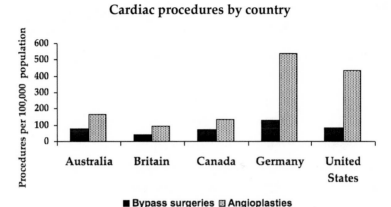

■ Bypass surgeries ▨ Angioplasties

PRIMARY CARE IN THE REST OF THE DEVELOPED WORLD

One of the important reasons Europe and other developed countries have better health at a lower cost is their commitment to primary care, particularly family medicine. Only about 30% of U.S. physicians are primary care physicians.[54] The proportion of doctors who are family physicians in the Britain (they call them general practitioners or GPs) is about 50%. Most developed countries have a ratio of generalists to ologists of about 50/50.

The British assume when their overall system needs improvements, the first answer is to improve primary care. Reforms in 2007 included improved access to general practitioners, felt to be a "massive investment in primary care provision [that] will benefit millions of patients across the country."[55]

Each year in the U.S., 32% of adults see an ologist[56] and 50% to 70% of those visits are for routine follow up that could easily be managed by a family physician.[57, 58] In contrast, only 14% of the population of Britain sees an ologist each year[56] and approximately 80% of patient contacts with the healthcare system are with primary care.[59, 60]

Countries with strong primary care systems are rated higher than other countries on many aspects of care, including their people's view of the healthcare system as not needing complete rebuilding, finding the regular physician's advice helpful, and providing effective coordination of care.[58] The U.S. scores poorest on all aspects of physician-patient care, including unnecessary tests, the number of people taking multiple medications, adverse effects, and patients' rating of the medical care they received.[58]

People in other countries spend more time with their family physicians each year. Estimates of annual exposure to primary care physicians in the U.S. (29 min.) is about half that of New Zealand (55 min) and one-third that of Australia (83 minutes). These differences are mostly explained by the observation that adults in the other countries visit primary care physicians more often.[61]

In part because U.S. patients see their family physicians less often, U.S. family physicians address two to three issues at an average visit,[62] six issues for elderly patients.[63] In contrast, patients in Britain are expected to present one problem to their GP at each visit and are reminded with signs that a consultation should last no more than 10 minutes.[64] This means British patients consult their GP an average of 5.5 times per year, though some of these visits are by telephone or with a nurse who works for the GP.[65]

Family physicians in the U.S. manage a narrower range of problems than their counterparts in New Zealand and Australia. In the U.S., 46 conditions account for 75% of the problems managed in primary care compared with 52 in Australia and 57 in New Zealand.[61] The availability of ologist physicians might also contribute to defining the range of problems managed in primary care. For example, compared to Australia and New Zealand, the U.S. has lower rates of visits to primary care for the management of reproductive problems in women (and no other country considers OB/Gyns to be primary care physicians).[61]

The U.S. is about the only developed country that provides most women with direct access to gynecologists.[58] The presence of general internists and general pediatricians among U.S. primary care physicians may also contribute to a narrower diagnostic scope of primary care physician practice in the U.S.[61]

U.S. primary care is not very convenient. Only 30% of U.S. respondents said they could get same day appointments with their primary care physicians when they were sick.[66] In contrast, half or more of patients in Germany, the Netherlands, and New Zealand reported rapid access to physicians, because there are more family physicians in the workforce.[67]

36% of U.S. adults visit an emergency room per year, the second highest percentage of all countries.[66] 40% of those said the visit was for a condition that could have been treated by a family physician if one had been readily available. Another study found the U.S. has the worst rate of ER visits for a condition that could have been treated by a family physician, had one been available.[68]

EFFECTS OF THE MULTI-OLOGIST U.S. SYSTEM ON MEDICAL ERRORS

The multi-ologist approach to healthcare in the U.S. is associated with more medical errors. Have you ever bounced around from doctor to doctor and felt like a mistake was made? If so, you're not alone. The more doctors you see, the more likely you are to experience a medical error.[68]

Figure 5 - Percent of patients reporting any error by number of doctors seen in last two years

Country	One doctor	4 or more doctors
Australia	12	37
Canada	15	40
Germany	14	31
New Zealand	14	35
Britain	12	28
U.S.	22	49

In a comparison of six developed countries, the U.S. had the worst rate of patients reporting the wrong medication or wrong dose given, a medical mistake was made in their treatment, they were given incorrect results for a diagnostic or lab test, and they experienced delays in being notified about abnormal test results.[68] A separate study found the U.S. had more patients who did not fill a prescription; skipped a recommended medical test, treatment, or follow-up; and did not visit the doctor or clinic because of out-of-pocket expenses.[67]

SATISFACTION WITH THE HEALTHCARE SYSTEM

In spite of the quickest access to expensive medical technology, Americans are the most dissatisfied with their healthcare system of all the major developed countries.[7, 15] In 2005, 34% of Americans said the system should be completely rebuilt and only 16% said minor changes are needed. In the Netherlands, 9% said the system should be completely rebuilt and 42% said only minor changes are needed.

The Gallup Company polled Canadians, Brits, and Americans and asked them if they have confidence in "health care of medical systems" in their country.[69] In Canada and Britain, 73% answered that they did. In the U.S., the rate was only 56%. Extra funding poured into the British NHS has led to the highest satisfaction ratings in 25 years[70] with 77% saying NHS care is "very good or excellent."[71]

I end this chapter with a reflection from Dr. Gil Grimes, who is an American family physician who moved from Texas to Canada in 2008.[72] He provides a few insights on why U.S. doctors and patients are more dissatisfied with our dysfunctional system.

> *The question in my mind is why am I less fatigued than when I was in Texas. I have been giving this a great deal of thought over the last weeks and I have come to a couple of conclusions.*
>
> *First, the ever present push in Texas to see more folks all the time felt like a weight on your back. The addition of three patients a day meant an additional 15 people a week,*

[which] really seemed to increase the workload (especially when you translate that into the additional dictations, labs, and pharmacy faxes). While I feel like I have the time to talk to folks here, I never really felt like that previously.

Second, the patients have a different level of expectation in Canada. In the U.S., I always had the feeling that patients wanted everything done all the time whether they needed it or not. I felt like I was always counseling patients about why they did not need antibiotics, an MRI, or a CAT scan. The sense of entitlement that I felt from the patients in the U.S. was always present as was a continuing concern that someone was going to file suit for the care that [I] provided. I am not saying these are rational feelings, but they reflect the feelings of the day when I was practicing. As well, my conversations with my colleagues during lunch confirmed that others felt the same way. The patients here do not demand that everything be done, and if you are sending them for extra tests, they do not fret if these tests take a couple of weeks to get accomplished. With the malpractice laws in Canada, the frequency of litigation is low, and patients do not seem to view it as a lottery like the chance for a big win.

Finally, paperwork here is not nearly as onerous as it was back in Texas. I know it goes against what I initially expected from a government run system, but the amount of paperwork that flows through the clinic is not nearly as copious. This burden was one I did not really appreciate until it went away and I do not miss it one bit.

PART OF THE SOLUTION

The British should be admired for objectively deciding which services the NHS provides. Other developed countries have slightly different processes that are also worthy of our praise, but the transparency of the British approach is especially admirable. Also in sharp contrast to the American Medical Association, the British Medical Association is leading the discussion of how to best set priorities,[73] not just complaining that doctors aren't paid enough.

To fully appreciate the efficiency of the British healthcare system, consider this. As a percentage of the GDP, if the U.S. spent what it currently does on just public healthcare programs (Medicare, Medicaid, and state and local programs), but developed a healthcare system as efficient as the British, that amount of money could provide healthcare to every single American.

When politicians say things like, "America has the greatest healthcare system in the world," I think they envision a Saudi prince flying to Houston to have some high tech test or procedure performed that is not available in Saudi Arabia. What the politicians don't seem to realize is convenient access to expensive technology doesn't define an excellent healthcare system.

By every measure except convenience for elective procedures, access to expensive technology, and visits to ologists, the rest of the developed world has better health at a lower cost than the U.S., and their citizens are happier with their healthcare systems. Therefore, we don't need to reinvent the wheel. We just need to learn a few important lessons from our friends and find the courage to make significant changes in our healthcare system consistent with some of our unique American values.

A more affordable health plan will require a strong base of family physicians. They should be so well supported by the greater healthcare system that a visit to a family physician's office is the most convenient way to access care. A patient should prefer to see her family physician because it is easier and less expensive than a trip to an emergency room or urgent care center. Convenience to ologists and expensive tests and procedures is less important.

If you asked citizens of European nations if their care is rationed, most would actually say yes. Their cultures expect individuals to tolerate health system limitations and a few personal inconveniences. But for the hassles, everyone in the country receives decent healthcare and is treated more or less equally by the healthcare system.

Perhaps the U.S. is still too wealthy a country to adopt an extremely lean British healthcare system. However, there could be a middle ground between the U.S. and British systems. In return for less expensive healthcare, would you be willing to voluntarily enroll in a health plan that explicitly listed healthcare services it would not provide -- simply because they cost too much, had no real proof of effectiveness, or were too rarely beneficial? Would you enroll in a basic healthcare plan if the trade-off meant you would receive more personal income or a more stable job? Part of an American solution is that a basic healthcare option must be made available to people who feel their lives would be better if they chose a more British-like healthcare system, and enjoyed greater personal income as a result.

7| WHY AREN'T THERE MORE FAMILY PHYSICIANS?

MANAGED CARE MEMORIES

Did you ever wonder why the managed care companies in the 1990s wanted their members to see primary care "gatekeepers" as the first contact with the healthcare system? The answer is simple. The HMO bean counters knew there was proof that primary care physicians, especially family physicians, provided low-cost care with high quality. They just didn't understand *why*.

I remember having a bad day at a clinic during the managed care era. I had several patients I tried to help, but the managed care industry frustrated me at every turn. We couldn't obtain pre-authorization for a test for one patient, and my nurse was kept on hold for 30 minutes, which was time and productivity I couldn't bill the HMO to recoup. Another patient kept getting the runaround on a referral and seemed to think I was the problem. Another wanted to see a therapist outside the HMO network and seemed to believe I had some special power to add benefits to the plan in which she had enrolled.

After my shift at the clinic was finally over, I drove down I-30, and a big billboard for an HMO caught my eye. A confident, middle-aged woman smiled at the camera and said, "You deserve health." I became nauseated.

The public revolted against managed care companies because they were dishonest. They promised comprehensive healthcare for nothing more than a few $5 co-pays. Their billboards said nothing about hassles, frustrations, and limits. Their billboards and brochures lied. Their slogans didn't disclose that the primary reason for the existence of managed care was that large companies wanted to pay less for their employee's health insurance premiums. The big employers share some of the blame. They would switch from HMO to HMO each year in search of short-term savings. The HMOs responded by obsessively focusing on market share – enrolling as many members as possible, even if that meant losing money in the short run.

As the HMOs became strapped for cash, they slashed the fees they paid family physicians. In spite of the HMO brochures touting the importance of primary care, during the managed care era, primary care physicians' incomes declined relative to the ologists,[1] and adjusted for inflation, from 1995 to 2003 primary care physicians' incomes decreased 10 percent.[2] If you were enrolled in an HMO and felt that your doctor was rushed, you were right. The difference in payment spurred by the HMOs persists, which means primary care physicians earn on average $3.5 million less over a career than ologists.[3]

As businesses played HMO roulette and family physicians dropped plans they previously accepted, patients were forced to find a new primary care physician every other year or so. With each new physician, patients had to explain their medical history, their healthcare preferences, and other vital information. An important contributor to the efficiency of primary care – knowing a patient well without having to review the chart every visit – was lost. Neither the bean counters at the HMOs nor the employers who paid the premiums understood the damage they caused when they forced their employees to bounce from one family physician to another year after year.

The managed care bean counters weren't so much evil as they were clueless. They simply did not know the characteristics of primary care that led to better outcomes. I disliked the word "gatekeeper" the first time I heard it. It implied family physicians were the bad guys, the ones who kept patients from receiving the best care. The HMOs never actually supported comprehensive primary care. They were too busy sacrificing family physicians by first squeezing their pay, then overloading them with patients, and finally not paying in a timely manner.

In the 1990s, family medicine became too intertwined with managed care in the minds of the American public. When Americans revolted against managed care, they simultaneously revolted against family medicine.

THE AFTERMATH OF THE COLLAPSE

Since the collapse of managed care and the resulting de-emphasis of primary care, ER visits have skyrocketed. In Texas, they jumped from 5.5 million in 1992 to 8.6 million in 2003.[4] Approximately half of those visits could have been addressed for less cost in a primary care office. ER visits in the U.S. jumped from 90 million in 1996 to 119 million in 2006, a 32 percent increase,[5] and the number of non-urgent visits to ERs increased 40 percent from 1997 to 2005.[6] The increase wasn't because the uninsured were using the ER more often for their primary care; people with insurance accounted for most of the increase. Those who earned more than 400 percent of the Federal Poverty Level (about $84,000 for a family of four) accounted for a growing portion of emergency room visits, while the number of ER visits by low-wage earners showed no substantial increase.[5] To reduce the burden on overcrowded ERs, America needs a stronger primary care foundation, not more ERs.

Massachusetts serves as another cautionary tale of the national shortage of primary care. After Massachusetts passed laws mandating nearly universal health insurance coverage, it tried to connect newly insured citizens with primary care physicians, only to realize the state lacks enough of them to care for everyone.[7, 8] Massachusetts' healthcare costs are higher than the national average and continue to climb unabated, and their ER visits have sky-rocketed.

To give the managed care devils their due, they did have some effect on cost control. The late 1990s were the only period in recent American history when healthcare inflation matched the general inflation rate. Since then, healthcare has increased from 13 percent of the GDP in the managed care era to 17.3 percent in 2009.[9] If that GDP percentage had held constant at 13 percent, Americans would have spent about $2.5 *trillion* less on healthcare from 1999 to 2009. Many smaller employers have responded to this incredible medical inflation by dropping healthcare coverage, especially for their lower wage employees.

THE EVIDENCE FOR PRIMARY CARE AND COSTS

The proof that primary care, especially family medicine, provides better health at a lower cost has continued to build. Ample proof exists to demonstrate regions with more primary care physicians have better health at a lower cost.[10] Studies compare counties to counties, states to states, and nations to nations, and almost all come to the same conclusion.

States with more primary care physicians have lower death rates overall, lower infant mortality, and lower death rates from heart disease, strokes, and cancer.[2-7] This evidence is especially strong for family physicians.[11] More ologists in a region are associated with higher death rates in some studies.[1, 2]

A comparison of counties in Florida found that a one-third increase in family physician supply was associated with a 20 percent lower death rate from cervical cancer.[12] The supply of OB/Gyns had no effect on cervical cancer deaths. Early detection of colon cancer and breast cancer is higher in areas with higher family physician supply, but not ologist supply.[13] (I know of only one study concluding more ologists are associated with higher quality care.[14] It measured only care processes, not disease outcomes or life expectancy.)

One of the reasons for these findings is that ologists are not good at making decisions in patients with common symptoms. They overestimate the likelihood of serious illness in the patients they see[13] and consequently order too many tests and treatments.

Researchers at Dartmouth examined the relationship between healthcare costs and quality in Medicare recipients.[15] States with the highest Medicare expenses per beneficiary had the worst quality of care and the highest supply of ologists. States with the lowest Medicare expenses had the highest quality of care and the highest supply of family physicians.

Family physicians manage new patient symptoms well and exercise restraint in deciding which ill patients can be treated as outpatients and which should be admitted to the hospital. Areas with more family physicians have lower hospitalization rates for diseases such as diabetes, high blood pressure, and pneumonia.[16] Ologists have 50 to 100 percent higher hospitalization rates than family physicians for the same condition.[15] In the U.S., for each 1 percent increase in primary care physicians in an average-sized metropolitan area, there is a decrease of 503 hospital admissions, 2,968 emergency room visits, and 512 surgeries.[17]

COMMITTING TO FAMILY MEDICINE

A few companies, healthcare systems, and states have taken this information on the strength of primary care, made a commitment to it, and reaped the rewards.

QUAD/GRAPHICS

Quad/Graphics is the largest privately held printing company in the U.S., and one of the largest in the world. Many of the magazines you read and catalogs you receive are printed in the suburbs of Milwaukee on a Quad/Graphics press.

In the early 1990s, the head of the company, Leonard Quadrucci, became frustrated with the expensive, dysfunctional healthcare system and decided to take matters in his own hands. He concluded he paid for sick employees anyway, even if they weren't injured on the job, because he paid for their healthcare as an employment benefit.

He started small and hired two doctors to work in a clinic near one of his printing plants. The clinic was intended as more than an on-the-job injury clinic. It was meant to be the primary care center for the employees and their families. Participation always was, and still is, voluntary.

His clinic system grew over time. The clinics became large, stand-alone structures that eventually included a variety of services such as primary care, counseling, a pharmacy, workers comp evaluation, a fitness center/rehabilitation facility, and a center for impaired employees. The clinics are separate entities of the company, and the physicians are given complete autonomy in their patient care.

Primary care physician visits are scheduled for 30 minutes. Patients and physicians feel less rushed and have time to deal with several issues in each visit. The physicians are paid a salary with bonuses based on quality of care and patient satisfaction. Their income is similar to other primary care physicians. Quad/Graphics' primary care physicians are a blend of family physicians, internists, and pediatricians with a few OB/Gyns for Pap smears and pregnancy care. Quad Med, the subsidiary that manages the clinics, provides these options because many of the families prefer a certain physician mix.

By investing in primary care, Quad Med achieves better health for its employees and families at a lower cost. Quad/Graphics spends roughly 30 percent less on healthcare for its employees than other large employers in the Midwest. This pattern has stayed consistent for 18 years.

Average Healthcare Costs per Employee

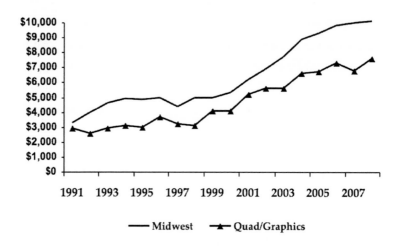

Quad/Graphics does not buy substandard care at a discount price. The vast majority of its employees choose the Quad Med clinics as their primary clinics. Like so many health plans these days, Quad/Graphics has a tiered benefit structure. Employees who choose to go outside the Quad Med clinic system pay more in premiums and co-pays. The Quad Med clinics deliver higher quality care than most other health care systems compared to national norms.

PERDUE FARMS

Perdue Farms is a large supplier of poultry products. It also built onsite primary care and ologist clinics at its chicken processing plants, and directly contracts with primary care physicians. Primary care increased from 6 percent to 30 percent of physician spending by 2005.[17] From 2002 to 2005, annual healthcare inflation for Perdue Farms was less than 1 percent.

GEISINGER HEALTH SYSTEM

Geisinger Health System in Pennsylvania implemented a primary care medical home approach that included many innovations to support primary care for 2.5 million patients. Preliminary data show a 20 percent reduction in total hospital admissions, a 40 percent reduction in hospital readmissions, and a 7 percent savings in total medical costs since this approach was launched.[18, 19] Patient and physician satisfaction is higher in the enhanced primary care sites.[19]

GROUP HEALTH PHYSICIANS

Group Health Physicians, located in the Seattle metropolitan area, manages about 250 primary care practices. The non-profit company made a substantial investment in its primary care teams and increased support staff by 30 percent. It decreased the number of patients per physician and increased the time each physician can spend with a patient from 20 minutes to 30 minutes. ER and urgent care visits dropped 29 percent in a one-year period,[20] and preventable hospitalizations dropped 11 percent.[21]

IBM

IBM has more than 350,000 employees in over 70 countries and spends more than $2 billion a year on healthcare. It discovered its employees in countries such as Denmark were happier with their healthcare system than its employees in America. Danes had easier access to their doctors and were given more time during visits. IBM realized it paid more for healthcare in the U.S. than all other countries, even after adjusting for other differences such as tax rates.

IBM concluded the reason its employees working in other countries were more satisfied with their healthcare and experienced higher quality and less costly healthcare was because those countries had stronger primary care systems. IBM approached the American Academy of Family Physicians in an effort to revamp healthcare for IBM employees in the U.S.

IBM's Martin Sepulveda, MD, MPH, explained, "We have a stake in addressing those root causes of the dysfunction in our healthcare system, and one of the most neglected and glaring root causes of that dysfunction is the crisis in the decline of primary care."[22] Added IBM's director of healthcare, Paul Gundy, "We are dissatisfied with buying episodic, noncomprehensive care – the human loss, the waste, the price we pay for that."

The two organizations are working together in a series of demonstration projects to enhance primary care for IBM employees and their families in the U.S.

NORTH CAROLINA

North Carolina in 2002 implemented a primary care management system for its 750,000 Medicaid patients, who account for about 10 percent of the state's population.[23] The approach relied heavily on primary care medical homes, community-based networks, and case management, with everything coordinated through the primary care physician's office. North Carolina saved $60 million from 2002 to 2003 and $120 million from 2003 to 2004 compared to what it would have spent in the old, uncoordinated non-primary care system. By

2006, North Carolina saved $161 to $300 million per year compared to 2000-2002. The biggest savings came from decreases in ER use (down 23 percent), outpatient care (25 percent less), and pharmacy (11 percent less).

WHAT TO EXPECT FROM YOUR FAMILY PHYSICIAN

Most Americans don't really know what family physicians do. Many Americans associate family physicians with treating colds and maybe a few cases of high blood pressure and diabetes. Others see family physicians only in the "doc-in-a-box" urgent care centers that have sprouted up all over America in the last 15 years. Family physicians can do much, much more.

Family physicians can be your one-stop healthcare experience because 90 percent of your healthcare needs can be met in a family physician's office. Here are some examples:

If you have symptoms like headaches, abdominal, arm, leg, toe, or finger pain, you should see your family physician.

If you have acne, eczema, dermatitis, phlebitis, ringworm, jock itch, toe itch, scalp itch, or any other itch ...

If you have angina, a previous heart attack, a previous cardiac stent procedure, heart failure, atrial fibrillation, or other heart abnormalities ...

If you have emphysema, acute bronchitis, chronic bronchitis, asthma, or bronchiolitis ...

If you have gastritis, esophagitis, irritable bowel syndrome, peptic ulcer disease, gastro-esophageal reflux disease, constipation, diarrhea, or hemorrhoids ...

If you have high blood pressure, diabetes, high cholesterol, thyroid disease, or any other chronic disease ...

If you need procedures like moles removed, skin tags removed, sun damaged skin removed, skin cancers removed, warts removed, or cuts stitched up ...

If you need birth control, if you have menstrual problems, pain down there, discharge down there, itching down there, rashes down there, you're urinating too much, you're not urinating enough ...

If you need Pap smears, mammograms, breast exams, vaccines, colon cancer testing ...

If you just don't feel right, are tired all the time, can't sleep, can't eat, have lost your pep, have lost your step ... see your family physician.

Family physicians can do even more than this, but you get the idea. Think of it this way. People make billions of visits to Target each year, often because most of what they need is there in one place and the prices are good. If family physicians were better supported in the U.S., they could become the one-stop healthcare shop for most Americans.

THE MAGIC OF FAMILY MEDICINE

We've discussed the excellent results enjoyed by regions with more family physicians, but what explains these outcomes? Not more prevention or wellness. We've already established that an ounce of prevention costs a ton of money. So, why do family physicians deliver better health at a lower cost? Simply put, they are better than other physicians at practicing medicine with common sense. The magic of family medicine is explained by excellent judgment.

Which patients with headaches need CAT scans? Which wheezing patients need to go to the hospital? Which patients who just don't feel right need thousands of dollars of tests and treatments versus a reassuring pat on the back? These are the kinds of judgment calls family physicians make dozens of times a day. They are good at taking complex and often conflicting information and making sense of it. They are more patient-centered than other doctors, meaning they are better at seeing the world through their patients' eyes. Family physicians are much more likely to adopt other approaches to make diagnoses, such as allowing more time to elapse for patients with non-specific symptoms before ordering a batch of costly tests.[24]

Family physicians are naturally excellent stewards of medical resources. They typically don't order tests or treatments of marginal benefit because they understand the effect on patients' time and finances. If family physicians need to order extensive tests or treatments, they will, but only if truly necessary.

Family physicians are more likely than ologists to consider patients' healthcare costs in their medical decisions,[25] including decisions about prescriptions, care settings, and diagnostic tests. Family physicians realize the only pill that has a chance of working is the one a patient will actually purchase.

THE FEDS DON'T UNDERSTAND

With all the evidence supporting the importance of primary care for an efficient healthcare system, why hasn't the federal government done more to encourage the growth of primary care? A group of researchers tried to answer that question. They interviewed the staff of members of Congress responsible for healthcare issues. These congressional staff members were generally aware of the declining interest in family medicine among American medical students, and the income gap between primary care providers and the ologists. But few were aware of the evidence showing that primary care improves health and reduces spending.

A few of the Congressional staffers who champion primary care noted the Congressional Budget Office (CBO) did not agree that investing in primary care decreases costs. The CBO is an independent research firm for the U.S. Congress. The CBO analysts were aware of the evidence that regions with more primary care physicians have lower death rates of common diseases and longer overall life expectancies. The few who were willing to talk confessed that they were concerned if the U.S. had more primary care physicians, people would live longer, and Medicare costs would increase.[26] The CBO understood more primary care physicians led to improved mortality rates, but they did not understand primary care accomplishes it at a lower cost.

In fact, the CBO's resistance to acknowledge the cost savings of primary care may have unfairly led to erroneous estimates of future costs for the healthcare law passed in 2010 – the Patient Protection and Affordable Care Act. According to some knowledgeable about the method used to calculate the estimates, the CBO took no account of cost savings that a strengthened primary care system would provide (Larry Green, MD, MPH, personal communication).

PART OF THE SOLUTION

When questioned about healthcare reform priorities, the first words out of a politician's or pundit's mouth should be, "We need more family physicians." When asked "How will we actually cut healthcare costs?", they should say, "More family physicians." All other reforms pale in comparison because no other healthcare services have been shown to actually improve health and reduce costs across large populations.

I have friends who have strong opinions about the kind of doctor they should see for various situations. One friend sees an OB/Gyn for all her symptoms and concerns, even though she is almost always referred to another doctor for non-reproductive issues. Another expects to see a dermatologist for every minor skin blemish. In all these cases, they assume they receive higher quality care. At the very least, I hope I've convinced you that, in most cases, they are wrong.

Would you be willing to give a group of well-supported family physicians a try? Would you be comfortable taking your entire family to see one physician who will diagnose and treat the vast majority of your healthcare needs? Would you be comfortable consulting a physician who won't order a battery of blood tests and X-rays every time you see him? If the answer to these questions is yes, you are in an excellent position to enjoy more affordable health care.

8 | THE NATIONAL BIGOTRY AGAINST FAMILY MEDICINE

I realize "bigotry" is a strong word, but no more accurate description exists for the forces that have stifled the growth of a vigorous primary care foundation for the American healthcare system. Many of the GIMeC members contribute to this united effort, and it starts in the medical schools.

WHERE DO DOCTORS COME FROM?

How much education is actually required to become a doctor in the U.S.? Before medical school, most doctors must complete a standard bachelor's degree. Any degree would suffice, but usually it's in one of the sciences. Toward the end of college, students apply to medical school. The ratio of applicants to medical school to the number of available medical school slots is currently about 2:1.

Medical school requires another four years of study. The workload is heavier than college, and medical students start to taste what it's like to be up all night caring for patients. This is known as being "on call."

Toward the end of medical school, students must decide what field they want to enter. At this point, medical students begin the journey to becoming surgeons, cardiologists, or family physicians. Choosing a medical field also is a competitive process, and some fields are more attractive than others. As you might imagine, the higher the pay, the harder it is to get into a field. Those in which patients develop diseases of a body part but rarely die from it also tend to be more competitive, such as ophthalmology and dermatology. Other competitive fields are the so-called "lifestyle" fields. In these, doctors work defined schedules and have little to no call duties when they leave the hospital. Examples include anesthesiology and emergency medicine.

The first year of training is commonly called an internship. This is an old term that's been around for probably 100 years. In the old days, doctors would essentially live in a hospital for one year after medical school before they went into the community and started their medical practices. Older physicians tell stories about being paid $25 per week with subsidized hospital meals and free laundry. They were interned in the hospital for one year – they entered the hospital July 1st and left June 30th.

Interns had almost no social life. I've heard many stories of women coming to the teaching hospital to visit their fiancées or husbands. They shared a meal between patients in the ER. That counted as a date. It was common for these doctors to treat patients most of the night every other night, working more than 100 hours per week.

These days, it's not quite as bad. Interns make about as much money as school teachers and have work-hour limits. They're not supposed to work more than 30 hours at one stretch and 80 hours per week, although occasional exceptions are allowed.

Most internships are directly tied to the ultimate field of medicine the young doctor wants to pursue. In other words, a medical student who wants to be a surgeon applies to a surgery program. If accepted, he just signed up for five years of training. The first year of that training is called the internship. The rest of the time he will be called a resident who is in his surgery residency.

Most residencies last three to five years, including the intern year. For doctors who want to narrow their ultimate scope and become an ologist, further training in a fellowship is required. For example, a cardiologist has to study general internal medicine for three years and follow that with three to four years of cardiology training. Similar expectations exist for doctors who want to become plastic surgeons, gastroenterologists, and the other narrow fields.

Even for a person who goes straight from high school to college to medical school to internship to residency and beyond, about the earliest someone could start his professional career is age 29. Many medical students had jobs before entering medical school, and some attended graduate school in other subjects. In that case, it is not unusual for doctors to be in their mid- to late 30s before starting their medical professional lives.

The other reality that hangs over the heads of many medical students is student loan debt. Doctors aren't paid until they finish college and medical school. A typical year of education at a state medical school might cost $20,000-$30,000 per year; and a private medical school can approach $50,000 annually. Also, remember that medical students are extremely busy with their studies and don't have time for full-time jobs, so they borrow money to cover living expenses, as well. Quite often, a person graduates from medical school with more than $200,000 in student loans to pay off. The average student loan

debt of a medical student graduating in 2009 was about
$155,000.[1] High debt load is one reason medical students don't
want to become family physicians, but not the only factor.[2]

OLOGIST TRAINING

The length of time required to become an ologist also
contributes to the distorted fee schedule. Ologists claim they
deserve more money because of the years of extra training and
the resultant "opportunity cost" – foregoing the opportunity to
make more money as a practicing physician instead of being
paid as a resident during their extra years of training. As well,
the ego thing plays into it. *The* expert on a single body part or
procedure *deserves* more money.

The ologists might say they need all the extra years of
training to be complete doctors. After all, that's how they have
been trained for half a century. If you want to be a heart ologist,
for example, you need three years of general adult internal
medicine followed by three years of a cardiology fellowship.
Additional fellowships are available after that.

This course of training is nonsense. Cardiologists, and
other ologists, use very little of their general training in their
practices. Cardiologists focus only on cardiovascular issues; the
culture of ologist medicine insists upon it. Some general medical
training before they focus on their favorite body part is good, but
three years of general medical training is a waste. Why is it
required? Mostly because during their training they are cheap
labor for hospitals , which are the entities that actually own the
residencies and fellowships. Even during some fellowships, the
fellows (trainees) might spend a year doing "research," which
commonly means they perform the grunt work for the

professors. They must learn something during that year, but it does little to prepare young doctors to care for patients when the fellowship ends.

The net effect of this culture is that ologists spend more years in training only to limit their final medical practices. Medical education ought to do the opposite. If all an ologist wants to do in her career is fix eyelids, why spend years learning about every aspect of eye care? Why not do a general medical training year, then one or two years learning how to fix eyelids? If she also wants to learn how to zap retinas with lasers, she could add another six to twelve months.

The surgical fields have a legitimate concern that young doctors in training need a certain number of cases before they are let loose on the world in private practice. It does take time to build up surgical experience. On the other hand, how many gallbladder surgeries must a surgeon in training perform to be competent? No one knows. The required number of surgeries to educate a young surgeon is based mostly on tradition. No studies varied the number of procedures in training and measured outcomes, such as complication rates and patient satisfaction, for surgical graduates in their early private practice years. Such research has never been attempted. The NIH funds research in miracles, not efficiency. No money is spent to determine the most efficient methods to train young physicians.

THE HYPEROLOGIST

The current system of ologist training has other negative, unintended consequences for the healthcare system. Ologists assume the best care is provided by the most narrowly focused doctor, the hyperologist, which means the standard of care in a community becomes one in which that hyperologist is expected to handle all potential cases. If a not-so-narrow ologist does a procedure on a patient when a hyperologist was theoretically available, and the patient has a less-than-ideal outcome, the not-so-narrow ologist could be accused of providing substandard care and be sued for medical malpractice.

Why shouldn't all cases go to the hyperologist? Consider a hypothetical example. Assume two doctors in a large city hold themselves out to be experts in thumbs. Thumbs are crucial; we need them to function well in our daily lives. These thumb doctors spend all of their professional time thinking about thumbs. They read the medical thumb journal religiously, which mostly contains studies of monkey thumbs, case reports on unusual thumb injuries, experiments on cadaveric thumbs, and other related thumb minutiae. The journal rarely publishes clinical trials providing definitive answers on the best way to manage different thumb maladies, because hardly any such trials are completed.

Even though these two thumb doctors live in a large city, the reality is that, in a given week, there aren't many serious thumb injuries. Therefore, minor thumb injuries that could be effectively managed by several other kinds of doctors are directed to the thumb doctors, who charge more for their services than the other doctors. Insurance companies convince employers – who pay for their employees' healthcare – that their health plans are excellent because they contain a huge list of participating hyperologists. Patients are convinced they are receiving the best care if their minor thumb sprains and lacerations are treated by the thumb doctor.

Additionally, the medical community creates additional pressure to send business to the thumb doctor. Local medical leaders will make statements such as, "We need to support the thumb doctors and send them all the patients we can. Otherwise, they may not see enough patients and will leave the community."

What's wrong with this approach? Let's turn our attention to the life of the thumb doctors. They have to take calls from all the hospitals in the region, which could be several dozen. They must be prepared to see a patient anywhere, any time, day or night. These doctors are always on call. They feel like they're always under the gun, because they are. Sometimes, to ease the burden, the two thumb doctors cooperate. They may agree to alternate weeks of call. They may agree to work together to schedule vacations and other coverage issues. Unfortunately, as many doctors' professional interests narrow, their egos increase. They become autocratic and demanding of the medical system around them. They are allowed to create local medical monopolies. Many of them do not play well in the sandbox with others, even their own kind.

Ten to 15 years into their careers – after 11 years of post-college training, after seeing nothing but thumbs for a decade or two – many burn out. They retire to their lake houses after relatively short careers because they were allowed to rake in exorbitant fees. This situation is not healthy for a healthcare system. The years of medical education, heavily subsidized by the taxpayers, were not fairly repaid by the thumb doctors.

And what happens if one thumb doctor retires and the other one leaves town? Now the entire medical community feels it must scramble to find another thumb doctor quickly, or now the more general orthopedic doctors, if there are any left, must try to remember how to care for the thumb maladies they haven't seen in years.

This drift toward hyperology in the medical profession affects more than the procedural doctors. In many communities, general OB-Gyns will refer any pregnancy with a hint of complication or co-existing medical condition to a maternal-fetal OB/Gyn. This means the general OB/Gyns deliver nothing but routine pregnancies their whole careers. Ophthalmology is the worst offender. For an organ the size of a ping-pong ball, they hyperologize into retina doctors, cornea doctors, glaucoma doctors, eyelid doctors, and more. It can't be *that* difficult to learn to care for the whole eye during four years of residency, but that's the system they've been allowed to create.

Researchers who study healthcare systems have observed that essentially no evidence exists to support the efforts of GIMeC to promote hyperology.[26] In other words, no one has proven the notion that a thumb hyperologist provides better care than a general orthopedic ologist. GIMeC just assumes it's true.

To be clear, the world needs a few thumb hyperologists – at medical schools. We need a few research-oriented doctors who spend their careers advancing the science of thumb care. That model, however, should not carry over into the broader healthcare system. The inflexibility it creates in the physician workforce negates any slight improvement in patient outcomes a thumb doctor might provide. Regional reliance on a few doctors who do limited work allows those doctors to create de facto mini-monopolies. If allowed to exist, these should be regulated like any other monopoly in a free market economy.

Family physicians can care for many thumb issues. General orthopedists should be able to care for almost all other thumb injuries requiring surgery. The very rare patient who has an unusual or devastating thumb injury could be referred to the thumb researcher at the regional medical school. In many cases, the patient wouldn't even have to make a trip. The local orthopedist could discuss the case with the regional thumb doctor, who could offer opinions on surgical approaches or other management issues. The expertise of the hyperologist at the medical school would still be put to good use.

Why does all this matter, and why should you care?

One of the reasons ologists are allowed to charge as much as they do is they claim they must be paid back for all their extra years in training. One solution is clear: decrease the length of training to the minimum necessary to deliver effective care of their favorite body part to the public. When that happens, the people who pay the bulk of the ologists' bills – Medicare and the insurance companies – can pay less for those services, and those savings will be passed along to employers, employees, and taxpayers.

In truth, some ologists have implicitly admitted the absurdity of the years of wasted training. Medical ologists, such as cardiologists or endocrinologists, used to be required to maintain their generalist board certification in internal medicine to maintain certification in their specific field. Many of the ologists complained it was silly to be tested on information they never used in their day-to-day practices. That requirement was recently removed. Now, a cardiologist has to retake only his cardiology board exams periodically throughout his career, which makes perfect sense, because taking care of cardiovascular disease is all he does.[27]

HYPEROLOGISTS AND FAMILY MEDICINE

The culture of hyperology in American medicine is ironic to this family physician. Any medical student who tells a professor she is considering family medicine as a career will hear something along these lines: "You mean you want to waste your brain by going into family medicine?" The bigotry against family medicine is deep and wide in American medical schools. Stories like this are common from coast to coast.

Family physicians have to master an enormous volume of medical information just to graduate from residency and start their medical careers. Afterward, they have to keep up with important advances in all fields of medicine for the rest of their careers. They must develop strategies to manage the mountain of information that will come to their attention. They must become comfortable allowing useless medical trivia to pass straight to the mental trash can, while retaining the nuggets of new information that should update their approach to patient care. Even more difficult, they must implement changes in patient care processes at their offices and hospitals to provide high-quality care based on the best available medical evidence.

For the ophthalmologist who sees nothing but retinas each day, or the OB/Gyn who sees nothing but uncomplicated pregnancies, or any other hyperologist who does the same thing over and over and over, professional life becomes simple and controlled, albeit boring.

Tell me: Who's wasting their brain?

ONE NIGHT IN A SMALL TOWN ER

The medical school and residency system has encouraged the growth of ologists and hyperologists to the detriment of family medicine. What follows next is an example of the misaligned incentives of the physician fee system once doctors finally complete their training and spread across America to care for patients.

A family physician in a small Texas town was called to see one of his patients when she showed up at the local emergency room. She was 89 years old with emphysema (also known as COPD) and a host of other medical problems. This doctor had cared for her for nearly 25 years. Her husband had died about four years earlier. She lived by herself, with some assistance, and was fairly functional for 89. She went to church, had friends, and was not at all depressed. She'd had a long life full of family and friends, but her breathing had worsened to the point she couldn't stand it anymore, so she called the ambulance.

It turned out her heart was failing. It still pumped, just not as efficiently, which caused fluid to build up in her heart and lungs and left her short of breath.

The emergency room doctor, although he shouldn't have, called a cardiologist first, and only later called the woman's family physician. The cardiologist agreed with the diagnosis of heart failure and wanted to take her to the catheterization lab and give her the heavy-duty diagnostic work up.

The family doctor arrived there, talked to his patient of 25 years, and asked the medical personnel assembled in the ER,

"Wait a minute, what are we doing here? Why do you want to put this lady through all that?"

The cardiologist was just following his usual routine. A sick heart came to his attention, which meant he took steps A, B, and C.

The woman didn't want any procedures, and her family physician knew that. (I don't know if she had already signed an Advance Directive documenting these wishes. Sometimes patients talk about their values and preferences with their family physicians, although they are intimidated by the thought of signing a legal document.) Neither the ER doctor nor the cardiologist had bothered to ask her wishes. The family doctor checked with her first, but he had known her so long that he already knew her answer. She wasn't suicidal; she wasn't depressed. She was a Christian who had lived a long and productive life and was ready to see her husband again. She wasn't afraid of death and didn't want a lot of medical interventions defining the last phase of her life. The family physician appropriately informed the cardiologist of her true wishes.

The family physician took care of her in the hospital. She stayed there less than a week. She received medicine to help her breathe better and make it easier for her heart to pump. She improved enough to go home, where a hospice service helped care for her. She died peacefully four months later surrounded by family and friends, including her family physician.

This may be uncomfortable, but let's review the financial implications of what took place. Because the woman's family physician applied his knowledge of this woman's spiritual life and personal wishes to her medical care, Medicare, which means our tax dollars, saved tens of thousands of dollars in unnecessary care. The cardiologist was paid for seeing her in the emergency room (probably about $240), but he missed out on the high-dollar procedures ($2,000) and subsequent follow-up visits ($130 per visit). Her hospital stay was shorter than otherwise, and no further hospitalizations followed because the hospice team, led by the family physician, did a great job caring for her at home.

The family physician was allowed to bill Medicare for seeing her in the hospital (about $150). In this kind of situation, where several doctors see one patient, each doctor can bill only for unique diagnoses. The cardiologist billed for the heart failure, and the family physician billed her other conditions, such as the emphysema. (Remember, though, that if a family physician takes care of more than two issues in the hospital, the rest of his services are essentially given away.)

But what about all of the extra time, energy, and liability risk the family physician accepted to ultimately do the right thing for this patient? By liability risk, I mean some relative could have popped up out of the woodwork after her death and accused him of abandoning her and providing poor care. After all, she had heart failure, and the family physician essentially called off the cardiologist. It is admittedly a small risk, but these cases do happen. How much of the tens of thousands of dollars he saved American taxpayers went into his pocket? NOTHING. Medicare paid him absolutely nothing extra for that effort, which all took place at about midnight one Saturday night.

Medicare has no codes for this sort of thing. The extra time he took to do the right thing doesn't fit the computer billing system. Medicare does not allow physicians to bill for extra time unless, in rare cases, it is a significantly large amount of time, and even then a lot of the Medicare plans and insurance companies deny the extra charge.

To be very clear, I am not suggesting family physicians be paid a percentage of potential tests and treatments they don't order. I am suggesting, however, that family physicians be compensated fairly for their time.

How did payments become so warped?

HOW MUCH SHOULD DOCTORS MAKE?

Doctors have a special obligation to their patients, called a fiduciary relationship, which means doctors are supposed to do right by their patients, especially in urgent or emergent situations, regardless of their ability to pay. However, doctors respond to incentives like anybody else, so incentives should be aligned with greater health system goals. A system that expects doctors to work when there are no incentives, or, even worse, disincentives, is not sustainable. I assume most people would agree it is reasonable for doctors to earn more than the average person. The difficult question is: how much more?

One way to answer this question is to compare the educational return on investment for doctors versus other professions such as lawyers, dentists, and business people. In other words, what kind of payback (higher salaries) do other professionals receive from their investments in extra education and lost income during the educational years? Other professions typically don't need as many years of education as doctors. Law school, for instance, requires three years of additional schooling after college. Dental school is four before most dentists start their careers (though some pursue endodontics and orthodontics, which require more training). One study calculated the annual yield on educational investment over a working life was 29.0 percent for business people, 25.4 percent for attorneys, and 20.7 percent for dentists, 20.9 percent for ologists, and 15.9 percent for primary care physicians. [3] A separate study estimated the rate of return for educational investment in family medicine at just 4 percent.[4] Ologists have much higher returns relative to family physicians: psychiatrists 17 percent higher, general surgeons 25 percent, OB/Gyns 50 percent, and radiologists 83 percent.[5]

In comparison to European doctors, American primary care physicians make about 30 percent more income, while ologists make about 65 percent more.[7] The disparity is not an apples-to-apples comparison because European doctors commonly graduate with no educational debt; other European professionals also earn less than American professionals; and European doctors are sued much less often. Correcting for these factors minimizes the income differential, but American doctors still probably have higher incomes.[8]

I'm sure there are other ways of looking at physician pay. My conclusion on the pay issue is that, on the whole, American doctors are probably compensated about right. They have similar rates of return on their educational investment as other professions, have to pay back so much medical school debt, have to spend so many years in training, and have to deal with stressful life-and-death decisions every day. The problem with the physician workforce in America is the imbalance between ologists' incomes and family physicians' incomes, which is one of the reasons few medical students choose to become family physicians.

HOW ARE DOCTORS' FEES SET?

Before the growth of employer-sponsored health insurance in the 1950s, supply and demand set the price for most medical services. If you had abdominal pain from a gallstone, you found out how much the surgeon would charge for the service. If you could afford the surgery, you got it, and if you couldn't afford the surgery, you just suffered with the pain. It was common in that era for doctors to charge on a sliding scale: wealthier patients paid more than those who earned less.

When Medicare was created in the mid-1960s, it paid based on the "usual and customary" fees doctors charged. The problem was, many times doctors didn't have a single fee because the fee would vary based on a patient's ability to pay. Once the government entered the picture, it essentially became the wealthiest patient with an almost unlimited supply of cash.

As you can imagine, fees took off. For years, Medicare didn't have the capacity to challenge the fees. It just paid them. Older physicians told me they gathered together and disclosed to each other what they charged for a certain procedure. The highest one then became the usual and customary rate for that area.

Medicare costs naturally skyrocketed in the early years. Also, technology was rapidly expanding and creating more expensive medical tests and treatments. Calls for Medicare reform, meaning cost controls, came as early as the Nixon administration, just a few years after Medicare was created.

During the next 40 years, many analyses were performed and new programs created to try to make sense of payments to physicians and hospitals. How much should a doctor be paid to see a patient with diabetes? How much should a doctor be paid to remove a gallbladder? Medicare faced a myriad of such fundamental questions in order to bring some sanity to the payment system.

The processes for determining doctors' fees go back decades, but the modern version really started in the 1980s. Medicare gave up trying to make a rational payment scheme based on usual and customary fees. The fees were too inconsistent across the country, and because of the growing presence of insurers in the market, fees were no longer influenced much by supply and demand. Medicare responded by putting out bids for someone to create a scheme to estimate how much doctors would be paid for thousands of services if a free market existed in healthcare. An economist at Harvard and his team won the bid and set in motion the approach that created the current fee system.

The Harvard team did a lot of good things. They brought some sanity to the system and reduced the variability of fees across America. While fees still vary a little, the cause is local factors such as cost of living and malpractice costs, not the whims of local physicians. Our current payment system is much more rational than it was 30 years ago; it just favors the ologists.

The last revision of the doctor payment rules was published in 1997.[6] These are the rules that list the steps a doctor must take to justify a certain billing level. In 2002, an Advisory Committee on Regulatory Reform of the U.S. Health and Human Services Department reviewed these guidelines because so many physicians, not just family physicians, howled at how onerous and ridiculous they were. The vote of the committee was 20-1 to eliminate the payment rules.[7] An advisor for Secretary Tommy Thompson concluded, "Documentation guidelines are the poster child for regulatory burden."[8] As might be expected, the federal government ignored the advice of its own advisory committee, and doctors are still forced to work under the 1995 and 1997 rules.

HOW ARE FEES UPDATED?

The system that updates physician fees is dominated by the ologists. The American Medical Association established the Relative Value Scale Update Commission (RUC) to advise Medicare how to update the payment system on a periodic basis. This commission has approximately 29 physician members, five of whom represent primary care.[9] Recommendations from RUC require a two-thirds vote.[13, 14] RUC's stacked deck is one reason procedures and other high-tech services are overvalued, and time spent talking to patients is undervalued. RUC's meetings are closed to the public; its deliberations are proprietary and not available for review.[10]

The RUC has a powerful influence on Medicare. Traditionally, more than 90 percent of the RUC's recommendations are accepted and enacted by Medicare.[2, 4] The Center for Medicare and Medicaid Services (CMS) is the agency that ultimately puts the fee schedule into effect. CMS sets fee schedules not only for physicians but for every other medical service, such as a day spent in the intensive care unit, the cost of a power wheelchair, and the fee for a nurse to visit you at home.

RUC is also charged with finding medical services that are either undervalued or overvalued, but the allowable charges are almost always increased. In 2006, based on RUC recommendations, Medicare increased allowable charges for 227 services and decreased them for 26.[10] When Congress agrees to pay more for procedures, especially new procedures, the money has to come from somewhere, and the loser is the fees Medicare pays doctors to spend time talking to their patients and deliberating on an appropriate course of treatment. [11]

Additionally, RUC does not consider other common cost trends. In the general economy, technology becomes less expensive over time. We've all experienced this trend with computers, cell phones, and flat screen TVs. Under the RUC system, physician fees for existing technological procedures were observed to increase 82 percent of the time over a 5-year review cycle.[12]

As far back as 1993, two leading health system experts noted the distortion in the physician payment system. Steven Schroeder, the head of the Robert Wood Johnson Foundation, commented, "Medicare is perpetuating existing distortions in the fee-for-service system that overpay the use of technology."[17] William Hsiao, the economist from Harvard who led the team that created the overall Medicare fee system for all services Medicare provides, concluded, "The misallocation of practice expenses . . . results in serious underpayment for medical services. We think it likely that physicians compensate by performing more lucrative services, such as diagnostic tests. Even if legislation is passed to deal with the misallocation of expenses, the [payment system] still produces unreasonably low levels of payment overall, which could dissuade those considering a career in medicine from entering the field."[13]

Obviously, GIMeC was warned that the physician payment system contained perverse incentives to overuse expensive technology, but ignored those warnings.

To be fair, a few people in the halls of government understand how warped the current payment system has become. Bruce Steinwald, director of healthcare for the Government Accountability Office, testified at the Senate Health Education, Labor, and Pensions Committee, "When I say primary care services are undervalued, that does not mean that just increasing the prices paid to primary care is the solution."[14] In Boston, for example, Medicare pays primary care $103 for a 30-minute visit, and $449 for a diagnostic colonoscopy, which supposedly should take about the same amount of time.[14] Other evidence finds that a screening colonoscopy actually takes just 14 minutes to perform.[15] Technological advances allow ologists to provide more services in a shorter amount of time, but the fees don't drop as they would in a free market.

The chair of the Medicare committee that ultimately recommends fee schedules to Congress also recently admitted the current fee structure "does not consider the value to patient or value to society or the shortage of various types of providers."[15]

The ologist bias in the RUC has influenced physician incomes in dramatic fashion. The bias of paying handsomely for procedures and not much for thinking and talking to patients – especially complex patient encounters involving multiple symptoms, chronic diseases, and social factors -- results in high fees for the procedure-heavy ologists. Physician income figures reflect the ologist bias for procedure fees and single-organ care.[16-18]

Annual Physician Income

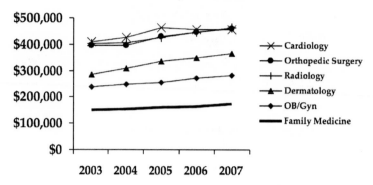

For doctors to thoroughly care for you in the manner you desire, Medicare and the insurance companies must pay doctors for the services you value. For family physicians, the reality is far from the ideal.

A FAIRER PAYMENT SYSTEM

Many people don't visit their doctors every time they have a health concern. They shouldn't. Most sniffles, aches, and pains go away on their own. Many people save up their more serious questions and concerns for the occasional visit to their doctor's office. Some even write lists (you know who you are) that they pull out of their purse at the beginning of the office visit. I think that's great. I would rather spend a lot of time with a patient and deal with as many issues as possible in one visit. The problem for family medicine is that after family physicians deal with more than two issues, Medicare and the insurance companies don't allow the family physician to bill for the extra time necessary to address the additional concerns. I don't mean they allow a little. I mean they allow nothing.

Sometimes these lists can be extensive. The following is a list of concerns one patient brought to one visit in our family medicine clinic:

- Tightness around ribs & waist
- Shortness of breath
- Eyesight not real good, even with glasses
- Can't hardly cough
- Can't strain to have bowel movement
- Have trouble swallowing – choke all the time
- Back hurts, especially when walking
- Hips hurt
- Left hand can't lift and grip
- Arm pain in big muscle of shoulder and numbness
- Left leg is very weak – right hip too
- Loss of some strength in right hand
- Trouble remembering things
- Very depressed
- Tired all the time
- Can't sleep
- Can't hardly turn over in bed – covers feel very heavy
- Trouble swallowing liquids
- Trouble chewing food
- Can't go up steps very good
- Can't hardly read a book
- Left hand and leg very numb and weak
- Take shots – sugar still high
- Blood pressure still high
- Some numbness along back of neck and shoulders

This was an actual list. There are too many issues in this list to cover in one visit, even if family physicians were actually paid for each concern they address.

On the other hand, there are times you might want one concern addressed quickly, and you don't want to spend a lot of time talking to your doctor about other issues. A fair primary care payment system would allow for either patient need: a long, complex visit that comes with a larger bill, or a quick visit with a smaller bill.

Have you ever seen your family physician for one service, to get your diabetes in better control, for instance, and then asked your doctor to investigate a new problem, like shoulder pain? Many times, your doctor might respond, "Your shoulder pain is very concerning to me, but I have other patients I need to see now, and your appointment was only allotted 15 minutes. Stop by the receptionist's desk on your way out and make an appointment as soon as possible so we can take a closer look at your shoulder." The reason he had to say this is primarily because any further time he spends caring for you is given away. Neither Medicare nor any other insurance company will allow him to bill for the extra time it takes to diagnose and treat your shoulder.

Similarly, if you've ever seen your doctor for a well-woman exam and asked about another problem, such as a rash, but were told to make another appointment, it's because some insurance companies won't pay the doctor for any service beyond the well-woman exam.

Family physicians are swamped as it is. Researchers looked at the guideline recommendations for 10 common chronic diseases and estimated the time it would take a family physician just to follow the guidelines for patients with those chronic diseases.[19] No new symptoms, no other preventive work, just manage those chronic diseases. They estimated it would take one family physician 2,484 hours per year, or 10.6 hours per day. Not only do Medicare and the insurance companies refuse to pay family physicians for all their work, under the current guidelines, there is too much chronic disease work to do.

All other professionals can charge for their time. If you see a lawyer for an appointment that was supposed to take an hour but took an hour and 15 minutes, the lawyer will charge you for the extra 15 minutes of his professional time and expertise. Accountants, counselors, plumbers – if they spend more time, they charge more. It's only fair to allow doctors to do the same.

INSURANCE COMPANY COMPUTERS

Sometimes, it's hard for family physicians to tell insurance company computers the services they provided, even when they address only one concern. Many issues patients discuss with their family physicians have no computer codes to describe them. This gap is important because almost all billing to insurance companies is electronic and based on diagnosis codes. The companies even have software that automatically denies claims if the codes don't make sense to the computer.

For example, different levels of chronic kidney disease have seven codes, but there is no code for a problem you might ask a family physician about, such as "My urine smells funny," "I just don't feel right," a runny nose, or scrotal pain. In contrast, there are codes for injury from a nuclear missile attack, or an "accident involving spacecraft injur[y]".[20] Perhaps a former head of the AMA was abducted by aliens.

The lack of codes appropriate for family medicine is a reflection of how ologists view the world. They don't handle uncertainty well. They don't like issues that are complex and messy. They want to reduce how you feel and what you experience into one cause that can be explained on a molecular or single-organ level. Unfortunately, many times it's not that simple.

This whole issue wouldn't be a big deal if the medical universe consisted only of you and your physician. Your physician could simply write down his diagnosis or assessment in the medical record and then proceed to order the appropriate tests or treatments. Medical visits don't happen in a vacuum anymore, however. Physicians have an army of people peering over their shoulders: insurance companies, quality inspectors, lawyers, etc.

For another example, say you felt weak all over for a couple of months. You gave it some time to go away on its own; you bought some vitamins but saw no improvement, so you decided to talk to your doctor about it.

How often does weakness occur with nothing else going on? No stress, no child issues, no spouse issues, no work issues, no weather changes, no missed medications, and so forth. Hardly ever. Your doctor has a tough job right out of the gate. This is a symptom that is common, but in spite of multiple tests, it also commonly defies simple explanation.

Typically, your doctor will listen to your story, ask many questions, examine the appropriate body parts, and begin to form a list of possible causes. The treatment plan at this point could follow a number of possibilities. It could be something as simple as a pat on the back accompanied by reassurance that it's unlikely there is anything seriously wrong. Or your doctor may advise you to rest a little more, get your husband to help around the house more (like that's going to happen), and come back if the symptoms don't improve. On the other extreme, your doctor might order a huge battery of tests and prescribe treatments after the first visit, even if the final diagnosis is still unclear.

Either way, your doctor can't communicate what just happened to the medical overlords. There is no code for "weak all over." Your doctor could put down something like "general physical exam." The insurance company would probably deny the claim; since there was no diagnosis, the doctor must not have done anything. She could enter something like "well-woman exam." But when the quality inspectors scan the computer records for evidence of a Pap smear or mammogram and find none, they will accuse her of either ripping off the insurance company for an incomplete exam or for providing poor care.

She could put down something like "arm weakness." There's a code for that. There are two problems with this approach. First, it doesn't accurately describe your concerns. Second, it is possible you might be denied health, disability, or life insurance in the future, because some paper pusher for an insurance company thought you had a stroke.

Your doctor could put down something that emerged in her conversation with you that wasn't the main issue, but that has a code. For example, you might have said you had a few headaches over the last two weeks. They weren't bad. The headaches went away with over-the-counter pain relievers. The weakness was more of a concern. Your doctor might put "headache" on the billing sheet because there is a code for that. This approach is also bad for several reasons. It inaccurately reflects your symptom. There is a small chance this issue will come up later in your life if you try to buy more insurance. But the bigger problem now is that the diagnostic plan will not make sense to a computer or other outsider. If your doctor decides to order a formal test of your muscle and nerve functions, it will catch the eye of the insurance company overlords. All they show on their computers is a visit for a headache and a request for a test of your muscles and nerves. Your doctor would risk having the claim denied or having some insurance company medical director hassle her.

THE HOSPITAL SETTING

When we return to the hospital setting, we find another failing of the current billing system for family physicians. Say an elderly male patient, Darryl Ward, is admitted for difficulty breathing, and his family physician takes care of him. Assume the primary cause of the difficulty is a severe worsening of his heart failure, which has been fully evaluated in the past. The heart failure is so bad Mr. Ward needs to be in a monitored unit and receive several powerful IV medications.

If that's the only issue the family physician handles, she can still bill the maximum amount Medicare allows for a physician visit each day. (The maximum allowable would decrease once the patient's condition improves.) But it's extremely rare a patient that sick would have only one problem for the doctor to monitor, diagnose, and treat.

A more realistic scenario is that Mr. Ward also has diabetes, high blood pressure, high cholesterol, and arthritis. For all of the medicines he takes, the family physician would have to make judgments about which ones should be continued at the usual dose, which ones should be stronger, which ones should be reduced or temporarily discontinued, or which ones should be permanently discontinued. Other issues would likely arise, as well. Treatment for heart failure commonly causes other problems. The potassium level in the blood could drop below normal, which increases the risk for sudden cardiac death. Sometimes, new symptoms occur during hospitalization, such as leg pain, stomach pain, mental status changes, and urinary difficulties.

Should Mr. Ward's family physician care for everything that arises during his hospital stay? This requires her to ask the right questions, examine the correct body parts, talk to other care providers, such as nurses and social workers, order the appropriate tests, and make the correct diagnoses and treatment decisions. Most of you would assume the bill she submits to the insurance company each day would look something like this:

Severe heart failure	**$XXX**
Low potassium level requiring treatment	**$XX**
Evaluation of new stomach pain	**$XX**
Diabetes – medicines adjusted for hospitalization	**$XX**
COPD – good control	**$X**
High cholesterol – good control	**$X**
Total	**$XXXX**

If you assumed this, you would be wrong. Under Medicare's billing rules, the time it took for Mr. Ward's family physician to deal with anything beyond the heart failure is not paid.

What if this same patient's treatment was approached in a different way, and the multi-ologist approach was used? Let's take the same scenario but assume Mr. Ward was admitted to a cardiologist service. Typically, one ologist asks for consultations from other ologists. The cardiologist might ask a nephrologist to consult for the potassium issue. A gastroenterologist or surgeon (or both) would be asked to deal with the stomach pain. An endocrinologist or diabetologist would be called upon to keep an eye on the diabetes. A pulmonologist would become responsible for the COPD, and maybe even a cholesterol ologist would be consulted about the cholesterol.

Medicare would pay each one of these doctors their fully allowable fee to see the patient. Multiple physician bills would not be denied because each would have a diagnosis within their particular field that they addressed. On top of the extra expense that the additional doctors' bills would cost taxpayers, each ologist likely would order tests above and beyond what a family physician would have, so the total cost of the hospitalization climbs even higher. And to top it off, the multi-ologist approach increases the risk for errors of communication, duplicated tests, and conflicting treatment plans in these complicated patients.

For that matter, the same inefficiency is promoted in the outpatient clinic setting. If a patient has high blood pressure, needs thyroid medication, needs a regular Pap smear and mammogram, has a painful shoulder, and hasn't felt quite herself lately, she has two basic choices. She could see a nephrologist or cardiologist, an endocrinologist, a gynecologist, a rheumatologist, and a psychiatrist; or she could just see a family physician.

The choice is straightforward. Would you rather try to keep up with five separate appointments, have your blood drawn at five different places, have several sets of X-rays, and come up with the co-pays on five different doctors visits, or would you rather have it all taken care of at one visit to one doctor? But for those keeping score at home, Medicare – and therefore all of the insurance companies – will not pay family physicians for the time and expertise required to do all that work in one visit. The system is flawed, to put it nicely.

EVEN MORE UNPAID SERVICES

The Medicare billing system ignores many other services provided by family physicians.

Suppose you suffered several chronic diseases. After a routine visit to your family doctor to check on your medications, you dug up the courage to talk to him about your wishes should you become terminally ill or in a persistent vegetative state. Your family physician can walk you through the legalities and paperwork specific to your individual situation. More importantly, your family physician needs to know your wishes, particularly if you have four chronic diseases and take eight different pills each day.

The result of that conversation, in the case of a patient who doesn't want to be hooked up to a breathing machine indefinitely in certain situations, is a likely savings to Medicare, and therefore American taxpayers, of thousands and thousands of dollars for ICU treatments the patient doesn't want. But how much does Medicare allow the family physician to bill for the extra 15 minutes spent dealing with this important issue? NOTHING.

Next, suppose you had trouble breathing and saw your family physician at his office. His nurse gave you several breathing treatments, but you felt no better and needed to go to the hospital.

When your family physician cares for you in his office, he must spend a fair amount of time asking the right questions, ordering the right tests, and making the right diagnosis – pneumonia, in this case. The medical-legal system expects him to fully document all of his findings in his clinic medical records, which is totally appropriate. So when you go to the hospital, can't he just copy his clinic note and send it with you? Unfortunately, no. Electronic medical record systems don't easily talk to each other. The hospital will insist he document his findings in its system. Plus, he will have to write the admission orders for your care and perform other paperwork for the hospital. He submits his bill for seeing you in his office and submits a bill for doing the hospital work to admit you. How much will Medicare pay him for the additional hospital work? NOTHING.

Now imagine you've been in the hospital for a few days and are breathing much better. Your family physician saw you in the morning and ordered one more test to address another issue that arose, and the test results become available that afternoon. The test results are reassuring and, by all accounts, it is reasonable for you to go home.

By this time your family physician has returned to his office and seen patients all day. He is tired from a long day and believes it is time to go home. The hospital, Medicare, and the insurance companies disagree. They expect the doctor to drive back to the hospital to discharge you. This argument has been going on for decades, and as you might guess, how much do Medicare and the insurance companies wish to pay the doctor for the extra time and hassle? NOTHING. The doctor would rather see you the next morning and discharge you then. He is paid for that trip to the hospital.

A complex web of payment rules and hospital regulations block efforts to pay doctors for extra work that ultimately saves the healthcare system money. Wouldn't it make sense to pay the doctor an extra $100 or so for the time and hassle of returning to the hospital and completing the discharge process in order to save the healthcare system $1,000 for an unnecessary extra night in the hospital?

In response to this conundrum, hospitals have encouraged the growth of doctors (hospitalists) who care only for patients in the hospital. The theory is a doctor who only works at the hospital can take care of these patients easier. Early research on hospitalist care found it may improve hospital efficiency.[21] Even so, the hospitalist approach frequently falls short of ideal. Tests are completed in the hospital, but the patient's family physician isn't told the results. Issues develop in the hospital that are not on the discharge paperwork, which also often isn't sent to the family physician. One study of two medical school-affiliated hospitals found that just 16 percent of pending tests were mentioned in the final reports of the hospitalists, the discharge summary.[22] Only 13 percent of the discharge summaries listed all pending tests.

By the time a patient is discharged, she may be on a completely new set of medications. The family physician has no way of knowing if the medication changes were made for a good reason like an intolerable side effect, or if they were temporary changes the hospitalist ordered with no intention of continuing in the long run. Complicating matters, hospitalists often work in shifts, so the patient has multiple doctors. If the family physician has questions, it is unclear which hospitalist has the primary responsibility, and when the family physician tries to call the hospitalist, the return call is slow and may not happen on the first attempt.

One study showed family physicians who care for their own patients in the hospital have lower overall costs than critical care hospitalists with no difference in health outcomes.[23] Research from another healthcare system found hospitalists provide no more efficient care than family physicians, except that an average hospital stay was shorter (0.4 days).[24] Hospitalists were found to provide slightly more cost-effective care than general internists – to the tune of $268 in the total cost of a hospitalization – but they were just equal to family physicians. The only attempt this study made to measure the downstream effects of hospitalists was the 14-day readmission rate, which also was similar in both groups.

In the end, the hospitalist movement has probably had a neutral effect on the overall healthcare system, neither helpful nor harmful. However, it illustrates one more work-around the greater system created that, in the end, undermines the relationship between family physicians and their patients.

In the tangled web that healthcare has become, sometimes family physicians serve their patients best simply by coordinating their care through the complex medical system. A recent estimate was that 13 percent of a family physician's time is spent coordinating care among different physicians and other health providers, such as physical therapists and home health agencies.[25] Other estimates indicate family physicians spend 30 percent to 40 percent of their day on work that is not paid by insurance companies or Medicare. Examples include filling out forms so the radiologists can be paid for an X-ray, ologists can be paid for a visit with the patient, and pharmacy benefits companies can take their cut of a prescription. How many businesses can thrive giving away up to 40 percent of their work?

PART OF THE SOLUTION

As professionals with a fiduciary duty to our patients, family physicians should rise above financial considerations and do the right thing. As a concession to realism, however, we should not have a system with so many disincentives for family physicians to go the extra mile for their patients.

At the risk of being redundant, let me review a few key points. For Americans to receive better bang for their healthcare buck, we must have more family physicians in America. Before that can happen, more American medical students must want to become family physicians. Before that can happen, medical students need clear incentives to become family physicians. It all comes back to the money. Family physicians should be paid more and, to balance the scales, the ologists paid less; the total outlay for physician's charges shouldn't increase.

The solution to this mess requires several changes. First, a coding system must be created that allows family physicians to inform insurance companies, the government, and the quality overlords exactly what they do at each office or hospital visit. Let the ologists keep the current medical coding system (called ICD-9 or ICD-10). They invented it for their own use, anyway. More family physician-appropriate codes should be added to the current codes. An existing alternative is the International Classification of Primary Care, which is already used by several European countries. Medicare and the insurance companies easily could adapt their computerized billing and coding systems to accept codes from this system.

Second, family physicians should be allowed to bill for additional time spent on patient care beyond a straightforward visit. I'm not talking about something simple; I'm talking about managing the care of a complicated patient or a complicated set of circumstances. That kind of care requires medical knowledge, so even if a nurse filled out some of the forms or made some of the phone calls, the physician must know what's going on and is ultimately responsible. These situations commonly include the physician making myriad decisions about symptoms or diseases and spending a lot of time counseling and educating patients and their families about the situation and their options. Currently, Medicare pays for one or the other, but not both at the same visit.

Third, family physicians should be allowed to bill for each issue they address in an office or hospital visit. The billing system must be additive. If the family physician is asked to address only one issue by a patient, the bill should only charge for that issue. If, however, a patient pulls out a list of six items to discuss, the family physician should be able to charge the insurance company or Medicare for six items (with some small discount for items two through six). Whether or not all six issues are actually addressed should be decided between patient and physician at that office visit. If you want to spend time talking about a lot of concerns, you can do that. If you would rather get in and out of the doctor's office quickly, you can do that, too.

In Britain, it isn't unusual for a patient to see a general practitioner 20 times a year. Generally speaking, one issue is addressed at each visit. Europeans are more accustomed to making multiple trips to merchants, such as shopping at several markets to buy food for that evening's meal. Americans aren't like that. We'd rather make the weekly trip to Wal-Mart and buy everything at one visit. The physician payment system should respect the busy schedules and purchasing preferences of American families.

Would you like a healthcare system that encouraged you to develop a relationship with one physician who is paid by the insurance companies and Medicare to spend an appropriate amount of time with you? Would you like to leave your doctor's office feeling that someone actually listened to you, rather than your doctor having to rush from one patient to the next? Or would you rather see multiple doctors in a series of office visits spread across town, each visit focused on only one part of your body? The current payment rules encourage the latter.

At the moment, there is nothing directly you can do to remedy the physician payment rules. But there is something you can do. If you must bring up three issues with your family physician the next time you see him, pat him on the back and thank him for spending some unpaid time with you. Then go home and contact your U.S. Senator and/or Representative and let them know you want the Medicare payment rules to change so that family physicians are encouraged to take total care of their patients and be fairly paid for their work. At least it's a start.

9 | EARLY DETECTION
YOU PLAY DOCTOR – ORDER TESTS

I once took care of a 63-year-old man who spent two months in the hospital following a prostate biopsy. Bacteria got into his bloodstream, traveled all over his body, and infected several major organs. He was on a breathing machine for three weeks and nearly died several times in the intensive care unit. Over the course of his hospitalization, his lungs filled with fluid, his intestines stopped working, he couldn't eat or drink for weeks, and he became extremely weak from lying in a hospital bed for so long. Finally, he was discharged to a rehabilitation facility.

The wife of a friend had a biopsy of a suspicious lung nodule. After the procedure, she developed pneumonia and other complications associated mostly with lying in a hospital bed for days. She died suddenly four weeks later.

A patient of a colleague underwent an operation to biopsy a small nodule detected in his kidney during an abdominal CAT scan performed for a completely unrelated reason. During the surgery, the urologist determined that the nodule could not be accessed with the laparoscope so he turned the patient over and reached the kidney through a traditional abdominal incision. The abdominal wound didn't heal well, leaving the patient with a large hernia that rendered him incapable of continuing his previous work, which involved heavy lifting. As of this writing, the patient is applying for disability. The nodule was benign.

The common thread is that all these illnesses started with a so-called "simple" test. The first man had a PSA blood test that was slightly high. That led to a prostate biopsy, which caused the bacteria to invade his bloodstream. The urologist did nothing wrong; infections are a recognized complication of the procedure. The woman had a chest X-ray ordered because of a cough. A small nodule was noticed and a biopsy was recommended. The surgeon did nothing wrong. In fact, the nodule turned out to be cancerous. In the end, however, the procedure killed her faster than the cancer would have. The last patient had a CAT scan just to ensure a severe disease wasn't causing his chronic abdominal symptoms.

Deciding which tests to order and when to order them is one of the hardest in medicine. GIMeC has convinced the American public no one would be injured or die if a complete battery of tests were ordered for every patient in every situation. Unfortunately, all tests are imperfect, especially the non-invasive ones such as blood tests, sonograms, X-rays, CAT scans, and MRIs. They can suggest a disease is present when it isn't; they can miss a disease when it's there. Earlier in the book, we discussed the POEM assumption that early detection prevents everything bad, which is usually attempted by some sort of test. The truth is, medical tests have their limits.

NOW YOU PLAY DOCTOR

Put yourself in a doctor's shoes. Imagine a 53-year-old female patient, Leah Martinez, comes to you complaining of chest pain. Which tests are medically necessary?

The first thing to do is ask Mrs. Martinez a series of questions to explore the nature of the pain, such as when it started, what it feels like, and how severe it is. After you've talked to her for a while, you examine her. Now, it's time to order tests. No universal medical test magically gives the diagnosis. The doctor has to determine the right tests to order based on the patient's story.

Chest pain can have dozens of causes. Some are immediately life threatening; some are life threatening, but won't kill her in the near future; and some are less severe. There is no "chest pain panel" of tests (a panel that will check every possible cause). Most doctors want to order the right number of tests, but doctors from different fields often disagree what that number is.

The appropriate number of tests is influenced by the likelihood your patient has the condition the test is meant to detect. In the ER, you learn that Mrs. Martinez has experienced two hours of severe chest pain in the middle of her chest, and she has a history of high cholesterol, high blood pressure, and diabetes. Based on that information and a relatively normal physical examination, a list of possible causes might look like this:

Heart attack	20 percent
Heart blockage without a heart attack	40 percent
Rib or chest muscle irritation	5 percent
Blood clot in her lungs	1 percent
Irritation of the lining of her heart only	1 percent
Collapsed lung	0.1 percent
Lung cancer	0.01 percent

(I realize the percentages don't add up to 100 percent. For the purposes of our example, we're leaving out a dozen other causes of chest pain.)

How many tests should you initially order? Reality is never this simple, but let's pretend each of the seven conditions requires one test to rule it in or out as the cause of her condition. Would you order seven tests initially, even for the rare causes?

All doctors would agree that tests to check for evidence of a heart attack are medically necessary for this patient. A blood test for heart attack (cardiac enzymes) doesn't show any evidence of one, but Mrs. Martinez is not out of the woods yet. About 50 percent of patients who come to ERs with heart attacks have normal initial tests.

It's possible she has a cancer near the lining of her lung. The tumor could suddenly start bleeding, which irritates the lung and causes a sudden onset of pain. Such a lump could be missed on a chest X-ray. If you were interested in pursuing lung cancer as a possible explanation for her chest pain, you might order a CAT scan of her chest, which includes injecting dye into her veins to make some of the internal structures more clearly visible on the computer screen.

Would you order the chest CAT scan immediately when she arrived at the hospital, since cancer is a possible cause, or would you wait for some of the other test results to come back first? Here's one of the risk/benefit trade-offs you must balance. A chest CAT scan could – in rare cases – injure or kill Mrs. Martinez if she has a severe allergic reaction to the dye injected into her. At this point, her chance of being harmed by the IV dye has entered the same ballpark as the chance that lung cancer caused the pain. Additionally, there are long-term risks to CAT scans. Some doctors believe CAT scans are ordered too often, and the unnecessary radiation may contribute to the later development of cancers, as we discussed earlier concerning President Obama's medical evaluation.[1]

The other rare, but possible, scenario is that Mrs. Martinez is having a heart attack that the first round of tests missed, and her condition could rapidly deteriorate while she undergoes the CAT scan. A CAT scanner tucked in a back corner of the radiology department is not a good place for your patient to lose her pulse and quit breathing.

Let's say you wait for a few sets of heart attack tests, and all return as "normal." The odds of lung cancer causing the pain you estimated at 0.01 percent, and a plain chest X-ray was normal, so you decide not to order further tests to look for lung cancer. For some symptoms, such as chest pain, no good test exists to determine causes such as sore ribs or pulled muscles. Doctors will often treat a patient for a less life-threatening cause even without proof of the cause. For chest pain, you prescribe Tylenol or another anti-inflammatory medication to take on a scheduled basis for a few weeks. If Mrs. Martinez feels better, you likely would conclude one of the unprovable causes explains her chest pain because of the way she responded to the treatment.

A FEW WEEKS LATER

On the other hand, what if Mrs. Martinez returns two weeks later and reports the pain is still there? The medicine helped a little, but the pain is not going away.

Back to our list of possible causes. We've ordered tests for heart attacks, heart blockages, blood clots, and a plain chest

X-ray for a collapsed lung. If the cause was a sore rib or pulled chest wall muscle, she didn't respond as expected. It's also possible she had one of the first diseases, but the initial tests missed the diagnosis. The fancy term for this scenario is a "false negative result." You could reorder the same tests to see if something shows up this time. Or, you could order different tests to look for the possible diseases in a different way.

Let's assume you decide not to re-test for the first group of causes, but instead start to hunt for rarer causes. If heart attack, heart blockage, blood clot, sore ribs, or pulled muscles are not likely, the chance the pain is caused by lung cancer has increased. It's not 0.01 percent anymore. Now it's in the single digits, maybe 5 percent. A CAT scan has become a more reasonable test, and the possibility a spot will be seen has increased, as has the chance the spot is the cause of the pain. The timing of a test has a great impact on how useful the test is, because the results of other tests influence the overall probability that another disease is the cause of the chest pain.

One last thought: notice that as we discussed different testing approaches, we didn't consider cost. Should the cost of a test be a factor you must consider in deciding the appropriate sequence of tests? If one of the possible tests cost $2,000 vs. $20, should that difference influence your decision? If we ever want to get healthcare costs under control, the answer to that question is a resounding YES.

In short, any new, more affordable healthcare plan must include agreements between patients and doctors that tests will be ordered only when there is a greater than minimal chance the test will find something important. An affordable plan simply must include an agreement that defines cost-effective testing.

These two principles, risk and cost, will serve as the foundation of a new definition of tests that are truly medically necessary.

GENERALISTS AND OLOGISTS

How do generalists and ologists view the medical necessity of testing? Very little research considers the outcomes of different testing strategies. The NIH doesn't fund much research to determine whether it is better for a doctor to order every possible test at the first opportunity, or to be selective initially and add tests only if compelling reasons exist.

Ologists typically take the first approach, while generalists typically take the second approach. Both groups' response is just part of the culture of their fields, but the situation sheds light on an important reason that family physicians provide better health at a lower cost. Under the care of family physicians, patients aren't exposed to the harms of excessive testing and hospitalizations, and the cost savings can be substantial.

This ologist/generalist divergence of opinion becomes even clearer in recent recommendations about children with ADHD who receive stimulant medications, such as Ritalin. The American Heart Association recommends EKG testing for all children about to be prescribed stimulants.[2] The American Academy of Pediatrics says this approach is unnecessary because it would expose healthy children to unnecessary and costly heart tests, which could limit access to effective ADHD treatments and thereby impact the children's mental health and school performance.[3]

GIMEC GROUPTHINK ON MEDICAL TESTING

The GIMeC members unite to support the belief that more testing equals better medical care. For many ologist professors in medical universities, the pursuit of the medical zebra – medical slang for a rare disease – gives them their greatest professional joy. The concept of the zebra in medical testing is known nationally and comes from the following aphorism, "If you hear thundering hooves in the distance, think horses, not zebras." Medical students are taught this wisdom by some professors, but the dominant culture among medical school professors is the belief that the ultimate professional achievement is diagnosing a rare disease. Pop culture reinforces the idea that the pursuit of the medical zebra is the pinnacle of achievement in television shows such as *House*.

Medical school administrations encourage and magnify this attitude. Their public relations departments send out press releases with stories of patients who came to their university hospital. Thanks to the thorough and caring ologists at the university medical center who put the patient through a complete battery of tests, the zebra was found. Now, the patient knows the diagnosis and is finally receiving the appropriate treatment. This story is repeated in fund-raising newsletters, and occasionally the lucky patient even gets to tell his own story to the annual meeting with the big donors.

The news media commonly becomes involved at this point. Zebra stories are easy to tell. There is conflict: either the patient is battling a symptom or the patient is in conflict with doctors. "I've been to several doctors, and no one can tell me what's wrong." And, of course, there is resolution: the patient receives a diagnosis and treatment, and all becomes right with the world. The rare patient for whom this scenario plays out feels lucky.

Certainly, for all physicians – ologist or generalist – the occasional zebra hunt is absolutely the right course. But the flipside of the obsession with zebra hunting appears in the medical schools, where the teaching professors demonstrate boredom to the point of disdain for diagnosing and treating common conditions. In teaching hospital rounds, many of the ologist professors will spend an hour pontificating about all the rare causes of a symptom. They insist the residents order a bunch of extra tests, whether to be thorough or just academic is unclear, and spend very little time teaching the best approaches to diagnose and treat common conditions. In many cases, the professors probably have no idea what those approaches are.

This attitude presents several problems. First, young ologist doctors are not taught common-sense diagnostic and treatment approaches. Even some of the professors who don't order every test possible often assume the young doctors will figure out more efficient ways of caring for patients once they enter private practice. A more likely result is that most physicians practice medicine in a style similar to their residency training.

Second, young ologist doctors are not taught how to handle uncertainty when they care for patients. An aphorism family physicians are more likely to follow is, "If it looks like a duck, walks like a duck, and quacks like a duck, it's a duck." This statement is almost always true. Rarely does the likely duck turn out to be a platypus. A confident family physician practices in a style that is efficient and patient-friendly. The family physician is not paralyzed by the fear of uncertainty when she orders tests selectively.

Trial lawyers also encourage the assumption that more tests equal better care, which is the foundation for many of their medical malpractice lawsuits and is the reason they earn billions per year in contingency fees.

A typical lawsuit story goes like this: A patient presents to a clinic or an ER with some symptoms, a few tests are ordered, a diagnosis is made, and the patient is sent home with some instructions for follow up with another doctor later. The patient gets home, feels worse, returns, and either ends up dying or having a prolonged hospitalization with long-term health problems.

In these cases, the patient has a rare disease or a very unusual presentation of a common disease. The defending doctor who is sued and her expert witness deal with a line of questioning in a deposition that goes something like this:

Lawyer: *Was there a chance the patient had rare disease X when he first showed up to the ER?*

Doctor: *Yes. (Of course it was possible. That's what the patient died of.)*

Lawyer: *Is there a test that could have been ordered in the ER to rule in or rule out rare disease X?*

Doctor: *Yes.*

Lawyer: *Could the test have led to an earlier diagnosis of rare disease X?*

Doctor: *Yes.*

Lawyer: *Is it possible that the patient could still be alive today if rare disease X had been diagnosed earlier?*

Doctor: *Yes, I suppose it's possible. (Anything is possible.)*

The underlying assumptions in this series of questions are: 1) No one would be injured or die if the offending disease was caught earlier, and 2) Over-testing does not harm patients. The potential harms of over-testing, such as excessive radiation exposure, are difficult to bring into legal proceedings, and issues of cost or cost-effectiveness are never allowed in the discussion. To address the costs associated with extensive testing would set up the defendant doctor for a slam-dunk drama moment by the plaintiff's lawyer.

"You mean, Doctor, you believe a life is worth less than a simple test?" Or, "Doctor, what price do you put on a human life?"

TORT REFORM

I will now attempt to deliver on a promise I made earlier in the book and reveal the secret to meaningful tort reform. The lack of attention to the issue of appropriate testing continues to stymie our nation's efforts to create an equitable medical malpractice resolution system. Too many times, the proposals for tort reform are based on limits of fees or awards. These solutions can have some effect, but they don't answer the most crucial questions of risk and cost.

Suppose a patient walks into an ER complaining of pain in her abdomen. The patient laughs, eats, and goes to the bathroom without difficulty. The pain has been off and on for a few days; the physical exam is essentially normal; a few basic tests are ordered and are all normal; and the patient is sent home with a diagnosis of something like indigestion or constipation. Do Americans feel the doctor did enough and provided decent care, or should that doctor have done more?

For the vast majority of patient visits, the answer is straightforward. The patients do fine and feel better with treatment and time. But for doctors who practice in the style of not ordering CAT scans and MRIs on every patient who walks into the ER, it is just a matter of time and chance until a patient with a similar story is sent home, returns later, and has a more life-threatening condition discovered at the second visit: a ruptured appendix, an ovarian abscess, a blocked intestine, and so on. Most of these patients will feel bad for a while but fully recover with treatment. Some of them, though, will have a stormier course and possible long-term health issues, and, rarely, a few will die. The GIMeC assumption is the patient would still be alive if every test was ordered at the first visit. After all, more testing equals better care. This is a false assumption. People can still die even if a disease is caught at the first opportunity.

What should be the relationship between American doctors and their patients in a more cost-effective healthcare system? A doctor should be allowed to exercise judgment on which patients will likely benefit from an aggressive diagnostic work up, and which won't, without worrying about being raked over the coals for missing the rare disease. Similarly, patients, insurance companies, legislators, and lawyers must recognize that aggressive testing also can lead to worse health than leaving a patient alone.

It all boils down to questions of risk and cost. Doctors and patients must agree that a disease's rarity justifies not testing for it on a first visit (or even second or third visits, in many cases). They also must agree that an all-out, gung-ho approach to testing, regardless of cost, is unjustified and often harmful in itself. When those things happen, meaningful tort reform finally will occur.

PART OF THE SOLUTION

For people who believe healthcare should be significantly more affordable, their doctors must be allowed to order fewer tests. Doctors must be discouraged from ordering tests for rare conditions, at least in the first few visits for a new problem. A new definition of "medical necessity" must include the requirement that a test has a greater than minimal chance of diagnosing the patient's symptoms. A medically necessary test must also meet cost-effectiveness guidelines. We must define when tests are too expensive to order, relative to their expected benefit.

Without these agreements, the NIH and private companies will continue inventing even more expensive tests; these newer and more expensive tests will be overused; and healthcare inflation in America will never be brought under control.

10 | YOU PLAY DOCTOR –
ORDER TREATMENTS

Because doctors' pens are the most expensive
technology in healthcare, doctors must change their method of
making decisions if meaningful healthcare reform is to take
place. Particularly, the habit of using the latest test, drug, or
device, even if it has limited proof of effectiveness, must change.

Don't misunderstand. I am not a Luddite, resisting
anything new. Many important medical advances have occurred
during the last 20 years. When I was in medical school, MRIs
were just becoming widespread. I also distinctly remember a
lecture by a professor who dismissed two Australian doctors'
theory that most stomach ulcers were caused by a bacterium. To
prove their theory, one of them went so far as to drink a glass
full of it. He developed a stomach ulcer. The Australians later
won the Nobel Prize in medicine for their efforts. Later, as an
intern, I saw one to two children a month admitted to the
hospital for meningitis. During my residency, a vaccine became
available to prevent the most common cause of early childhood
meningitis. The rate of meningitis plummeted. And in my early
career, cholesterol-lowering drugs called statins were
introduced. All of us in family medicine had to decide which
patients should be tested for high cholesterol, and which of those
who registered high should be treated. Over the years, a series of

national guidelines from the National Cholesterol Education Program provided detailed instructions for diagnosing and treating high cholesterol.[1] Similar panels occasionally update guidelines for other chronic diseases such as asthma, emphysema, and high blood pressure.[2-4]

What I do oppose, however, is the POEM assumption that newer treatments or more treatments equal better care. Specifically, let's consider how much proof is required to demonstrate that a treatment actually works before a doctor should order it.

Many published medical studies are broadly called "observational studies." These could include anything from the microscopic (observing how cells react to different drugs) to the macroscopic (seeking connections between smoking and cancer in large populations). Observational studies make no attempt to change anything. They simply look for statistical associations between one factor and another.

The media loves to report the results of these studies because there are many of them out there, and they generate a lot of drama and fear. These stories almost always end with a statement about risk. A hidden danger in your own body could put you at risk. Something you enjoy eating, drinking, or doing could put you at risk. We're all familiar with the tale.

HORMONES

The post-menopausal women and hormones controversy provides an excellent example of the weakness of observational studies. The Harvard Nurses Study involved tens of thousands of nurses who completed surveys every two years about their health. The researchers asked questions about the nurses' personal habits, new diagnoses received in the last two years, and what medicines they took. The study found an association between women who took hormones after menopause and a decreased risk of heart attacks.[5, 6] They sliced and diced these results many different ways, performed fancy statistical analyses, and kept coming to the same conclusion: women who took hormones around and after menopause were much less likely to die from a heart attack.

OB/Gyns, some of whom were paid by drug companies that manufactured female hormones, exhorted other physicians to administer hormones to all women at menopause because it would significantly cut the rate of heart attacks. As an added bonus, the hormone pills also would do many other magical things, such as decrease moodiness. One particularly dramatic speaker made the following point: Doctors treat other forms of organ failure, such as kidney failure and heart failure. Therefore, only sexist doctors would refuse to treat ovarian failure (the ovaries stop producing enough hormones, which causes menopause).

Treating menopausal women with hormones was the accepted standard of care in the 1990s. Successful malpractice lawsuits claimed their victims died from a heart attack because the family physician or other doctor elected not start the women on hormones. In their closing arguments, the lawyers surely chanted the GIMeC mantra that early detection and treatment prevents everything bad.

I had a patient in the mid-1990s who was a healthy 52-year-old woman, except for high blood pressure that was well controlled on one medication. Her cholesterol wasn't elevated. I encouraged her to start taking hormones on a regular basis so she could enjoy all of their magic benefits. She was a nurse and knew that all the medical and nursing publications said to put women like her on hormones, so she readily agreed. A month after she started taking the hormones, she had a small heart attack. One of the branches coming off one of her main coronary arteries became blocked, causing some of the heart tissue downstream from the blockage to die, which is what happens in a heart attack. She made it to the emergency room quickly and was administered one of the clot-busting drugs.

The cardiologist put an angioplasty balloon in the blocked artery and started to blow it up. As the balloon expanded to push the cholesterol blockage away from the center of the artery, the artery ruptured. The cardiologist did nothing wrong. Sometimes, things just happen. She was rushed to the operating room to have her chest cracked open for heart surgery to bypass the now-ruptured blood vessel. She survived the whole ordeal with no long-term ill effects, other than a big scar down the middle of her chest and daily medicines she must take as a heart-attack survivor.

I remember thinking two things at the time. First, it seemed odd she had a heart attack so soon after she started medication (the hormones) to prevent a heart attack. Second, I thought she was probably lucky she was taking the hormones. She could have had a bigger heart attack if the preventive medicines had not been in her system.

With this background, let's return to the research. During the hormone hoopla, some careful observers noted that clinical trials using hormones to prevent heart attacks already had been conducted, and these studies found hormones were useless for this purpose.[7, 8] However, the studies were limited because they enrolled almost exclusively white men.

Critics of these studies correctly pointed out that just because female hormones did not prevent heart attacks in men did not mean they would prove ineffective in women. To fill this knowledge deficit, a series of studies was launched during the Clinton administration called the Women's Health Initiative. The NIH committed hundreds of millions of dollars to study important health issues for women, including the use of hormones in post-menopausal women.

The hormone advocates went ballistic. Instead of appreciating that a clinical trial finally would answer these important questions, they accused the federal government of wasting taxpayer money. They said we already knew hormones prevented heart attacks. We didn't need additional studies to confirm the obvious.

By now, most women know the punch line of this story. The clinical trials showed female hormones did not prevent heart attacks, but did increase the risk of significant blood clots, gallbladder disease, and breast cancer.[9, 10] The truth turned out much differently than the observational studies had predicted.

TREATING PATIENTS WITH LITTLE EVIDENCE

Suppose you were a doctor with an adult patient, Michelle Enmon, who has a flare up of low back pain. Of course, Mrs. Enmon needs pain medicine, but which one? For simplicity's sake, assume that just two different treatments have been shown to ease low back pain in clinical trials. You try both treatments at different times. One treatment helped a little, while the other didn't seem to do much. Reasonably, you advise your patient to discontinue the second treatment.

Mrs. Enmon returns to your clinic and says she can't work or drive because she is in constant pain. She says, "Doc, you gotta do something. I'm miserable." You search the medical journals and other sources, but nothing else is proven to make a difference for her pain. However, many articles, blogs, and ads claim an experimental treatment helped two patients with low back pain, providing near-miraculous results. Do you prescribe or recommend an experimental treatment proposed by a potential charlatan? No? Then how many amazing personal anecdotes would it take to convince you a treatment is reasonable to try – one testimonial, ten testimonials, a hundred? If you tried a few without success, how many attempts at experimental treatment would it take before you told Mrs. Enmon, "I'm sorry you still have significant pain, but we've tried everything within reason. Medical science has found nothing better for your back pain"?

These are very difficult questions with no right or wrong answers. One thing is certain, however. In the balance between medical aggression and humility, GIMeC always chooses aggression.

WHICH INNOVATIONS SHOULD THE HEALTHCARE SYSTEM ADOPT?

When to adopt a new technology is always a challenging decision. Many new healthcare technologies come to market each year, and they typically are expensive. Reasonable doctors differ on the amount of proof they believe is required to conclude a new technology is better than an older one.

One of the sayings handed down by the wise physicians who proceeded the current generation was, "Never be the first doctor, nor the last doctor, to use a new drug." This approach made a lot of sense. It allowed most physicians to have some reassurance that a new drug was safe and effective before it became widely used. It also discouraged physicians from being stubborn and holding onto old ways even if better treatment options were available.

Unfortunately, this axiom is too simplistic. Someone has to be the first one to use a new drug, and someone has to be the last. The better question is: How much proof should we require before a new treatment is determined to be superior to the existing treatment and is widely adopted by the general medical community? It's an extremely complex question, but it deserves an answer.

The first step toward a judicious reply is to consider that a drug company may spend $800 million to bring a completely new drug to market.[11] That astronomical figure includes the cost of drugs that did not make it to large human trials. Understandably, the FDA is under pressure from the pharmaceutical companies and their allies to release drugs to the market as soon as possible so the companies can begin recouping their research costs.

PROOF OF EFFECTIVENESS

Let's say a pharmaceutical company announced it invented a new drug that works in a completely different way than any existing drug, and this new drug was found to reduce cholesterol build-up in the arteries of mice hearts. Should the drug go on the market at this point? Most scientists would say no.

A few years later, the new drug has been tested successfully on several different animals. In each animal, the drug reduced cholesterol build-up in the heart arteries, and no obvious damage to other parts of the body was observed. The drug also was given to a few humans. Ultrasounds of their heart arteries showed the cholesterol build-up shrank by 25 percent in half of them. Should the drug be widely sold now?

To prove the effectiveness of a drug, several types of studies must be completed that build on the results of previous studies. Even for human trials, the FDA requires different phases of study. In a Phase 1 study, a research subject is given just one dose of an experimental drug, and afterward a lot of blood work is done to test the effect of the drug on the body. In a Phase 3 study, hundreds to thousands of patients are given either the experimental drug or a placebo to see if the drug improves peoples' health.

It's relatively easy for a company to show a new drug changes something measurable like a cholesterol level, the size of a tumor, or the amount of a protein in the blood stream. It's much harder to show a new drug improves a person's health, such as reducing strokes, heart attacks, or death.

For example, the ILLUMINATE trial tested an experimental drug (torcetrapib), which raised the good cholesterol (HDL) level by 72 percent and lowered the LDL level by 25 percent in patients who received it compared to the group that received placebos. However, the overall death rate was higher in the group receiving the experimental drug.[5] Better cholesterol levels didn't result in less heart disease or fewer deaths.

In the ENHANCE clinical trial, a combination of two drugs to lower bad cholesterol (LDL) was compared to therapy with just one of the drugs.[6] The combination pill, which goes by the brand name Vytorin, contained the drugs ezetimibe and simvastatin. Patients who took Vytorin were compared to patients who took simvastatin (Zocor) alone. The LDL was lowered more in the Vytorin group than the simvastatin group, but the heart attack rate and overall death rate was no different in the two groups. Cholesterol levels further lowered by the additional drug did not result in better health.

Vytorin was already approved by the FDA and on the market when the ENHANCE results were published. How could the FDA have approved Vytorin with no proof that it actually saves lives compared to other cholesterol treatment options? The FDA already had made a policy decision that a new cholesterol drug would only have to prove it lowered bad cholesterol. It assumed the health benefits would follow. The FDA wasn't necessarily irresponsible to approve Vytorin. Many doctors would have made a similar mental leap of faith that lowering bad cholesterol could only have good results for patients.

The movement in modern medicine that concerns itself with these issues is called "evidence-based medicine." Its underlying philosophy is there should be proof that a patient's health improves with a new drug or device before a new technology is widely adopted. Improvements in blood test numbers or scan results do not constitute adequate proof of benefit.

Other examples exist, as well. Just because a test shows a person's lung function is better with a drug doesn't mean the person will feel better, go to the hospital less often, or live longer. Just because a drug is shown to delay the start of microscopic kidney damage doesn't mean the drug delays the start of dialysis. Just because a test finds a smaller cancer does not mean a person is less likely to die from the cancer.

There is a spectrum of choices for widely adopting a new technology. On one end, we could adopt a new technology at the slightest hint of its effectiveness. On the other end, we could adhere to a strict evidence-based standard that insisted upon ironclad proof of a new technology's benefit before it was used outside of a clinical trial.

The danger of the evidence-based approach is that it delays the introduction of important new drugs and devices. Patients who could have benefited will continue to suffer or die waiting for some elusive final level of proof.

The danger of introducing drugs and devices too quickly into the market is that new products are adopted even though they later prove ineffective, as in the ENHANCE trial, or even harmful, as in the ILLUMINATE trial. Using an ineffective drug presents problems because new technologies are almost always more expensive, therefore wasting precious medical resources.

Unfortunately, the reality of technology development means we have no way of knowing in advance which drugs or devices that change a measurement in a lab will actually improve people's health. Either approach is potentially justifiable: approve drugs early and make them available with no solid proof of effectiveness, or wait for definitive proof. But as a society, we need to realize that the former approach has an enormous impact on healthcare costs. Aggressive adoption of expensive new technologies increases the cost of care. Cautious adoption keeps costs down. The choice is ours. We just need to understand the implications of that choice.

GIMEC GROUPTHINK AND LOW BACK PAIN

The following story illustrates what can happen when special interest groups push for aggressive adoption of new technologies, especially when politicians become involved.

In 1994, an agency of the federal government called the Agency for Health Care Policy and Research (AHCPR) published guidelines on "Acute Low Back Problems in Adults: Assessment and Treatment."[12] In that era, many patients with low back pain were advised to have surgery. MRIs had just come into widespread use and, like today, millions of people had low back pain. When they went to their doctors seeking relief, millions of MRIs were ordered to investigate. Millions of people were found to have bulging disks and other irregularities, so millions of people had surgery to correct the problem.

In this surgery, a neurosurgeon or orthopedic surgeon cuts out the cushion (the disk) between two back bones (lumbar vertebrae) and puts a piece of bone on top of the two back bones (with or without things like metal screws and plates), which then causes those two back bones to fuse together. These two now move as one unit.

Over time, the fused back bones put more stress on the disks above and below them. The patient may report either continued or worsening back pain, so another MRI is ordered and – lo and behold – one or both of the disks above and below the fused back bones bulge. Back to the operating room to have another disk removed and another back bone fused onto the set that was already fused.

After more physical therapy and more medications, the patient still complains of back pain. The surgeon operates again, and again the patient has no significant relief. At this point the surgeon declares the patient is not a surgical candidate anymore; therefore, the surgeon has nothing else to offer and essentially banishes the patient from his office. The current name for this situation is "failed back syndrome," which might be better named "failed surgeon syndrome." Family physicians have legions of such patients that the back surgeons refuse to treat any longer, even with medical therapy.

AHCPR noticed billions of dollars being spent on low back MRIs and surgeries in the late 1980s and early 1990s. They reviewed the medical literature to decide if these surgeries were helpful and to determine the kind of medical care, both tests and treatments, that really relieved low back pain.

AHCPR concluded many tests and treatments had little to no proof they actually relieved pain. AHCPR further concluded there was no evidence to support spinal fusion surgery and commented that such surgery commonly had complications. Its findings included statements such as, "In the absence of dangerous signs and symptoms, special studies (like MRIs) are not necessary, since 90 percent of patients will recover spontaneously within four weeks."[12] It concluded that unless the patient had serious symptoms other than the pain, there was no reason to order even a plain X-ray, much less a $1,500 MRI. According to AHCPR, billions of dollars per year were wasted on ineffective tests and treatments on millions of patients.

Needless to say, the ologists were not pleased.

OLOGISTS AND THE CONGRESS

The lucrative practices of orthopedic surgeons and neurosurgeons were threatened. Being smart, aggressive, action-oriented people, they did not cower and quietly slink into the night.

The North American Spine Society (NASS) created an ad hoc committee that attacked the literature review and subsequent AHCPR practice guideline. In a letter published in 1994 in the journal *Spine,* the committee not only criticized the methods used in the literature review and expressed concern the conclusions might be used by payers or regulators to limit spinal fusion procedures, it also accused AHCPR of wasting taxpayer dollars on the study.[13]

Neil Kahanovitz, a back surgeon from Arlington, Va., founded a group called the Center for Patient Advocacy to lobby on the issue.[13] It organized a letter-writing campaign to gain congressional support for its attack on AHCPR. Kahanovitz used personal contacts to gain the support of a Rep. Bonilla (D-TX), whose staff member was one of Kahanovitz's patients. Representatives Bonilla and others led the effort in the House to end the agency's funding, energetically supporting the NASS/Kahanovitz argument that AHCPR supported unsound research and wasted taxpayer money.

At a Ways and Means subcommittee hearing, other representatives attacked AHCPR for wastefulness and unwarranted interference with the practice of medicine. Another Congressman proposed an amendment to eliminate AHCPR by stopping its funding. After intense behind-the-scenes negotiations, that amendment was withdrawn. A joint conference set the funding at $125 million, a 21 percent cut from 1995.

The final compromise was that AHCPR would disappear. It was reborn with a new name: the Agency for Healthcare Research and Quality (AHRQ), whose new mission was limited to matters of healthcare safety and quality. It was forbidden to ever write another medical care guideline.

EPILOGUE

After the near extinction of AHCPR, independent researchers published studies further supporting its original position. In 1994, researchers measured how often normal people have abnormal MRIs.[14] They enrolled 98 middle-age adults with no back pain and ordered MRIs of their lower backs. Sixty-four percent of the subjects had abnormal disks; 52 percent had at least one bulging disk; and 27 percent had at least one protruding disk. Additionally, 38 percent had an abnormality of more than one disk. All of this in people with no reported back pain. This study was conducted and published years after MRIs became widely used.

Slowly over the next 10 years, the tide shifted in the surgical community to recognize the limits of major low back surgery. An editorial published in a leading medical journal in 2004 expressed concern about the overuse of spinal-fusion surgery.[15] Another observer described a 15-fold increase in complex spinal fusion surgeries among Medicare beneficiaries from 2002 to 2007, despite higher morbidity, mortality, and costs.[16] I suspect the surgeons truly believed the complex approaches were better at the time, although increased income to the surgeons and hospitals, a lack of cost-awareness on the part of the patients, and aggressive marketing by the device companies played a role in the procedures' growth.[17]

A study published in 2010 found that workers' compensation patients in Ohio with a variety of low back ailments were much more likely to return to work if they didn't have surgery (67 percent without surgery versus 26 percent with surgery).[18] Additionally, patients who had surgery experienced a 41 percent increase in the use of narcotic painkillers. Other studies found that back surgeries either didn't help or made the pain and function worse.[19] Today, a qualified orthopedic surgeon or neurosurgeon will bend over backwards not to perform surgery.

The final ironic twist in this story is that a new set of back pain guidelines was published in 2007.[20] It offered many of the same recommendations AHCPR had put forward 13 years earlier. It recognized that 85 percent of patients with acute back pain do not have a simple explanation for that pain, no matter how many tests are ordered. Even the North American Spine Society called these new guidelines "extraordinarily educational."[21]

So, it turns out AHCPR died needlessly. Being right didn't matter. Publishing diagnosis and treatment guidelines that questioned the POEM assumptions of GIMeC sounded the death knell for AHCPR.

Low back pain is a prime area where all of us, doctors and patients, need a large dose of humility. Many people suffer debilitating back pain, but it is rare that a simple explanation is found that is easily and permanently fixed. Human beings walk the earth with back structures that just can't take the pounding.

Taking the GIMeC approach in this area almost never helps, but wastes billions of healthcare dollars a year.

PART OF THE SOLUTION

There is actually proof that GIMeC has successfully convinced the American public that more treatments and more expensive care is necessarily better. A study published in *Health Affairs* in 2010 asked a representative sample of Americans with private insurance about their attitudes towards medical guidelines and evidence-based medicine.[22] Less than half felt that insurance plans should provide the best treatments at the lowest cost. Said one anonymous participant, "I don't see how extra care can be harmful to your health. Care would only benefit you." When participants were presented the term "good value for the money," many equated it with bargain-basement pricing and low quality.

For people who want healthcare to become radically more affordable, their relationships with their doctors must change in the area of treatments. Doctors and patients must agree that if no solid proof exists that a certain treatment will be successful – only theory and speculation to support the notion – the treatment won't be offered. Patients will always be free to enroll in clinical trials separate from a basic healthcare plan, or to pay for experimental treatments on their own.

Experimental cancer treatments are a particularly thorny issue. I can't say for sure how I would react if a family member had cancer not cured after one or two rounds of traditional treatment. Nevertheless, I and some other doctors wouldn't opt for an aggressive experimental treatment journey. We have seen too many patients experience prolonged suffering for themselves and their families because they put too much faith in toxic experimental treatments that didn't cure anything. If a treatment might extend my life three months but make me miserable for six, it's not worth it. With rare exceptions, experimental cancer treatments can't promise cures, only a few more months of survival at most.

For a healthcare system to be more affordable, a medically necessary treatment must meet two criteria: 1) It has greater than a tiny chance of being successful, and 2) It doesn't cost more than an amount agreed to by everyone in advance. Doctors and patients must humbly accept that there are many symptoms and conditions for which there are no good answers, and spending thousands of dollars on treatments unlikely to be effective doesn't change this reality.

As daunting as this proposal might sound, there is an upside. If your family physician practices evidence-based medicine, it also means when he recommends a test or treatment, there is a good chance it will work. You can be sure the physician is not proposing a series of office visits or procedures just to milk money out of you and your insurance company.

In the future, when well-meaning friends and family ask patients who enroll in more affordable health plans why a treatment they heard about wasn't prescribed, patients must be willing to tell their friends, "My doctor didn't prescribe that treatment because it's very unlikely to work," or "My doctor didn't prescribe that treatment because it isn't cost-effective."

11 | AN OUNCE OF PREVENTION COSTS A TON OF MONEY

In chapter four, I presented the reality that almost all preventive tests and treatments in healthcare don't save money, either in the short- or long-term. Because this is such a radical thought to the ears of most Americans, I felt I should spend a little more time explaining this important concept. Possibly more than any of the other POEM assumptions, GIMeC heartily promotes this special brand of voodoo medical economics.

GIMEC AND PREVENTION

GIMeC loves an inspirational prevention story. Promoting more spending for preventive medical tests is an area where the government and the media actually cooperate. A couple of examples:

A U.S. Representative from Florida lined up 350 sponsors on her bill to spend taxpayer money to promote early detection of breast cancer in young women.[1] The bill proposed spending $45 million over five years to do things such as teach young women breast self-exams and educate them about the availability of genetic testing, among other things. The problem with this approach is there is no proof these interventions actually save lives, though genetic testing of very highly selected women might make sense.

A Manhattan advertising agency designed an ad for a thyroid cancer advocacy group after one of the ad agency's employees was diagnosed with thyroid cancer.[1] An ologist on the advocacy group's board wanted the campaign to encourage busy family physicians to routinely check for the disease. The ad agency convinced national magazines to donate $800,000 worth of advertising space to the cause. The problem with this campaign is there is no evidence that early detection of thyroid cancer saves lives.

THE TALE OF TWO HOUSES

To further illustrate the reasons prevention doesn't save money in the long run, consider the following story. Imagine two houses were built several decades ago. Both houses were well constructed, but have started to show their age. The women in both houses were tired of the cracked tiles and stained walls in their bathrooms and wanted to remodel, but money was tight.

In the early detection house, the woman of the house looked for any excuse to remodel her bathroom. She diligently inspected the tile and grout every day and even hired a handyman who claimed that for $200 he would be able to detect a leaking pipe with a fancy electrical gadget. She hired him to test her house every three months and sure enough, one day his gizmo erupted in a cacophony of flashing lights and sounds. These readings meant there was a chance the pipes behind the tile had rusted through, causing a small leak that could lead to disaster if not fixed early. Because this was a non-invasive test, he couldn't be sure there was a leak.

She was committed to finding a leak, so she hired the handyman to directly inspect the pipe. The handyman ripped off some tile and sheetrock but to his surprise the pipe was only moderately rusted and there was no leak. $500 later, he patched up the damage and left the house, never to be seen again.

Because this woman believed early detection equals early cure, a few months later she answered the next ad of someone who claimed that an old leaking pipe could be detected at the earliest possible stage. This handyman appeared at her house with a different device that bounced sound waves off the pipe. After collecting his $200 testing fee every three months, one day his machine whizzed and purred, suggesting a leak behind the bathroom sink. The handyman ripped off the tile and sheetrock and sure enough, this time there was a small leak in a rusted pipe creating a small water puddle with a little wood rot and mold below the pipe.

Now it was proven this bathroom needed repairing. All the tile and sheet rock had to be ripped off and replaced, most of the piping had to be replaced, the electrical outlets had to be brought up to modern code, the sink and the linoleum flooring had to be replaced. $10,000 later -- not including the thousands of dollars she had already paid for leak detection and minor handy work -- the early detection woman had a brand new bathroom with updated colors and fixtures.

She was so enamored with these gadgets she told all her friends about her great experience with these products. Thirty of her neighbors had their pipes tested for $200. None of them had evidence of a leak, which greatly reassured them. Now early leak detection companies were set to make tens of thousands of dollars per year scanning for trouble in this neighborhood.

In the wait-for-symptoms house, the woman knew eventually the piping in the bathroom would rust to the point it needed to be replaced, but she would wait for a really good reason to go through the hassle and expense of repairing the damage. She would keep her eyes open for an indication something was wrong, but she refused to let the worry consume her.

About a year later, she noticed the linoleum floor under the sink was buckled a little. She poked and prodded the slightly warped flooring and noticed a wet spot. She called a handyman to investigate.

He agreed with her assessment and recommended ripping out some of the wall and flooring to check the pipes. He tore out the damaged section and found a leaking pipe behind the bathroom sink with a moderate-sized amount of rotten wood and some mold growing on it. The tile, sheet rock, sink, and linoleum flooring had to be gutted and replaced, along with most of the pipes, and the electrical outlets had to be brought up to modern code. Along with a bill for $10,200, the wait-for-symptoms woman had a brand new bathroom with updated colors and fixtures. A little more wood had to be replaced in the walls and the flooring than the first woman, otherwise the two jobs were essentially the same. Early detection of the leak did not save money.

Five years later both women had equally healthy houses, though the wait-for-symptoms woman was in better financial shape, because she refused to pay the quarterly $200 leak detection fee.

The moral of this story is in healthcare, early detection does not often change the list of treatments needed to address the detected disease. Labs must be drawn, X-rays must be taken, biopsies must be done (which are technically easier in larger masses), surgery must be performed, chemotherapy and radiation must be given, complications must be addressed, and follow up visits must occur. The overall treatment costs hardly differ, whether a lump is pea-size or golf ball-size when first detected. The cost of screening for disease with no symptoms is much greater than savings generated in reduced treatment costs in the future.

SMOKING CESSATION

Another example where conventional wisdom on the true costs of prevention is usually wrong is the effort to get people to stop smoking. A smoker has a life expectancy up to 10 years less than a non-smoker.[2] Smoking increases the risk of lung cancer, emphysema, heart attacks, strokes, and many other forms of cancer. Wouldn't the U.S. healthcare system save billions of dollars a year if people gave up smoking? Actually, no. That line of thinking has two problems.

The first problem is money must be spent on the smokers who want to quit for items such as pills, nicotine patches, nicotine gum, and counseling sessions. These interventions help a few people, although most people keep smoking. The majority of studies conclude the initial cost of these treatments is more than the savings generated later from reduced cases of lung cancer and heart attacks.[3-7]

The second problem is even if all smokers magically quit one day without spending a dime, one comprehensive study published in the *New England Journal of Medicine* estimated there would be short term savings but probably greater long term costs.[8] This conclusion contradicts the conventional wisdom people are accustomed to hearing, so let me explain.

The fundamental reality of long-term healthcare costs is everyone has to die of something. The amount of money spent on a person in the last year of life might be in the $50,000 to $150,000 range. No matter what you die of, there is a good chance some big bucks will be spent on your behalf.

It turns out that smokers can die of relatively inexpensive diseases. Some people who ultimately die of heart attacks generate a lot of costs in their last year of life for things like coronary artery bypass procedures. But other heart attack victims die suddenly, sometimes in their sleep. Lung cancer is another relatively inexpensive way to die, because for many forms of lung cancer there are no great treatments.

Other causes of death are much more expensive, especially Alzheimer's disease. Alzheimer's probably doesn't cost much more than other diseases in the last year of life but it includes many years of expensive care, mostly for nursing homes. That's why getting everyone to quit smoking would not save healthcare costs. In the long run, all we'd do is replace less expensive ways to die with more expensive ways to die. (I acknowledge that at least one study predicts total costs would be reduced. The differences in the estimates depend on which costs are included and assumptions of how smoking-related deaths are replaced by non-smoking-related deaths.)

My message to smokers is this: smoking has major harmful effects on your life and increases your risk of heart attacks, strokes, lung cancer, and many other forms of cancer. You know you should quit. You don't need me to tell you that. Several therapies can help you quit smoking, but ultimately you have to find the courage within yourself to quit. On the other hand, if you love smoking so much you feel your life would be worth living only if you had cigarettes every day and you accept you will die perhaps ten years sooner than you would if you didn't smoke, I respect your right to make that decision.[2] Just don't smoke around your wife, children, or any other nonsmokers. It will harm their health and isn't fair to them.

COST-EFFECTIVENESS OF COMMON TESTS AND TREATMENTS

The subject of cost-effectiveness in healthcare is tangled and difficult because this is the point where we begin to talk about lives and dollars in the same breath. As I discuss the cost-effectiveness of a few different scenarios, you might imagine a loved one or even yourself in the examples. That's okay; we are talking about human lives here. We must not shy away from difficult truths.

When informed of cost-effectiveness realities, I've heard some people respond along these lines: "You're talking about populations, but doctors still have to make individual treatment decisions." The fallacy of this position is it assumes doctors have crystal balls and can predict which individual will suffer harm in the future that could have been prevented earlier. For instance, if I treat 100 patients for high blood pressure to reduce the chance of stroke by 1% over 10 years, there is no way for me to know which one of the 100 is the one in whom the stroke is prevented. For the other 99, the bottom line is they were treated unnecessarily. All had to be treated to prevent the stroke in the one. Populations must be tested and treated for a few individuals to benefit.

Let me be very clear about another point. It is not my place to pronounce what a human life is worth or how much should be spent to improve a patient's quality of life. As I continue to develop my positions throughout the book, a recurrent theme is that GIMeC has unilaterally forced Americans into expensive healthcare with no prior approval from the American people. A radically more affordable healthcare option will require some cost-effectiveness realities to be considered, but where to draw the line is for you to decide -- not GIMeC, and not me.

The examples I present below show the cost of prevention in two ways. One category is prevention in people with no known disease. Examples include tetanus shots and mammograms. The other category is the reduction of the long-term effects of chronic diseases, for example treating diabetics with more medicines to lower their blood sugars to near normal levels. Many commonly provided preventive tests and chronic disease treatments can be very expensive. Remember, these costs include the cost of the interventions, such as medications or tests, minus the savings resulting from fewer hospitalizations and other future costs. Note also the costs listed are to extend one *year* of life, not the whole life as in the tetanus example in chapter four.

Intervention	Increased life expectancy	Cost to extend a year of life
Prevention in people with no known disease		
Medication to help quit smoking[3, 5-7]	1.4 years	$1,000 to $10,000
Mammograms[9-12]	3 to 20 days	$33,000-$134,000
Reduction of long-term effects of chronic diseases		
Medication (statin) to prevent heart attacks in different patient groups (1997 dollars):[13, 14]		
50-year-old man who already had a heart attack	(not explicitly stated in the	$15,000
40-year-old woman with no risk factors except high cholesterol	source articles)	$1,500,000
Aggressive diabetes control compared to less aggressive control (2000 dollars. This model assumes aggressive control extends lives, which is not necessarily true.)[15]		
60-year old	1.5 months	$71,800
70-year old	3 weeks	$154,000
80-year old	5 days	$402,000
90-year old	16 hours	$2,100,000

Just in case the take-home message of this table isn't clear, look at the cost-effectiveness of the 40-year-old low risk woman treated with a statin drug to lower her cholesterol. The dollar figure at the far right means it costs approximately $1.5 million dollars for each year her life is extended by the medication. That figure takes into account all treatment costs minus any future savings from fewer hospitalizations and procedures.

COST-EFFECTIVENESS TAKE-HOME MESSAGES

The cost-effectiveness conclusions listed in the table run counter to common misconceptions about prevention and healthcare costs. Here are the realities:

Reality # 1: Expensive care for sick people can be very cost effective

Imagine two 60-year-old women who suddenly become very ill. Their hearts and lungs stop working well, they have serious infections, and they are admitted to an ICU. The expected likelihood of survival of this sudden illness is 50 percent. The doctors treat both women equally well, but the seriousness of the disease means one will die. The day both are admitted to the hospital, the doctors have no way of knowing who will be the survivor.

Let's estimate the cost of this prolonged stay in the ICU is $200,000 for each of them. One lives and one dies. Therefore $400,000 is spent to extend one life ($200,000 times the two women treated.)

The woman who lives recovers to about her same quality of life before she fell ill. She lives another 20 years and dies of something else at age 80. Therefore, in simple terms, the cost-effectiveness of the ICU stay was $400,000 divided by 20 years, which equals $20,000 per year of life extended. Compare that figure with some of the preventive cost-effectiveness values in the preceding Table.

**Reality #2: Aggressive preventive care for
low-risk people is very expensive**

The second reality of cost-effectiveness is the less likely a
person is to have a disease, the less cost-effective the preventive
test or treatment. Certain results, such as cholesterol levels, can
tell us who is at slightly higher risk than another person, but
doctors don't have the ability to predict which individual will
have the heart attack in the future. It could actually be the
person with a lower cholesterol level. Many other factors
contribute to the risk.

It is extraordinarily expensive to do a lot of aggressive
testing and treating in younger people. By younger, I mean
people from about 18 to 45. The exception to this rule is a few
interventions for young women who may become pregnant. One
is a public health measure, not a medical intervention: fortifying
flour with folic acid to prevent certain types of birth defects.
Another is traditional medical care: prenatal care to prevent
birth defects and neonatal deaths. (Although the NIH rarely
funds studies to determine which interventions in routine
prenatal care really make a difference.)

**Reality #3: Preventive care becomes less
cost-effective in the elderly**

All of us have to die some day. The older we get the
more likely it is to happen sooner rather than later.

Imagine two elderly individuals: a 70-year-old man and
a 90-year-old man. Each has a new diagnosis of cancer. The
recommended treatment will cost approximately $250,000.
Assume both men survive the cancer and live out a relatively

normal lifespan. The 70-year-old lives another 18 years, so the cost-effectiveness value of the cancer treatment is $14,000 per year of life extended. The 90-year-old lives another four years, so the cost-effectiveness value of the treatment is $58,000 per year of life extended.

The higher expense in the 90-year-old is a reflection of the reality that 90-year-old people have shorter average life expectancies than 70-year-old people.

Reality #4: Improved chronic disease care increases costs most of the time

Diabetes is an example of a chronic disease with significant yearly healthcare costs. Published cost-effectiveness studies of treating people with diabetes by adding new expensive drugs to generic drugs have assumed this will extend their lives, in the range of a few months.[15-17] Even assuming this benefit is real, the cost of treatment is greater than savings from reduced disease burden (see preceding Table). On the other hand, different studies have found giving people more diabetes medicine in order to lower their blood sugar levels has no impact on life expectancy.[18-21] Therefore, the cost-effectiveness of more diabetes medicines would be extraordinarily expensive, because most lives aren't extended.

The reality that improved chronic disease care doesn't save money in broad populations of people with those diseases has a few exceptions. For patients with severe chronic diseases who are prone to suddenly get worse to the point they might go to the emergency room and be admitted to the hospital, good primary care can help keep those people feeling better longer and prevent many of those ER visits or hospitalizations.[22-24]

For people with diabetes, the cost of aggressive blood pressure treatment, which means more daily medicines, is paid for by savings from reduced hospitalizations for heart attacks, angina, and strokes.[15, 25, 26] In fact, in terms of staying out of the hospital and improving life expectancy, it is better for a diabetic to focus on her blood pressure than her sugar levels.

The take home point of these examples is better health costs more money. It works like every other aspect of our lives: If you want better health, it will cost you. How much money you devote to healthcare, as opposed to other things that bring you health and happiness, should be your decision.

WHAT ABOUT OTHER DEVELOPED COUNTRIES?

Many other developed countries have a completely different attitude about cost-effectiveness than the U.S. These countries use the cost-effectiveness medical economic literature to guide decisions on which tests and treatments should be covered by their provincial or national healthcare systems. This attitude is demonstrated in a quote from Iona Heath, the President of the Royal College of General Practitioners in Britain, who wrote an editorial criticizing the comments of a previous author in the prestigious medical journal, *BMJ*.[27] (For those of you who dismiss anything written about British healthcare because it is just "socialized medicine", please keep your mind open for one page.)

> *"[B]y making the same mistake and appearing to believe that by investing in prevention the service can reduce the cost of disease, you endanger the enduring social solidarity [of the National Health Service].*

Medical science does not save lives, it defers death. No one lives for ever, and, on average, a quarter of a lifetime's cost of health care is incurred in the last year of life. Preventive health care, when it lengthens lives, exposes people to other health risks and cannot reduce costs. [The other author] implies that preventive health screening is an entirely benign endeavour and [the other author] makes absolutely no mention of the well recognized harms of screening. When those who consider themselves healthy submit themselves to screening, they confront the possibility of serious disease and inevitably this can cause a burden of anxiety that varies from the trivial to a severity amounting to disease in itself. Every screening test gives both false positives and false negatives: the one dangerously reassuring, the other leading inevitably to further investigations that become increasingly invasive and risky.

[C]ostly procedures and treatments are put in place to minimize the risk[s of disease] with the confident assumption that the incidence of the disease will thereby be reduced. Sometimes this happens, more often it does not. Too often, particularly in old age, one disease is prevented only to be replaced by another."

American doctors or politicians rarely speak from this point of view. GIMeC wants everyone to believe they could live forever if only the appropriate test could be ordered in time, with an aggressive and usually expensive treatment regimen to follow. To my ears, the British have a much more realistic and humble attitude about the role of medical care in society. They view it as a right, but a limited one. It's something everyone should have access to, but the healthcare system can't make outrageous promises. There are other public goods competing for society's resources that also impact health: clean air and water, safe transportation, safe neighborhoods, and good schools.

FINAL PREVENTION REALITY CHECK

The U.S. actually does quite well in the area of providing expensive medical preventive interventions. Compared to five other developed countries, the U.S. had the highest rate of women who had a Pap smear, women ages 50-64 who had a mammogram, adults who received a reminder for preventive care, and adults who received advice from a doctor on diet and exercise.[28] The U.S. was second best in other preventive categories such as elderly citizens who received a flu shot, doctors who provided all appropriate care to diabetic patients, high blood pressure patients who received blood pressure and cholesterol checks, and chronically ill patients who received self-care plans.[28] Our outrageous healthcare bills are not caused by a lack of preventive tests and treatments

In contrast, the U.S. doesn't do well in the area of non-medical prevention. We are more sedentary, drive our cars when we could walk, eat too much, and let our children exercise their thumbs on video game controllers when we should be telling them to go outside and run around.

PART OF THE SOLUTION

To significantly reduce the cost of healthcare, America needs less aggressive medical prevention, particularly in young people and the elderly. Americans must work with the medical establishment and other GIMeC members to define when preventive tests or treatments cost too much, or when the benefits are too rare to justify the hassle and expense.

On an individual level, I encourage you to dismiss the comments of any politician, pundit, or reporter who declares more prevention will lower healthcare costs. When the healthcare system spends money to prevent something, with rare exception, it makes healthcare more expensive for everyone, and those costs come from your wages and taxes.

12 | REALLY EXPENSIVE DRUGS AND DEVICES

One of the most difficult decisions health policy makers must make is how to handle new pharmaceuticals and medical devices that may cost more than $100,000 per treatment or device. Because these therapies are so new, today's planners have few precedents to guide them.

EXPENSIVE CHEMOTHERAPY

One of the most expensive therapies is cancer treatment.[1] Chemotherapy has become so expensive that the National Cancer Institute, a branch of the NIH, projects chemotherapy drugs will consume almost a quarter of all drug expenditures in the near future.[2]

Many widely used chemotherapy agents were invented in the last decade. Older chemotherapy agents are relatively simple compounds that work by killing fast-growing cancer cells. Hair follicle cells and intestinal cells also normally grow fast, which is why two common side effects of traditional chemotherapies are hair loss and nausea.

The newer generation of chemotherapy drugs more precisely target and kill cancer cells and cause fewer side effects. Some drugs work by bonding to the cancer cells and killing them. Other drugs work by inhibiting the growth of new blood vessels that feed the cancer as it grows. Such drugs are highly complex molecules, neither easy nor cheap to manufacture. They cost a fortune, but how well do they work? Let's look at two examples.

AVASTIN (GENERIC: BEVACIZUMAB)

One cancer drug drawing attention for its cost is Avastin, which cuts off a tumor's blood supply. Avastin has the potential to become a "cure-all" cancer treatment because all fast-growing cancers need new blood vessels to supply the new cells. Avastin does help, but not dramatically. Studies of patients with colon or kidney cancer show Avastin only prolongs life by a few months.[3-5] Newer studies suggest Avastin might be less effective than its manufacturer, Genentech, reported to the FDA when it was approved.[3] The largest clinical trial of Avastin for colorectal cancer showed that early positive results were transient. With longer follow up, Avastin was found to improve neither overall survival nor even disease-free survival.[4]

The average wholesale cost of Avastin to treat one type of lung cancer is $56,000 annually, although it can cost up to $100,000 per year, depending on the type of cancer.[1] In spite of this expense, oncologists were observed to prescribe Avastin for patients in whom its benefit is unproven.[5] Genentech sold $3.5 billion of Avastin in 2008.[3]

HERCEPTIN (TRASTUZUMAB)

Genentech also manufactures Herceptin, which is used for women with a certain kind of breast cancer. About 20-30 percent of breast cancers have a receptor on the outside of the cancer cell called a HER2 receptor. These breast cancers are more aggressive and more lethal than breast cancers that lack this receptor. Herceptin is an artificially manufactured antibody that binds to the HER2 receptor and thus inhibits tumor growth.

Initial results of Herceptin studies were positive, but modestly so. One trial reported that after two years, 3.5 percent of the women treated with Herceptin had died, compared to 5.3 percent of the women who received a placebo treatment.[7] Another study found no significant difference in survival after one year,[6] and yet another saw only a modest decrease in deaths after three years.[7]

The Herceptin researchers later were accused of hiding damaging clinical trial results.[7] One arm of a clinical trial found the drug worked well for women with a certain form of breast cancer, but another arm of that same trial with less promising results was not publicly reported. Critics of the Herceptin trials believe the missing data could have an important impact on the assessment of its cost-effectiveness.[8]

A single course of treatment for Herceptin costs about $50,000. A patient receives injections of the drug for a year, and then the treatment is complete. Herceptin is estimated to cost $80,000-$200,000 per year of life extended at U.S. prices.[9-11]

MORE ABOUT COSTS

Even having private insurance or Medicare does not spare people from enormous pharmaceutical costs. Medicare requires a 25 percent co-pay on some of the newer cancer drugs. In the case of a drug called Gleevec, that 25 percent portion can reach as high as $40,000 per year.[9] But expensive drugs aren't limited to cancer treatments. Conditions such as rheumatoid arthritis and some forms of anemia also can cost $25,000 to $85,000 per year to treat.[10]

The reality GIMeC doesn't want publicized is that many of the new cancer drugs do not cure cancer; they just turn it into a chronic disease. The cancer doesn't get worse, but it doesn't go away. How much should we pay each year for an individual patient to keep a cancer frozen in its current state: $20,000, $50,000, $200,000? American oncologists are not leading this discussion. When asked if cost should be a consideration in treatment, 78 percent of them stated patients should have access to "effective care," regardless of cost.[11] If no price is too expensive to justify, how will we ever gain control over healthcare costs?

CANADIAN DRUGS

Other developed countries, such as Canada, have developed processes to balance the needs of individual patients with the greater society. Patented drugs in Canada cost about 60 percent of what we pay in the U.S.[11, 12] The provincial governments of Canada directly negotiate with drug companies for the right to supply drugs. No entity in the U.S. has similar clout, except perhaps for the VA system, which has also been successful in negotiating favorable rates. Canadian regulators are slower to approve new drugs than the U.S. FDA, but fewer drugs are later recalled for safety reasons (2.0 percent in Canada compared to 3.6 percent in the U.S.).[12]

Canadian provincial governments use pricing guidelines the U.S. lacks, which contributes to the disparity between U.S. and Canadian drug prices. Here, we spend $728 per capita each year on drugs, while in Canada it is $509.[13] At the same time, pharmaceutical consumption is higher in Canada, with about 12 prescriptions filled per person each year in Canada vs. 10.6 in the U.S.[13] The price differential for brand-name drugs between the two countries has led Americans to purchase approximately $1 billion in drugs per year from Canadian pharmacies.[14] The difference is far less dramatic for generic drugs, which may actually cost more in Canada than in the U.S.[12]

Patent protection also doesn't last as long in Canada as it does in the U.S., where a drug patent may be extended five years to make up for time lost in development. Therefore, some drugs are available earlier on Canadian shelves as generics.[15]

The primary reason Canada's patented drugs cost less is very simply this – the Canadians are willing to tell the drug companies "no." It doesn't matter if a new drug works well for a handful of patients. Each province has a limited healthcare budget, and if the drug costs too much, the provincial government may conclude it can't afford the drug. Money not spent on expensive drugs for a few people is money available for other goods and services for the greater community.

EUROPEAN APPROACHES TO EXPENSIVE CANCER DRUGS

European countries, such as Britain, also have processes to evaluate which new drugs should be purchased. Sometimes, they choose a middle ground between making a new drug available for everyone and not using it at all. The British NHS, for example, doesn't use one of the new expensive cancer drugs as the first-line treatment for colorectal cancer.[2] If traditional treatment doesn't effectively treat the cancer, however, combination therapy with one of the newer, expensive agents is likely the next step. This approach reduces the number of colon cancer patients receiving the expensive drug by half with little to no effect on the overall success of treatment.

NICE analyzed Avastin for treatment of metastatic colon cancer. NICE concluded the cost-effectiveness of Avastin plus the standard treatment regimen (compared to the standard treatment regimen by itself) was likely to be about £62,000 per year of life extended.[16] That cost per year of life extended was more than the allowable limit, so the NHS did not approve it.[16]

Drug companies don't necessarily give up when a drug-purchasing agency concludes a new drug is too expensive. NICE similarly declined to support coverage for bortezomib to treat multiple myeloma, which is a form of blood cancer.[17] The manufacturer of bortezomib, Johnson & Johnson, returned with a counter offer – not an offer to reduce the price, but to refund charges for patients who did not respond adequately to the drug.[17] As of this writing, the NHS is still considering the offer.

MEDICARE AND EXPENSIVE TREATMENTS

In contrast to European and Canadian systems, Medicare lacks the clear legal authority to take costs into account when determining which services are covered.[18] Since its inception in 1965, the language in Medicare's founding act says it covers "items and services which are reasonable and necessary for the diagnosis or treatment of illness or injury or to improve the functioning of a malformed body member."[19] Medicare has never explicitly considered costs in making coverage decisions.[20]

Medicare officials have attempted to include cost in their coverage decisions in the past. In 1980, Medicare drafted a policy proposing criteria based on economic, safety, ethical, and other considerations.[19] According to some observers, the rule was suppressed in part by the medical device industry. Nearly 10 years later, Medicare announced it planned to issue a rule including considerations of appropriateness and cost-effectiveness in coverage decisions. That rule was also defeated. In a recent revision of the process for making coverage decisions, Medicare stated, "Given that there are substantial competing interests about the coverage criteria, we believe it best not to pursue rulemaking. In the meantime, as we have done in the past 35 years, we will continue to make coverage decisions and to interpret what is 'reasonable and necessary.' "[19]

Medicare does push back against the constant pressure to bust its budget, but in sneaky ways. A perfect example is the saga of the left ventricular assist device (LVAD), a mechanical device used in people who have heart failure so severe the heart muscle can barely pump. The LVAD is a small artificial heart primarily used to keep these patients alive while they wait for a transplant.

The problem with the LVAD is its cost. Implantation centers charge around $200,000 to implant these devices. On top of that, the companies charge about $65,000 just for the LVAD, which is a tube and motor about the size of a large pickle. A decision by Medicare on whether and under what circumstances it would cover the device was repeatedly postponed because of concern about the cost. But in October 2003, Medicare agreed to provide coverage for the LVAD if the operation was performed in selected heart-transplantation facilities that agreed to a stringent set of guidelines to determine which patients received the device.[19]

Medicare agreed to pay about $70,000 for the whole procedure (with the cost of the LVAD device included in that amount).[19] Medicare set the payment so low that doctors and hospitals would lose a substantial amount of money offering the service.

About 5,000 Medicare patients were expected to qualify for the device initially, although Medicare officials feared the number could rise to 100,000. Because of this wide variation, the expected cost to Medicare ranged anywhere from $350 million to $7 billion per year.[19] As part of the approval process, Medicare set a goal of 50 percent survival at two years and minimal time in the hospital after LVAD implantation as a prerequisite for widespread adoption of this treatment.[21] Real world experience has not met this goal.

As computed by Blue Cross Blue Shield, the cost-effectiveness of the LVAD ranges from $500,000 to $1.4 million per year of life extended.[22] This cost is astronomically higher than any Canadian or European health service is willing to pay.

PART OF THE SOLUTION

I absolutely believe in the power of innovation and am proud of America's history of innovation fueled by the profit motive. I also acknowledge that many biomedical researchers, both in and out of industry, are committed to their missions for altruistic reasons. Risk-takers willing to invest their time, money, and sweat gave us the light bulb, the intermittent windshield wiper, personal computers, and an amazing array of software. Drug companies, likewise, should have a financial incentive to innovate.

However, both the general public and state regulators expect U.S. insurance companies and Medicare to provide any service that might possibly improve someone's health, no matter how expensive. Given the situation, the drug companies can set virtually any price.[2]

A middle ground exists between the absolutes of full coverage and no coverage. A certain drug might be cost-effective for one kind of patient with one kind of cancer, but extraordinarily expensive for a different patient with a different cancer. A decision by a more affordable health plan never to pay for a drug would sometimes be too crude. An efficient system would not limit new tests and treatments to an all-or-nothing proposal. Rather, it would allow new tests and treatments proven to be cost effective for certain patients in this system to work; doctors and patients must live within limits. Would you be willing to be a member of such a system? Would you willingly accept vastly lower healthcare costs, knowing you might be among the few with a form of cancer for which one potential treatment is just too expensive?

For the new, ultra-expensive drugs, the ethical dilemma for me is not necessarily treating a patient riddled with cancer; it is treating a patient with a condition such as rheumatoid arthritis. For some patients, these drugs can be the difference between living with constant pain and virtually disabled versus occasional manageable pain and being fully functional. But is it right for any health plan to spend more than the average American earns in a year for this result? Perhaps there is a middle ground here, as well. A new, expensive drug could be tried on many people with rheumatoid arthritis for a few months. For those with dramatic improvement, they could continue taking the drug. For the people whose pain and function improved only modestly, further use of the expensive drug is not justified. People in the latter group would not go untreated; they just wouldn't receive the expensive medication any longer.

13 | SUGAR DIABETES

Most Americans probably have at least one family member or friend who has diabetes. Imagine a favorite relative, Aunt Taylor, has diabetes and needs your help. What significant changes must she really make in her life? Be careful what she eats, exercise on a regular basis, take a bunch of pills every day, stick needles in her skin to check her blood sugar levels, and maybe give herself insulin? Which of the long-term consequences of diabetes – blindness, dialysis, foot ulcers, amputations, heart attacks – are really preventable, and by how much?

Although diabetes will be the focus of this chapter, it's only one example of an expensive, chronic disease. The contribution of chronic diseases to the cost of American healthcare can't be overstated and is one of the fundamental issues that must be addressed. GIMeC has controlled this discussion for decades, and it applies the erroneous POEM assumptions to many of its communications. Even when some of the POEM assumptions are technically true, their impact on your health is minimal.

THE COST OF CHRONIC DISEASES

By far the biggest factor driving healthcare costs in America, and the rest of the developed world, is chronic disease, especially in the elderly. About 80 percent of Medicare beneficiaries have at least one chronic disease, and they account for about 96 percent of program spending.[1,2] The total costs increase exponentially as the number of diseases increase (Figure).[1]

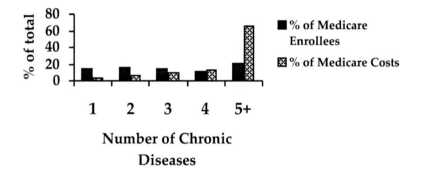

Medicare Enrollees and Costs

Medicare spends so much on patients with five or more chronic conditions because they fill an average of 49 prescriptions in a year, have an average of 37 physician visits, see 14 different physicians, and spend roughly seven days in the hospital each year.[2]

An amazing amount of money is spent on drugs for chronic diseases each year. The top prescription drug expenses for U.S. citizens in 2005 included[3]

- Drugs to lower blood sugar, reduce cholesterol, or help control other metabolic problems: $36 billion.
- Cardiovascular drugs for high blood pressure and heart conditions: $33 billion.

- Central nervous system drugs, including pain killers,
  sleep aids, and attention deficit disorders: $26
  billion.

The CDC estimates chronic diseases account for 70
percent of all deaths in the US and 75 percent of the $2.5 trillion
spent on annual medical care costs.[4] These conditions cause
major limitations for more than one in every 10 Americans, or 25
million people.[4] An estimate of the impact on the workplace
concluded three chronic diseases – asthma, diabetes, and high
blood pressure – result in 164 million days of absenteeism each
year, costing $30 billion.[4]

To a large degree, increasing numbers of chronic
diseases are an inevitable consequence of living long enough for
them to develop. But we still have choices how we respond to
these new diagnoses. For example, adhering to a Mediterranean
diet may provide long-term cardiovascular benefits.

BACK TO SUGAR DIABETES

Diabetes provides a classic example of the difficult
trade-offs inherent in deciding the best overall approach to
caring for people with chronic diseases. All four POEM
assumptions are applied regularly to diabetes by GIMeC, though
recent studies have raised questions about these assumptions. By
way of background, diabetes is usually classified as type I,
which is usually the kind children get; and type II, which is
usually the kind middle-aged adults get. More than 10 times as
many people have type II diabetes as type I. Aunt Taylor has
type II diabetes.

The ologists who consider themselves diabetes experts have long believed that the lower a diabetic patient's blood sugar, the better off the patient. Observational studies find an association between higher average sugar levels and increased risk of diabetic complications. Recently, three large studies were conducted to see how low the sugar levels should be pushed with medicine.

One study enrolled 10,251 adults with type II diabetes who were randomized into two groups: the intensive treatment group and the usual treatment group.[5] The goal for the intensely treated group was to keep a measure of blood sugar called the hemoglobin A1c below 6.0, which would be near normal. The less intensely treated group was given enough treatment (medicines mostly) to keep the hemoglobin A1c below 8.0.

Everyone's blood has sugar (glucose) in it, which we need for energy. The sugar sticks to some of the hemoglobin in the red blood cells. The higher the sugar level in the blood stream, the more sugar sticks to the hemoglobin. The hemoglobin A1c measures the percent of hemoglobin with sugar attached and is considered the best measure of average blood sugar over time. ("A1c" doesn't really stand for anything special.)

To give you an idea of possible ranges, a normal person's hemoglobin A1c falls in the range of 4 to 6. The American Diabetes Association currently defines the goal for diabetes control as a hemoglobin A1c less than 7.0. A person with poorly controlled diabetes has a hemoglobin A1c in double digits. The highest hemoglobin A1c I have personally seen is 19.

In the study, the goal for the intensely treated group was to push the hemoglobin A1c below 6.0 by a combination of whatever treatments were necessary. A review board demanded the trial be stopped early, because 20 percent more people had died in the intensely treated group than the less intensely treated group – 257 patients in the intensely treated group compared to 203 patients in the other. Additionally, the intensely treated group was more likely to gain more than 22 pounds and develop severe hypoglycemia (low blood sugar). Two similar trials were published about the same time.[6, 7] In both of these studies, as well, there were similar rates of cardiovascular disease, death, and most other complications between the intense and standard treatment groups. Intensive treatment did not change health outcomes that patients care about.

It was reasonable to conduct these experiments. It was fair to ask what is the best target hemoglobin A1c for people with diabetes? Some reviewers concluded the results of these three clinical trials should change our treatment goals for patients with type II diabetes to higher hemoglobin A1c targets,[8-10] including the National Committee on Quality Assurance,[11] though the American Diabetes Association did not change its recommendations.[12]

Others feel the hemoglobin A1c target of 7.0 is partially a result of drug company influence. Drs. David Aron and Leonard Pogach, writing in the *Journal of the American Medical Association*, stated that "publicly available information suggests that an industry-driven campaign was successful in coalescing numerous organizations, key professional opinion leaders . . ., business leaders, and politicians around a national goal of hemoglobin A1c level of less than 7 percent for glycemic control."[13] They also point out that other experts on medical guideline development concluded "a review of existing North

American and United Kingdom diabetes guidelines rated the
two U.S. professional societies – the American Diabetes
Association and the American Association of Clinical
Endocrinologists – as having significantly less evidence-based
development processes than other professional society and
government guidelines."

LONG-TERM OUTCOMES

Another line of evidence shows Aunt Taylor won't have
much difference in her long-term health if she has good control
compared to fair control. An international group of investigators
took a hypothetical group of newly diagnosed 51-year-old
patients with type II diabetes and projected their health
outcomes over 20 years.[13] The hemoglobin A1c in the less tightly
controlled group in their study was 10.0 percent, which was very
high by current standards. A difference in long-term health was
evident, but the differences were in quality-of-life measures and
also were fairly small. There was no difference in overall
survival.

Health outcome	Patients with a hemoglobin A1C of 10 percent	Patients with a hemoglobin A1C of 7.2 percent
Legal blindness	10 percent	2 percent
Kidney failure requiring dialysis or transplant	3 percent	1 percent
First amputation of at least part of the leg	2 percent	1 percent
Overall survival	55 percent	55 percent

LONG-TERM HEALTH OUTCOMES IN PEOPLE WITH DIABETES: LOOSE VS. TIGHT CONTROL

Another study in Italy found similar results in type II diabetics and also measured the development of kidney failure, which was 0.1 percent per year (1 per 1,000 per year).[14] Another study looking specifically at heart disease found intensive glucose control had no effect on stroke or life expectancy, although it did reduce the non-fatal heart attack rate by 17 percent.[15]

COST-EFFECTIVENESS OF DIABETES TREATMENT AND PREVENTION

The cost-effectiveness of diabetes treatment is consistent with the realities of cost-effectiveness we reviewed earlier. Some studies estimate the cost to extend a year of life by adding medicine to a diabetics' regimen is not that bad, approximately $10,000-$40,000.[16-20] Others estimate the cost to extend a year of life in the hundreds of thousands to millions of dollars for certain patient populations.[17, 21]

If treating diabetes once it's developed is expensive, what about screening for the disease to catch it earlier or preventing the disease in the first place? Screening for diabetes is estimated to be of marginal cost-effectiveness at best, costing more than $50,000 to extend a year of life.[22]

Prevention is another matter, but the study results are confusing. The hope is that lifestyle changes, such as medically supervised improvements in diet and exercise, will delay or even prevent the development of diabetes. Cost-effectiveness estimates of diabetes prevention vary widely, from around $1,000 to nearly $150,000 per year of life extended, depending on many assumptions.[23-26] If an overweight person without diabetes decides to eat better and exercise more on her own, these actions might even prove cost saving. On the other hand, if a company or health plan spends $1,000 per family on gym memberships and cooking classes but few people change their behavior and actually lose weight, almost no diabetes is prevented. This scenario explains the higher cost-effectiveness estimates.

The main problem with preventing diabetes is that few medical interventions are proven to help people lose a significant amount of weight or body fat. Nothing really works well. Look at it this way. If there were a magic medical solution for weight loss, there would be no fat doctors. Clearly, this is not the case.

On the other hand, some researchers estimate that lifestyle improvements such as bike paths, parks, and better grocery selections in low-income neighborhoods actually would save money because fewer people would develop chronic diseases such as diabetes in the first place.[27]

The cost-effectiveness results for more aggressive diabetes prevention and care are disappointing. At least three reasons show why better sugar control doesn't save money.

- *Drugs are expensive.* Some diabetes medicines cost $2,000 per year for one medicine, and many patients take three or four diabetes medicines.
- *High sugars can't necessarily be reduced to ideal levels.* It's a fallacy to assume a high hemoglobin A1C means the doctor's care is substandard, or a patient isn't doing what she should. Many patients just have a bad case of diabetes, particularly if they've had it for many years.

- *Health outcomes aren't much different for patients with good control of their blood sugar than those with less-ideal control.*

COMPARISON WITH THE WESTERN EUROPEANS

We've looked at diabetes in detail as an example of the difficult trade-offs of costs and outcomes for chronic disease care. Since the Western Europeans have lower healthcare costs overall and chronic disease care obviously drives up many costs, let's examine differences in disease care between the U.S. and Europe more broadly.

Lower European healthcare costs are not explained by their doctors aggressively ordering more tests and treatments. Americans age 50 or older report they are in overall poorer health than their European counterparts, are more likely to have been diagnosed with a chronic disease, and are more frequently on treatment for a chronic disease.[28, 29] For instance, 21.8 percent of adult Americans say they have been diagnosed with heart disease, and 60.7 percent of those are on medications. In contrast, 11.4 percent of Europeans have been diagnosed with heart disease, and 54.5 percent of those are on medications.

Prevalence of Chronic Diseases

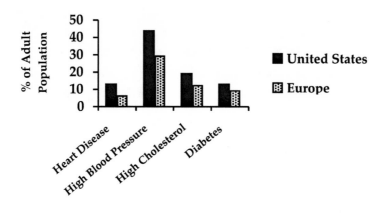

The U.S. has a higher rate of chronic diseases in large part because disease screening is much more aggressive. We covered the differences in British and U.S. guidelines for treating high blood pressure and cholesterol earlier. Part of the difficulty of determining the best approaches to detecting and treating these diseases is they can be detected decades earlier than they begin to cause noticeable health problems. Any population will have more people with high blood pressure if it's defined as 140/90 instead of 160/100. Incidence rates of diabetes will increase if it's defined as a hemoglobin A1c greater than 7.0 instead of 8.0.

Cancer rates between the U.S. and Europe also suggest that differences of disease prevalence are largely explained by aggressively testing to detect them. The prevalence of diagnosed cancer in U.S. adults is more than double that of Europeans – 12.2 percent vs. 5.4 percent of adults.[29] Are Americans really more likely to develop malignant tumors, or are they just screened more intensely than Europeans are? Comparisons of breast cancer screening rates and five-year cancer survival rates suggest the aggressiveness of screening explains the difference.[29]

PART OF THE SOLUTION

In the U.S. over the past two decades, lowering the numbers that define diabetes, high blood pressure, overweight, and high cholesterol increased the number of Americans with these diagnoses by 14 percent, 35 percent, 42 percent, and 86 percent, respectively.[30] GIMeC wants everyone to believe the answer to America's healthcare crisis is more screening, more prevention, more testing, more drugs, more scans, and more doctors' visits for patients with chronic diseases. Unfortunately for our wallets, the reality is the opposite.

The solution for more cost-effective chronic disease care in America is *less* aggressive care. We should allow sugars higher than current standards to diagnose diabetes, for example, and doctors should be less aggressive in asking patients to load up on medicines to lower sugar levels.

A reasonable approach to diabetes that considers both costs and outcomes might go something like this:

Aunt Taylor could be diagnosed with diabetes if her hemoglobin A1c is over 7.0, but treatment with drugs will not start until it surpasses 8.0. (Remember the table of health outcomes earlier in the chapter compared hemoglobin A1c levels of 7.2 to 10.0, and the results were not that different. The long-term health differences between people with A1cs of 7.0 and 8.0 will be even smaller.) Generic medications would be used to keep the hemoglobin A1c in the 7-8 range, particularly if she has no trouble with low blood sugars affecting the quality of her life.

As her diabetes naturally worsens and becomes harder to treat over time, more generic drugs will be added. The newer, more expensive drugs will be added only to keep her hemoglobin A1c below 9.0 And she would not often be asked to prick her finger at home to check her blood sugar, because there is evidence this practice makes little difference in glucose control.[31]

If one of Aunt Taylor's great joys in life is to have a little extra chocolate a few times a week, even if it means her sugar moderately rises that evening, a less stringent approach to diabetes care would allow her to have the chocolate without a doctor fussing in response. It seems pointless to live 30 years deprived of chocolate just so she can reduce her risk of future complications by single-digit percentages.

To lower healthcare costs, the treatment of other chronic diseases should be similarly relaxed. More tests and treatments result in higher healthcare costs. Fewer tests and treatments result in lower healthcare costs. It's that simple.

14 | KEEP THE GOVERNMENT OUT
OF MY MEDICARE

In the early 1990s, John Breaux, a senator from
Louisiana, was in his home state speaking about healthcare
reform during the Clinton presidency.[1] An elderly constituent
begged the Senator, "Whatever you do, keep the government out
of my Medicare." In case you don't understand the irony,
Medicare *is* a federal government program – one of the largest.
This concern was repeated during the Obama presidency at a
healthcare town hall meeting in South Carolina in 2009.[2]

The U.S. government pays for a lot of healthcare. The
largest single program is Medicare, which in 2010 cost the U.S.
government $521 billion.[3] Next is Medicaid, a program shared
by the federal government and the states, which cost the
combined governments $425 billion in 2010.[3] The U.S.
government also funds veterans' health care, military health
care, almost all kidney dialysis, and a few other smaller
programs. These numbers translate into government spending of
more than $2 billion *per day* for healthcare.

The other significant cost for the U.S. government is not
a direct cost, but lost income. Health insurance is a tax-
deductible cost for businesses and some individuals. If
healthcare costs weren't deductible and the U.S. government
collected these tax revenues, about $200 billion more would

enter the government's coffers.[4] Once that lost income is included in the mix, the U.S. government funds more than half the cost of U.S. healthcare. Socialized medicine has been a reality in this country for nearly half a century, whether we recognized it or not.

THE VETERANS AFFAIRS SYSTEM

The VA system wasn't originally intended to be the primary healthcare provider for most veterans.[5] It was created to care for war-related injuries, such as blindness, paralysis, and loss of limbs. Only about 2 percent of veterans have service-connected disabilities, and roughly 90 percent have other insurance coverage. The majority of patients treated at VA hospitals receive care not because of service-connected conditions, but because they are poor.[5]

The VA has pioneered some cutting-edge approaches to care. It has, for example, incorporated some disease management approaches in its clinic systems, leading to above-average chronic disease care. In the 1990s, the VA made a commitment to improve its delivery of primary care and reaped the expected rewards of decreased hospitalizations and higher quality care.[6] Other aspects of the VA system are less positive, however.

I, like many medical students across the U.S., spent some of my training years in a VA hospital. I worked in two different facilities and since then have compared notes with other students who likewise worked in VAs across the country. My experiences, validated by more recent medical students, had a powerful effect on forming my belief that a healthcare system completely run by the federal government isn't a good solution.

In medical school, one of our jobs was to do "scut" work. That's the routine, unglamorous work all medical students perform to learn how the healthcare system works and pay their dues. One of those jobs was to round up X-rays for my superiors on my medical team to review during morning rounds.

The X-ray file room commonly would have only one file clerk who worked at one pace: slow. Nothing could make this guy speed up beyond a deliberate crawl. Lines of medical students would form at the checkout window as they pretended not to notice pages from their professors demanding the X-rays NOW! Woe to the student who happened to reach the file room window when the clerk decided it was break time. He would sit down in full view of the students and refuse to move. We would offer to pull the folders ourselves. As far as we were concerned, he could sit forever and we would gladly do his job, but he refused. He held onto his one bit of control with an iron grip. He refused to unlock the door and let us into the file room. The window had thick glass and a narrow slit. We had no choice but to wait.

One time I had a patient admitted to the hospital with urinary problems. One of the important pieces of information we needed was the amount of urine he produced over a certain amount of time. He went for two days without anyone collecting a single urine sample, which meant several thousand dollars of taxpayer money was wasted.

Some government waste and inefficiency I could have tolerated. No organization is perfect. I know that my own personal organization, my immediate family, can be rife with chaos and poor communication. At the VA, I didn't expect perfection, but a slight bit of effort would have been nice.

One of the real disappointments of the system was the data reported by VA administrators, which bordered on outright lies. For example, they would present data suggesting the hospital length of stay for their patients was in line with other hospitals. What really happened wasn't quite so neat and tidy.

Many times we had a patient who needed a CAT scan. It was typically a patient who had a lump that, when biopsied, turned out to be cancer. In normal patient care, one factor in determining the best treatment is the extent the cancer has spread, which is assessed with a CAT scan. The patient was physically fine and didn't need to be in a hospital bed. He just needed a CAT scan. The problem was the VA's limited capacity for doing CAT scans. Hospitalized patients received priority over clinic patients, who could wait nine months for a CAT scan on an outpatient basis. If you were that patient's physician, what would you do? Probably what we did – admit him to the hospital.

Now, the interns and medical students had to do the paperwork to actually admit the guy into the hospital. The admitting diagnosis was always serious enough, cancer in this case, to prevent the utilization overseers from questioning the appropriateness of the admission. The guy would be admitted during the day, get his CAT scan that evening or the next morning, then be sent home. Long-term management could be worked out in the clinic, though the waiting time for an appointment might be several months. To the paper pushers in Washington, however, the entire episode smelled like great care: a hospital stay of only two days for cancer.

With just one more CAT scan machine, many thousands of hospital bed days could have been avoided, along with countless labor hours by nurses, medical students, residents, and attending physicians completing all the hospital admission paperwork.

The saddest aspect of the VA system was its soul-sucking effect on new employees. Several times I saw this scenario. A nurse would be hired to work in a unit, let's say a cancer ward. Several of these new hires had personal reasons for wanting to work at a VA hospital. Some of them were retired military and wanted to continue serving veterans. Others might have had a relative, a father or uncle, who needed the VA system. This type of nurse had a passion to ensure people like her father were given the care and respect they deserved. These new hires knew what they were getting into, to an extent. Asked how they planned to deal with the hassles, they would make statements such as, "I was in the military, I'm used to it," or, "I know, it's just part of the job. I can deal with it." Their spunk usually lasted about six months. They would enthusiastically show up for work each day and begin battle with the VA system. Slowly, the overwhelming inertia ground them down as they tried to motivate suboptimal employees or improve system inefficiencies. It was like being caught in a bad psychological movie. After a while, that formerly idealistic, energetic nurse would either be driven away, go crazy, or become "one of them." The system really was that oppressive.

In fact, one of the big-shot cardiologists at the medical school I attended told people his greatest career accomplishment was actually having a VA employee fired. The employee did something amazingly brazen, like saying point blank he would not do something within his job description. The cardiologist got mad enough to start the process of documenting the rude and inappropriate behavior and pursuing some sort of disciplinary action on the employee. After two years of appeals, hearings, grace periods and union interventions, the employee finally was fired. That, in a nutshell, represents probably two-thirds of the VA's problems. It can't do anything to substandard employees and simultaneously drives away good employees, so all that is left are a cadre of unmotivated people who know they can't be fired unless they do something blatantly illegal.

Other doctors I know who currently work in VA clinics report hassles built into the system that, in effect, ration care (without a larger ethical understanding of which care should be limited and why). For example, it is nearly impossible in some VA centers for otherwise healthy veterans to receive a colonoscopy to screen for colon cancer. There aren't enough gastroenterologists to provide the service, and they won't let family physicians perform the procedures.

Approximately 79 percent of VA-eligible veterans go outside the system to receive care, most commonly from Medicare.[7] The failings of the VA aren't fully expressed, because veterans have alternate ways to receive care, thereby letting the VA off the hook.

The VA has other troubles that recently made the national news. Officials said more than 3,000 patients at a VA hospital in Miami had colonoscopies with equipment that wasn't properly sterilized.[8] Because of this, the VA officials told the veterans who had the procedure they should be tested for HIV and other diseases. More than 6,000 patients at a clinic in Tennessee were told they may have been exposed to infectious body fluids during colonoscopies. The VA also admitted 1,800 veterans treated at an ear, nose, and throat clinic in Augusta,

Ga., were alerted they could have been exposed to an infection due to improper disinfection of an instrument.[9] Surprise inspections found that fewer than half of VA centers had proper training and followed guidelines for common endoscopic procedures.[10]

PART OF THE SOLUTION

I have worked in other government health systems, mostly county hospitals. They aren't perfect, but they function better than the VA system. The main reason the VA system is so toxic is that its final place of accountability, Washington, D.C., is 1,500 miles away. Local control of a healthcare system prevents some of the extreme dysfunctions I've experienced in a federal system.

However, I also realize that a radically more affordable U.S. healthcare system probably must adopt some aspects of the VA system. These include the Spartan nature of its facilities; its reliance on some treatment protocols that limit care in some situations; and its culture of being slow to adopt expensive new technologies. The key difference between the VA system and an *ethical* basic healthcare system is transparency. We deserve a system with transparent criteria that spell out which services will and will not be offered, and those criteria should be based on sound data, *not* the whims of politicians and federal government bureaucrats.

A healthcare system run by the U.S. government is not part of the solution.

15 | GET YOUR MOTOR RUNNING

Get your motor runnin'
Head out on the highway
Lookin' for adventure
And whatever comes our way

. . .

Like a true nature's child
We were born, born to be wild
We can climb so high,
I never wanna diiiee
- Mars Bonfire of Steppenwolf

Healthcare decisions almost always involve risks —
identifying who is at risk for a life-threatening condition,
treating someone at higher risk for a serious condition, or
balancing the risks and benefits of different treatment options.
Life has risks. There is no avoiding it. Perfectly normal and sane
people take risks all the time, and no one accuses them of
treating life as anything less than precious.

When you pull out of your driveway to head out on the
highway, do you think to yourself, "This could be my last
adventure"? Or when you get your motor running, do you feel
more like a teenager experiencing the freedom and wild
abandon of the open road? If it's the latter, you are still normal,
even if you don't consciously think about the inherent danger of
a one-ton object hurtling at 70 mph.

PUTTING RISK INTO PERSPECTIVE

It's easy for news outlets to exaggerate risks, though they may not intend to. Simply publicizing the story of a person with a rare injury or disease makes it seem more common than it is. For example, the media commonly runs stories on sudden deaths of young athletes. These stories invariably include an interview with an ologist who says it probably could have been prevented and who recommends that you bring your child to her office to test for the disease.

The media rarely questions whether the ologist could be biased, even though the ologist makes money performing the screening tests. The media never mentions how rare sudden cardiac death is. A study of 12 years of it in Minnesota found three sudden cardiac deaths among 651,695 student athletes.[1] None of the deaths were girls. Only one death could have been prevented by standard non-invasive testing.

The media rarely mentions the concept of competing risks. A recent study attempted to measure the phenomenon.[4] The authors compared the death rate of people running in marathons with the fact that roads have to be shut down for many hours in order to run a marathon. Traffic fatalities are a function of miles driven and time spent exposed to the possibility of accidents. The authors concluded the rare deaths in marathon runners were less than the deaths saved by closing down roads in order to run the marathon.

Other rare events the media loves to talk about are drug side effects. Researchers tried to measure the risk of a few known drug side effects with other risks people commonly take. The following table gives a few examples of their findings:[5]

Risky event	Cause of death	Fatality risk per 100,000 person-years
High school and college football	Death on the playing field	0.058
Riding on a train	Train crash	0.11
Bicycling	Bicycle crash	2.1
First-generation antihistamine taken during the day four months per year	Injury caused by being sleepy	2.8
All on-the-job injuries	Variety of causes	3.9
Driving a car or light truck	Car crash	11
Construction work	On-the-job death	29
Heart attack from taking Vioxx	Heart attack	76
Cutting down trees for a living	Crushed by a falling tree	358
Riding a motorcycle	Motorcycle crash	450

Comparing apples to apples in these kinds of analyses is difficult, and reasonable people can disagree on how to calculate these numbers. The football numbers, for example, are for all football players in a given year. They're not playing football most of the time during that year, so the actual risk per hour is much higher when they're practicing or playing.

The point is not to quibble about the exact numbers but to look at the overall patterns and what we can learn from them about our choices. Should motorcycles be outlawed because the risk of death riding them is about 40 times higher than that of driving a car?[6] What about mandatory motorcycle helmet laws? They decrease motorcycle crash deaths 38 percent, yet helmet use is not required in all states.[7] Many motorcyclists would fight long and hard against this proposal. To them, increased personal freedom outweighs the increased risk of injury and death.

Should the job of cutting trees be outlawed because it's dangerous? Lumberjacks and their families would disagree. Loggers might like their jobs to be safer, but they realize it is a practical impossibility. The job pays well, and consumers buy the lumber they produce. It's a trade off. Loggers accept the risk in return for more pay, and society accepts the risk in return for necessary lumber.

MOTOR VEHICLE DEATHS AND SUBCONSCIOUS RISK

News stories commonly state that diseases or toxins increase your risk of becoming ill or dying. How do those risks compare to other risks we accept without much thought?

Motor vehicles kill a lot of people. Each year, nearly as many Americans are killed in motor vehicle accidents as were killed in the entire 25 years of U.S. military action in Vietnam,[8, 9] yet no one calls for the elimination of motor vehicles to reduce the horrible carnage on our nation's streets and highways. I don't mean to be silly about this. It is impossible to reduce transportation risks to zero. Nevertheless, the number of deaths we accept is staggering: 33,800 Americans were killed in motor vehicle accidents in 2009, and 2.2 million were injured.[10] Motor vehicle crashes are the leading cause of death for almost every age from 3 to 34.[11] Roughly one out of every 136 Americans will be injured in a motor vehicle crash each year.[11]

Despite the overall risks, some Americans make choices that increase the risk of injury and death. If all passenger vehicle occupants over age 4 wore seat belts, the National Highway Traffic Safety Administration (NHTSA) estimates an additional 5,024 lives could be saved each year.[11] Just 65 percent of vehicle occupants currently wear their seatbelts. Fines and driving restrictions for not wearing seatbelts could be made more severe, but we choose not to strengthen existing laws.

Many of us also drive faster than we should, even though speeding was a contributing factor in 31 percent of all fatal crashes in 2006.[13] Some people encourage the use of smaller cars to promote fuel efficiency, even though these cars pose more risk than larger cars.[14] Driving while talking on a cell phone increases the risk of accident – and there is no difference between hand-held and hands-off units – but few states comprehensively outlaw cell phone use while driving.[15, 16] Texting is more dangerous. Texting drivers take their eyes off the road for 4 ½ of 6 seconds, which brings with it a 23-fold increase in the risk of a serious crash.[17]

Yes, people need to travel, but we could choose safer ways. The risk of death on buses is roughly 90 percent less than cars,[5, 12] and trains may be even safer.[5] We could force everyone to ride buses or trains, thereby saving tens of thousands of lives per year.

But we don't.

Americans have shown they are willing to trade a small risk of death for other desirable outcomes. In particular, we trade a small risk of death for convenience. Americans go about their business with little thought for most of the risks they take. Let's call the level of risk people accept without thinking about it *"subconscious risk."*

By subconscious risk, I don't mean Americans never think about the risks they take. A few folks probably remind themselves of the risk of driving when they put on their seatbelts before they start their cars. My hunch, however, is fear of getting a ticket is the primary motivation for most Americans to fasten their seatbelts.

Perfectly sane, normal, moral people are willing to accept small risks of injury or death in order to achieve other goals. We allow rare risks of death to occur, even though we could reduce those risks, because millions of people feel their quality of life is better with risk-taking activities. People should have the same freedom with their healthcare.

RARE MEDICAL RISKS

How do these subconscious risks compare to those discussed in healthcare? The number of deaths from cervical cancer has dropped from 26,000 per year in 1941 to about 4,900 in 1996.[18] This drop is mostly because women have regular Pap smears. The current mortality rate means the risk each year for a reproductive-age woman of dying from cervical cancer is approximately half that of dying in a motor vehicle accident. A woman who rides a motorcycle has 50 times more chance of dying on her bike as she does from cervical cancer.

Why should the risk of dying from cervical cancer be lowered any further, if it's already roughly the same as a common risk? How much should the medical system spend to reduce that risk further? Those aren't questions for GIMeC to answer. Those questions should be answered by the American public.

BACK TO BREAST CANCER

Now that we've put a few common risks into perspective, let's go back to the breast cancer controversy mentioned at the beginning of the book. The U.S. Preventive

Services Task Force calculated the impact of mammography in women ages 40-49 and concluded that 1,904 women must be tested every year for 10 years to save one woman from dying of breast cancer.[19] Other reviews reach similar conclusions.[20] More women than this will be diagnosed with breast cancer, but most will survive or die regardless of whether they received a mammogram.

To put this number in perspective, during the same 10-year period, one in 1,348 women age 40 to 49 will die in motor vehicle accidents.[21] Put simply, the theoretical risk of dying of breast cancer by not receiving mammograms from age 40 to 49 is lower than the subconscious risk women accept from driving their cars each year. This reality in itself doesn't mean mammograms shouldn't be offered. It does, however, mean the acrimony with which GIMeC attacked the government task force's recommendations lacked perspective. Any woman is in her right mind to decide to forgo the hassle and expense of annual mammograms in her 40s.

PART OF THE SOLUTION

If anyone wants to expend every dollar they have on traditional, aggressive medical care, they should have that right. Conversely, Americans also should be able to apply their resources to any aspect of their lives they believe will maximize their health and happiness.

If doctors' pens are the most expensive technology in healthcare, then *medically necessary* is the most expensive phrase. How likely must a condition be to justify an expensive test looking for an abnormality? Isn't some level of risk just too low to be worth the time, hassle, and expense? How much evidence in the medical literature is required to justify an expensive treatment as *necessary*? These are the questions organized American medicine hasn't put to its fellow citizens.

Doctors who care for patients willing to accept a small amount of risk to achieve more affordable healthcare can devise new approaches to medical care that respect those wishes. This level of risk should approximate subconscious risk. Here are some examples of what I mean:

- Women will not receive screening mammograms until they are 50, and afterward only every other year.
- Young people with classic migraine headaches, and no other worrisome issues, will not have CAT scans or MRIs of their heads.
- Minor injuries will not be X-rayed.
- Joints that look like classic arthritis in older patients will not be X-rayed.
- Few patients with low back pain will receive MRIs.
- Antibiotics will not be given for a cold, and rarely for sinusitis.
- People with low-risk chest pain will receive less aggressive testing.
- Patients who come to emergency rooms with mild or chronic symptoms will receive little testing or treatment.

All of the above conditions should be treated in family physicians' offices. In addition:

- Experimental treatments will not be offered.

- Patients whose cancer has spread throughout their bodies after one or two treatments, depending on the type and location of the cancer, will not be offered further curative treatment, but will be kept as comfortable as possible.

These are broad examples, and obviously many details remain to be ironed out. The final decisions of which services should be offered, and to whom, should be determined by a collaborative process between doctors and patients. Of course, for each of these examples, a rare set of circumstances could be imagined to make the counterpoint that a patient could be harmed by not providing the mentioned service. However, the more important question is: What is the level of risk you are willing to accept to create a more affordable healthcare system? Put another way, now that you know more about the risk of motor vehicles, will you stop driving your car and take the bus instead?

Perhaps an intermediate step on the road to affordable healthcare could be a new choice for women on Medicare. Women who feel the hassle and expense of mammography isn't worth the small chance of benefit could forgo mammograms and have those savings to the Medicare system rebated to them, roughly $200 every other year (the cost of the mammograms themselves plus further evaluation for a false positive mammogram). They could use that money for other things that might bring them more health and happiness. They should have that choice.

16 | A FEW MORE ISSUES

Before I propose solutions to the healthcare crisis, let's discuss a few more topics recently tossed around in healthcare debates.

ELECTRONIC MEDICAL RECORDS

Electronic medical records (EMRs) have been touted by everyone from President Obama to Newt Gingrich as the solution to America's healthcare woes. When President Obama appeared on *Meet the Press* soon after he won the election, he was asked about healthcare reform. EMRs were the first thing he mentioned.

Computers are amazing. I never want to go back to a world without word processing, spreadsheets, the internet, or search engines. Computers and the web clearly have made our lives better. But computers are just tools – tools with limitations and their own set of problems. Just as paper records have limitations, they also have benefits. Paper systems don't crash, don't catch viruses or Trojans, and don't need upgrades.

Researchers have studied the impact of EMRs on healthcare quality, and the results are mixed. Some studies find quality of care goes up, and some don't.[1-5] One clinic system found that EMR use led to more orders for diabetes tests, but the results of the tests did not improve.[6] Other studies actually found that family medicine offices using EMRs delivered lower quality care for patients with diabetes than offices using paper records.[7, 8] Some studies found that medical errors are reduced; some found they aren't.[8-10] In one hospital, the EMR created a whole new set of medication errors that didn't exist with the paper system.[9] Some studies in clinics found preventive interventions improved; some found they didn't.[10-13] Physicians who use EMRs may have paid fewer malpractice claims,[10] but EMRs didn't improve their job satisfaction.[11]

Implementing electronic systems that allow physicians to input orders directly is difficult.[12, 13] The doctors' experience with computerized order entry was so bad at Cedars Sinai Hospital in Los Angeles that the system was abandoned.[14] EMR systems also have difficulty interacting with Medicare computers.[16]

Reminder systems are another area of potential benefit for EMRs. Doctors forget things like everyone else. If it has been more than a year since a 55-year-old woman had a mammogram, the doctor may forget to order one, especially if the woman has an appointment for an unrelated problem. A computerized system can automatically remind the doctor to order another mammogram.

Similarly, disease registries are another method for improving chronic disease care. Disease registries are lists of patients with a certain chronic disease. If it's been longer than a year since a patient had a routine test, such as a hemoglobin A1C, the EMR can inform the doctor and send a reminder letter or e-mail to the patient to come to the clinic for the test.

Unfortunately, at least three reasons prevent these tools from fulfilling their promise.

First, EMRs don't work so well in general. Besides the obvious problems, such as crashes, there are more subtle barriers that involve technical and legal issues of the handling of sensitive information.[15] No clinical record-keeping system is ideal, and each of the commercially available EMRs has its own strengths and weaknesses. Some evidence exists to show these systems can reduce, though not eliminate, medication errors. However, the old error of "I couldn't read the doctor's writing" is now replaced with "I pushed the wrong button," "The system had erroneous information," "The EMR crashed," or "This EMR won't talk to the other EMR." EMRs introduce medical errors, as well.[9] Studies of doctors who purchased EMRs discovered many believed the alerts and reminders interrupted their workflow, so they turned off these features.[2, 14]

Second, patient expectations often conflict with EMRs. Many times, a patient doesn't want to deal with the litany of things an EMR might remind the doctor to do. If a new patient shows up at a clinic and her agenda is a simple refill on blood pressure medicine, is the doctor now responsible for all the current and future healthcare needs of that patient? The answer depends on the patients' expectations, and EMRs cannot adjust for patients' wishes.

The third, and most important, reason is time. EMRs can produce meaningful information, but if the doctor or patient doesn't have the time to deal with the information, they will not act on it. It really doesn't matter if a physician maintains a list of diabetic patients electronically or has it is written on a notepad stuck in a drawer. The information is the same. The EMR may be better at capturing every diabetic patient who appeared at a clinic in the last two years. The notepad is better at reflecting the doctor's judgment about which patients are really his long-term patients.

EMRs will not save healthcare costs. Whatever savings are realized from preventing medical errors and reducing duplication of tests are matched (if not exceeded) by the cost of acquiring, implementing, and constantly updating the technology. Even when EMRs help doctors improve the quality of care, through things such as reminders to order mammograms or other preventive services, overall healthcare costs still increase. As you've learned, an ounce of prevention costs a ton of money.

DOC-IN-A-BOXES

Urgent care centers have sprung up all over America. Many in the healthcare industry refer to them as a doc-in-a-box.

These centers have filled a niche. A person can walk in without an appointment and be seen relatively quickly, even without insurance. These centers have become relief valves for overcrowded ERs and primary care clinics. Some employer-sponsored health plans even encourage their employees to frequent these places. They view the doc-in-a-box as a cheaper alternative to ERs.

Why have these businesses become so successful? Show me the money. Let's take the example of a mom who is called from work to pick up her 8-year-old daughter from school because of a sore throat and a fever. She might call her family physician or pediatrician first. Perhaps the doctors can squeeze the daughter into their busy schedule. Perhaps not. If they can't, now the mother has three choices: take her daughter home and treat her symptoms with over-the-counter medicines, take her to an ER, or take her to a doc-in-a-box.

Insurance companies will typically pay about $150 for an urgent care center visit. An ER bill might total $400 to $500. However, the insurance company will make no allowance for a family physician's office that hustles to see this acutely ill child. They still only pay about $80, which includes the charge for a strep test.

Armed with this example and the knowledge that there is a massive lack of support for primary care in America, an entrepreneur looking to build a general care clinic has an easy choice. Invest in the place where he can charge $150 for a relatively simple visit, or in the one where he can charge $80. Which would you choose?

Generalist medical care provided outside of the Monday-Friday, 8-5 clinic schedule can be scant. Out-of-office-hours coverage is a physician workforce issue that primary care systems throughout the world wrestle to handle.[18, 19] Patients have needs that arise at any hour of the day, but individual doctors can't work 24/7. If primary care ever gets the support it deserves in America, part of the plan must include family physicians to cover patients' needs outside of normal office hours. Currently, barely 29 percent of U.S. primary care doctors have after-hours arrangements for patient care, compared to 89 to 97 percent in Europe.[16]

Two huge problems come with the doc-in-a-box, though. First, even though they are commonly staffed by generalists, including family physicians, they function as limited ologist clinics. The patient is allowed to bring up one concern, and one concern only. Any more, and it's too bad. Check in again and pay a separate bill, and the doctors will deal with that issue next. The doctors at doc-in-a-box clinics take no responsibility for the long-term or chronic disease care of their patients. They have effectively created patient care walls within the house of generalism, and they cherry-pick the easy stuff for themselves.

The next problem with the doc-in-a-box is that the quality of care is frequently awful. They have become so customer-focused that they have prostituted their medical training to the whims of paying customers. A family medicine resident moonlighted in one of these places recently. A patient came in one evening who clearly had a mild cold but demanded antibiotics. ("Early detection means early cure," the patient complained). The resident patiently explained why antibiotics were not necessary, would not speed his recovery, and would only contribute to antibiotic-resistant bacteria in the community. The resident did not write a prescription for antibiotics, but did write a prescription for some long-acting medicines to help with the symptoms. The patient called the next day to complain to the doc-in-a-box office manager. That afternoon, the medical director of the doc-in-a-box called the resident and fired him over the phone.

Some patients believe medical facilities are like hamburger joints. Walk into the clinic and order what you want. From a patient satisfaction point of view, it makes perfect sense. From the point of view of managing healthcare costs and protecting the public from irresponsible medical practices, it is an awful approach.

Family physicians – all physicians, for that matter – must be supported when they make medically appropriate decisions that aren't what a patient wants to hear. Second opinions are always appropriate. No doctor is perfect. But turning a medical practice into a McClinic is not the path to a better American medical system. Excellent customer service sometimes results in lousy medical care. If we ever move toward a family medicine-based healthcare system, these irresponsible doc-in-a-boxes must be among the first things to disappear.

GENOMICS

Much has been made of the potential of the human genome project to deliver amazing advances in medicine. As with EMRs, the potential is over-hyped.

Proponents of genomics suggest that in the future we can personalize healthcare.[21-24] For example, patients will receive a complete gene analysis saying which high blood pressure medicine will work best for them. There are at least two problems with this. First, gene analyses only comment on risk. They might point out increased risk for this condition and decreased risk for that condition. What are you supposed to do with that information? If you you bought a gene analysis as a 40-year-old and learned of a 10 percent increased risk of Alzheimer's disease, what have you gained? There is no evidence you can do anything in your 40s that will decrease your chance of developing Alzheimer's at 70 or 80, other than the usual list of common sense approaches – eat right, exercise, don't smoke, and keep your mind active. Some people might view this information as empowering. They might feel some control over their future, even if nothing they do in response to the information actually improves these risks 40 years later.

Meanwhile, the genetic testing companies have been allowed to make contradictory claims, saying on the one hand that their products help patients "take charge of their health," while on the other claiming they don't provide medical advice.[17]

Second, there is the cost. A report stated it cost one lab $200,000 and took eight months to completely document a single person's DNA.[18] Although in 2010 a company claimed to be able to sequence an entire genome for about $10,000, it is still a very expensive test.[19]

Third, reliability remains an issue. In many cases, little evidence backs the validity of genetic tests because there is generally no FDA requirement for the premarketing submission of such data.[17] The Government Accountability Office issued a report in 2010 citing deceptive marketing practices, erroneous medical management advice, and a lack of standardization among consumer-marketed genetic testing companies.[20]

Companies today offer less comprehensive gene analyses. These run in the range of $400 to $2,500 for an assessment of 100-200 diseases and health risks.[21, 22] The gene analysis companies also claim a person's healthcare can be personalized with their products. There are more than 1,000 genetic tests on the market,[23] although, like other laboratory tests, they enter the marketplace without any prior regulatory review.[24]

Other observers are cautious about the potential for genomics to impact the nation's health. As they point out, only some genomic tests provide clinically important information,[23] and the increased risk to an individual patient who tests positive for a genetic marker is often minimal.[24] As well, much is unknown about how to apply genomic medicine to common chronic diseases.[25]

Genomic tests will continue to generate further costs because abnormal results spawn more tests. A small increased risk of cancer or heart disease, as predicted by a genetic test, will certainly be followed by heart tests, CAT scans, and MRIs.[24] This follow-up testing is guaranteed to increase healthcare costs.

Some research into the usefulness of genomic information has been undertaken. One study examined patients who take a blood-thinning drug, warfarin, and divided them into two groups: one group had their doses of warfarin adjusted with the help of genomic information; the other was adjusted with standard laboratory data.[26] No difference was found in the success rate for reaching appropriate treatment levels between the two groups. A review by AHRQ that included results from other studies also concluded we have insufficient evidence that testing patients for genetic mutations prevents deep vein blood clots or other bad outcomes.[27]

Even if a case can be made that some genomic tests are helpful, it is unlikely Medicaid would ever cover these tests for poor people. If these tests are demanded by large numbers of people, however, insurance companies will face pressure to cover them. Should that happen, you can bet these costs will be passed on to you and your employer, along with a 25 percent mark-up for administrative costs.

For personalized medicine, I have a better idea. Instead of spending $2,500 for a test to predict which blood pressure medicine will work best, I'll prescribe a few dollars worth of blood pressure medicine and see if it works. If it works for you, which it typically does even on the first attempt, we have our answer.

MID-LEVEL PROVIDERS

Mid-level providers are nurse practitioners, physician's assistants, and such. Anyone who thinks mid-levels are a cheap alternative to family physicians either has no idea what family medicine can do, an inflated view of what mid-levels can do, or they live in a geographic region where the family physicians are so beaten down that they function at about the capacity of a mid-level.

Mid-levels provide high-quality care as long as the problems they face are relatively simple and straightforward. They are good at following protocols. They are good at educating patients. They tend to have excellent relationship skills, and patients are often satisfied with their care.[28] Mid-levels also can excel at chronic disease management. For instance, one study concluded mid-levels provided the same quality of care for diabetes, asthma, and high blood pressure as primary care physicians.[29] Reviews of the role of mid-levels as primary care providers find they see fewer patients per hour, work fewer hours per week,[30] and order more tests and other services.[30, 31]

Because their training is shorter and less intense than physicians, mid-levels aren't comfortable with complicated cases. Many times, they may know what to do, but they don't fully understand why. This limits their ability to deal with patients for whom a cookbook treatment approach may not be the best. Their knowledge base is not as broad as physicians', nor are their procedural skills.

About 15 years ago, the county hospital system where I work had an adult medicine clinic staffed mostly by experienced nurse practitioners. It was supervised by an internist, but the nurse practitioners saw most of the patients, who tended to be middle-aged to elderly and had multiple chronic diseases. At the same time, a similar clinic was staffed by family medicine residents fresh out of medical school. These residents were supervised by the teaching physicians of the family medicine department. The populations of the two clinics were similar, except that the residency patients were a little older and a little sicker.

We compared the performance of the two clinics over a one-year period. The patients of mid-level clinic went to the emergency department and were admitted to the hospital twice as often as the residency patients. The patients of the mid-level clinic were consulted to ologists three times as often as the residency patients. These outcomes occurred even though the mid-levels saw about half as many patients per day as the residents. Clearly, mid-level care was proving itself more expensive overall, not less. When we presented these findings to the hospital and clinic administration, they accused us of fabricating the results! The mid-level clinic was their baby. After emotions calmed down about a year later, that clinic was shut down.

OTHER PRIMARY CARE FIELDS
OB/Gyn

GIMeC promotes the idea that first contact primary healthcare should be provided by 2-½ doctors: a pediatrician, an internist, and an OB/Gyn for female issues. This attitude propagates needless expense in the healthcare system.

For starters, OB/Gyns are not primary care physicians, even though they claimed that title when their patient visits were threatened in the managed care era. As soon as the managed care pressure went away, the primary care rhetoric in the OB/Gyn community went with it.

Medical students choose OB/Gyn because they are concerned with women's issues. The other deciding factor is that many of them want to do a little medicine and a little surgery, but nothing too complicated. Their world revolves around medical issues with a definite end point: a pregnancy that ends with a delivery, or vaginal bleeding that stops with a surgical procedure. Many of them don't feel comfortable caring for patients with chronic issues not easily managed or cured, especially if it falls outside the reproductive track.

Many women bring up other symptoms with their OB/Gyns, not just female issues. The way most OB/Gyns handle concerns more serious than runny noses is to order a few tests, sometimes make the diagnosis, then refer the patient to another ologist for long-term care. The culture of OB/Gyn is not to take care of long-term problems or take responsibility for the whole person, but to refer non-female medical concerns to their ologist colleagues. This is the antithesis of primary care.

General internal medicine

General internal medicine is dying. Recently, about 90 percent of medical students choosing internal medicine want to become ologists.[32] Internal medicine and family medicine have more in common than there are differences. However, general internal medicine training does not equip its graduates to care for the whole patient as well as family medicine.

Typical internal medicine training doesn't teach its trainees to care for women's healthcare needs. This statement doesn't include just prenatal care and deliveries. The culture and training of internal medicine does not encourage its trainees to care for women with vaginal symptoms, menstrual issues, breast symptoms or lumps, pelvic pain or even contraception. They refer all that to OB/Gyns.

Internists usually have almost no formal training in psychiatric, psychological, or behavioral issues. They are taught to send patients with those concerns to psychiatrists. Internists have no training in sports or emergency medicine dealing with strains, sprains, and fractures. If a patient with a painful joint doesn't have osteoarthritis, rheumatoid arthritis, or lupus, they are at a loss. Even for the last two diseases I mentioned, they are taught to refer them to rheumatologists.

Internists spend very little time in clinic settings during their training because they spend almost all their time in the hospital. They graduate from their programs with little experience developing long-term relationships with patients and managing complex problems in the clinic environment. Internists are commonly discouraged from learning procedures.

Perhaps if the climate for generalism improved in the future, general internal medicine would make a comeback. But a strong force works against this: the cultures of medical schools and residencies. Any medical student who intimates she wants to be a general internist will, at some point, be bombarded with statements from ologist professors or residents similar to those they throw at students wanting to become family physicians: "So, you want to waste your brain and just do general internal medicine?"[33]

Because the majority of family medicine residents train in facilities away from the university-associated tertiary care hospitals, many of them have a safe haven from ologist abuse and learn in a more supportive environment. More than 90 percent of doctors who complete a family medicine residency remain committed to primary care.[34] Most general internists don't have supportive settings in which to train. The vast majority of internal medicine residencies are in the university hospitals, where they are bombarded by negative attitudes about generalism the entire three years of their training. In that environment, the epitome of being a doctor is to become an ologist.

Pediatrics

General pediatricians still are coming down the training pipeline, although their numbers are shrinking, too. In 2007, about half of the graduates of pediatrics programs became generalists.

If any primary care field is susceptible to takeover by mid-level providers, it's pediatrics. The majority of visits to pediatricians are for well-child care. These visits lack complexity. Family physicians consider them as nice breathers between their elderly patients with five chronic diseases.

As a practical matter, though, general pediatricians will be around for a long time. Generalist pediatricians are still going into practice, generations of families have taken their children to pediatricians, and they will always have the elitist appeal of marketing themselves as experts in children's health. Other countries, such as Britain and Canada, have pediatricians as part of their physician work force, but they are consultants for the family physicians. Routine children's healthcare is provided by the family physicians. Only complicated cases, such as children with significant ADHD, severe asthma, or developmental delays, are seen by pediatricians in these countries.

PRIMARY CARE BOTTOM LINE

The first bottom line is that family physicians can do everything internists and pediatricians can do, and more. They can take care of most women's issues, and some family physicians even provide complete maternity care, including C-sections.

The second bottom line is that practically all other developed countries do not split their primary care system into 2-½ doctors. They rely on one doctor to perform the primary care. They are called family physicians in Canada and general practitioners in much of the rest of the world. As healthcare planners think about America's future, they should imagine an America with a similar army of well-trained, well-supported family physicians to provide the bulk of healthcare for America.

17 | GOD AND AMERICAN MEDICINE

The Serenity Prayer, long version[1]
God grant me the SERENITY to
accept the things I cannot change;
the COURAGE to change the things I can;
and the WISDOM to know the difference.

Living one day at a time;
enjoying one moment at a time;
accepting hardships as the pathway to peace;

taking, as He did, this sinful world
as it is, not as I would have it:

Trusting that He will make all things
right if I surrender to His Will;
that I may be reasonably happy in this life
and supremely happy with Him forever in the next.

Amen

When the Frenchman Alexis de Tocqueville visited the young nation of the United States of America in the 1830s, he initially crossed the Atlantic to learn more about the American penal system. But as he traveled across the young nation, he also learned how the new American democracy worked and developed keen insights into the American people. One of the differences he noted between the cultures of America and Europe was the religious nature of America compared to the secular nature of Europe.[2] I mention this to recognize that any proposed changes to the American healthcare system must be mindful and respectful of the religious values that guide the daily lives of most Americans.

I am not a theologian. I am a Christian and a member of the United Methodist Church. I attend church the majority of Sundays in a year. Theologically, I consider myself a middle-of-the-road Methodist – not leaning toward an extreme on either side of the political or theological spectrum. To be clear, I am in no way trying to influence anyone's religious views. I will, however, try to establish an ethical and spiritual foundation for people of faith to imagine American healthcare in a slightly different way, to allow them to see other possibilities for what the system might look like.

ETHICAL FOUNDATION

One of the landmark legal cases that shaped modern medical ethics for end-of-life care was that of Helga Wanglie.[3, 4] She was an 84-year-old woman with many medical conditions, including heart failure, that contributed to an intensive care unit admission for many weeks with little hope of recovery. She could not speak because she was sedated and had a tube down her windpipe attached to a breathing machine. She could not breathe on her own. After many weeks passed with essentially no progress, her doctors and the hospital believed further care was futile.

She and her husband were religious people, members of the Lutheran church. The husband disagreed with the doctors' and hospital's assessment. He concluded she was alive on life support; therefore God wanted her to be alive. According to their beliefs, to do anything to cause her to die would be abhorrent to God.

The hospital took them to court, and the judge sided with the Wanglies. Some side issues were present, but the ethical principle affirmed in this case was individual religious beliefs of the patient are paramount, and any medical treatments necessary to keep the patient alive must be administered in this case. The hassle and expense of keeping Mrs. Wanglie alive was not an issue. The hospital appealed the decision, but Mrs. Wanglie died before the case could be heard, in spite of all attempts to keep her alive.

The Wanglie case, as well as several others, established the principle that patients have the right to determine the amount of aggressive care they receive. Almost without exception over the last 30 years, American courts have ruled there is no higher moral or legal authority defining appropriate treatments than the individual beliefs of the patient.

The problem with these rulings is that they ignore the issue of cost. Aggressive treatment of patients who are extremely unlikely to have a meaningful recovery is extremely expensive. By meaningful recovery, I mean patients who recover to the point they can independently interact with their environment – appreciate beautiful days, interact with family members, and not be completely dependent for all aspects of their self care.

However, if the courts say patients have the right to accept aggressive treatment, they also say patients have the right to refuse aggressive treatments. A classic example of this principle is the right of adult Jehovah's Witnesses to refuse blood products, even if this means they will die. (The courts consistently rule that the children of Jehovah's Witnesses have to receive life-saving blood products even if their parents object.) But again, I am not defending people with extreme religious views who choose to pray about their children's illnesses instead of giving them standard treatments (for example, not giving insulin to a child with diabetes).

Futility

The previous case study evokes the concept of futility. Why provide a futile medical service? It is a question that unfortunately has no answer. Many thoughtful people feel medical futility is indefinable, given the current medical/legal culture in America. Futility is distinguishable from completely inappropriate care, though. Patients rarely request a treatment that is at best worthless and at worst harmful. It's inappropriate and medically indefensible, for instance, to operate on a patient who doesn't have a disease curable by surgery.

The practice of medicine is less about absolutes than it is about probabilities. There are too many unusual and rare reactions to medical tests and treatments, making certainty in medicine unobtainable. The fundamental role of a doctor is to maximize the chance your health will improve and minimize the chance your health will decline.

The cases reasonable people might label as futile are often patients with massive strokes or brain injury who are still technically alive because they have minimal brain function. Other examples include patients with severe dementia and those with prolonged multiple organ failure unable to survive without mechanical life support.

While many doctors hate to admit it, we are lousy at predicting the future. American doctors have been observed to miss the mark on the high and low side, but the tendency is to be too optimistic – to assume patients will live longer than they actually do.[3] In contrast, at least one British study found their ICU doctors were too pessimistic in predicting outcomes in patients with emphysema.[4] The authors speculated the reason for this pessimistic pattern was the doctors worked in units with a limited number of intensive care beds. Some extremely sick patients were kept out of the ICU because the physicians felt the likelihood of recovery was too small, and the ICU beds were better used for people with better chances. I'm not aware of any ICU doctors in America having to make this difficult decision, except perhaps in extreme situations such as New Orleans in the aftermath of Hurricane Katrina.

Scoring systems have been created to help doctors estimate which critically ill patients will survive and which will not.[5, 6] These prediction systems work fairly well at grouping patients into prognostic categories. For example, a young patient who has severe pneumonia, but all her other major organs are working well, has less than a 5 percent predicted chance of dying. An elderly person with dementia, chronic kidney disease, heart failure, emphysema, hypertension, anemia, and liver damage who is in septic shock from a bacterial infection in the blood system might have greater than a 90 percent chance of dying. But not 100 percent. It's never certain.

This is as good as these prediction systems get. They can predict a person has a low chance of dying, but not zero percent. They predict another person has a high chance of dying, but not 100 percent. Unusual events do occur; miracles do happen.

Other scoring systems try to predict which patients with brain injuries will die or be left in a persistent vegetative state.[7, 8] Even in these systems, all bets are off in the first three days. There are too many cases of people who seem brain dead a day after an injury who perk up the next day and eventually walk out of the hospital with minimal long-term health problems. People who seem in a persistent vegetative state more than three days after an injury are much less likely to wake up. Most of those who do survive have minimal interaction with the world and, at best, survive the hospitalization only to spend the rest of their lives severely incapacitated in a nursing home. Still, miracles do happen, and no medical scoring system can predict which individual patient may experience a miraculous recovery. The currently accepted definition of a persistent vegetative state is no sign of higher brain function for more than one month.[9]

How many people in the U.S. are in a persistent vegetative state, and how many of them wake up years later? No one knows. To my knowledge, the NIH has never funded a study to answer that question.

SANCTITY OF LIFE

There are some religious traditions that hold very dearly the belief that life is a gift from God and must be preserved by sparing no hassle or expense. Many Orthodox Jews, Roman Catholics, and conservative Protestant Christians share this belief. But as much as some American religious leaders talk about the sanctity of life, the fact remains that, no matter how much technology we provide a sick patient, eventually that patient will die. Every human life may be sacred, but every life also must come to an end.

One of the fundamental sources of the tension many Americans feel about letting go of loved ones is that Americans value life. This national value is expressed not only in religious circles. Our military branches have a credo that no one is left behind. A captured or wounded soldier who knows that his buddies will never give up their search is sustained by that thought. We are also captivated by stories of little girls pulled from a well or rescued from the rubble of a building collapsed by an earthquake.

To reach an affordable healthcare solution that fits American values, we have to find a middle ground between squeezing out every minute that technology can accomplish and the reality that all life must come to an end. A fundamental difference exists between rescuing an otherwise healthy person trapped in a building and keeping a person who has minimal functioning brain tissue alive for years on life support.

FEEDING PEOPLE WITH MINIMAL BRAIN FUNCTION

One of the difficult issues in end-of-life care is feeding people who can't feed themselves. Many patients and families believe food and water are not medical therapies, but basics of life. They are legitimately concerned that withholding any nutrition is tantamount to inflicting misery on a loved one by starving him or her to death.

Medical research doesn't support the belief that withholding nutrition inflicts pain and suffering – for certain patients. When patients with metastatic cancer who have exhausted all reasonable curative treatment options become mildly dehydrated, their comfort actually may increase.[10] The changes in their body's fluid and salt balance may act as a natural anesthetic. Other effects of dehydration, such as a dry mouth and lips, can be treated with low-tech comfort care such as ice chips or small amounts of food or water.[11]

To feed someone who can't swallow well, we can perform a surgical procedure where a plastic and metal device is pierced through the skin, several layers of muscle, and the stomach or intestinal wall. A processed homogeneous liquid is poured down a plastic tube through the hole into the digestive system. These artificial feeding tubes don't result in better health for most terminally ill patients. Of Medicare patients who received feeding tubes, 24 percent died in one month and 63 percent in one year.[12] Two-thirds of feeding-tube patients developed pneumonia after some of the liquid nutrition worked its way into their lungs. Patients hospitalized with advanced dementia who received feeding tubes had no better survival at six months than those who did not receive a feeding tube.[13] Patients with feeding tubes and advanced dementia, compared to those without feeding tubes, have no better outcomes for malnutrition, pneumonia, other infections, bed sores, comfort, or overall survival.[14]

Some people only require feeding tubes temporarily. They may have had a large stroke but stand a reasonable chance of recovering their ability to swallow. Plus, they are aware of their surroundings and can interact with their family. Another example is a person who needs a feeding tube after throat surgery.

For most of human history, people who had massive strokes, severe brain injuries, and digestive system cancers died, in part, from the disease process making it very difficult to ingest food and water. People died naturally this way even 60 years ago, before the invention of modern life support. It is ethically permissible to withhold artificial nutrition and hydration from patients who do not desire it.

AN ALTERNATIVE WAY TO LOOK AT END-OF-LIFE CARE

Other Americans have different beliefs about aggressive care at the end-of-life than the Wanglies. I have met many deeply religious people who don't want a lot of aggressive care if they develop severe, irreversible illness. When asked how they're doing, they say, "I'm blessed," and they mean it. Of course, they want to be handled with care and compassion and have their medical ailments appropriately treated. But if the day comes when they have a serious medical condition that causes their heart, lungs, or brain to stop working, they simply want to be kept comfortable and allowed to die naturally.

We rarely hear about such people in the media. There's no conflict, so it's not an "interesting" story, according to the common media definition. No one is fighting to stay alive, fighting to find a cure, or seeking out the one doctor in America who could possibly save her.

Nevertheless, there are people in America who have humble expectations of services the healthcare system should provide. They take care of themselves as much as they can without visiting doctors or hospitals. They don't expect the healthcare system to fix every ache and tingly sensation. They realize bodies change as they age, and they humbly adapt their lives to those changes. They don't expect to run marathons at 80, but they don't want to be miserable every day, either. They just want to be able to take care of their personal needs and share intimate moments with their family and friends.

One of the real tragedies of the American healthcare system is that people with these values are lumped into the same health insurance pool as people who expect the healthcare system to fix every problem and keep them alive forever. The humble population has its resources transferred to the aggressive population without any debate or consent that such a transfer of resources should take place.

The humble population should be allowed to keep their resources and use them in other ways. They should receive a little more money in their Social Security check, or pay a little lower tax rate (the Medicare income tax, e.g.). They ought to be able to use the savings to take a vacation every year, not have to pinch every penny, help the grandchildren pay for college, and so forth. The humble population might believe other things in life can contribute to their health, things that have nothing to do with the healthcare system. These values should be respected as much as the values of people who want every advantage of technology, no matter how expensive the treatment or rare the benefit.

WHAT IF IT WERE ME

My personal religious beliefs differ from the Wanglies. Still, I know I don't have all the answers. I believe life is a precious gift from God, but He intended us to die one day. We have no guarantees when or how that death will occur, and it might come like a thief in the night. For most of the existence of human life on Earth, when people suffered severe brain injury or disease, they died from it. If God intended a different reality, He would have done something about it thousands of years ago. This doesn't mean we shouldn't use medical care. The oldest parts of the Bible mention treatments for medical conditions.

Personally, I wouldn't want to be kept alive in a persistent vegetative state for at least two reasons. (I say this knowing recent research shows it is a difficult diagnosis to make with certainty.[15]) First, it would represent a huge emotional drain on my family to watch me just lie there staring off into space. I would feel selfish to put so many demands on their time and emotional energy. They should be allowed to grieve my death and then get on with their lives. Second, there is the cost. Estimates from the early 1990s pegged the figure at roughly $100,000 per year to care for a person in a persistent vegetative state. Without doubt, it costs more now. Although no one knows long-term outcomes with certainty, a crude back-of-the-envelope estimate is possible. Let's say there is a one-in-a-thousand chance that keeping someone alive in a vegetative state for five years results in one person waking up enough to interact with her family again. We have now spent $500 million to allow the one person to wake up. In my view, that is just too much. Think of how many people could benefit from a sum that large. If I were in a vegetative state and could magically talk to my loved ones for one hour only, I would say to turn off the technology and let me go. I would feel too guilty for taking those resources from the greater society.

If I'm in a persistent vegetative state, or even a state of minimal brain activity that isn't technically vegetative, my family knows my wishes. I want the artificial feeding stopped so

I can die a natural death, just as billions of humans have done before me. I will not experience hunger or thirst, because I will lack the brain function to have those sensations. In my view, God is trying to call me home. Don't stop Him.

PART OF THE SOLUTION

Ask yourself if you could join a health plan supporting a different set of values than mainstream American medicine espouses. The agreement between you and your fellow health plan members is, for example, that if any of you suffer severe irreversible brain damage with miniscule hope of meaningful recovery, your doctors will discontinue life support but keep you comfortable until you die. You agree to this proposition because it is consistent with your inherent ethical and religious values, and also because you believe it is unfair that so many medical resources are used on you and therefore taken from others. You accept that life is sacred in the eyes of God, but also that God intended your life on Earth to end one day. You believe that just because a medical technology is available doesn't mean it has to be used. You believe if God wants to perform a miracle, He doesn't need man's machines to accomplish it.

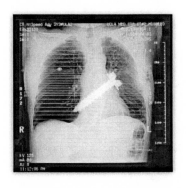

Part 3

Solutions

18 | SOLUTIONS

INTRODUCTION

America needs a fresh approach to fix its healthcare system because we pay too much and receive so little in return.

There are no easy solutions, no pat answers, to our healthcare mess. Rather, I propose solutions that actually cut to the heart of why American healthcare costs more and more and delivers less and less. My solutions aren't concerned with benefit packages and co-pays. Countless past reforms have tried to manipulate these aspects of insurance coverage with minimal impact on the overall cost or quality of healthcare.

I don't intend to nationalize healthcare or even to take away your current health plan, if you are satisfied with it. Instead, I propose to create more choices for healthcare consumers. I'm talking about more effective choices, choices that alter the basic formula for what drives up the cost of American healthcare.

The difficult changes I propose naturally will have human and ethical consequences. Let's first consider the effects of my solutions on an imaginary extended family.

- Mom: 39, just had a baby, no major health problems.
- Dad: 40, may have high blood pressure.

- Baby: 2 months old, developing normally.
- Child: 6 years old, moderately severe asthma.
- Uncle: 62, diabetes, high blood pressure, high cholesterol, early kidney disease, heart attack three years ago.
- Aunt: 60, kidney cancer two years ago, currently disease free.
- Grandmother: 65, heart failure under good control, otherwise active for her age.
- Great-grandmother: 85, assisted living home with moderate Alzheimer's dementia, high blood pressure, high cholesterol, heart failure, diabetes.

Assume that mom or dad has a job and is the primary breadwinner who works for a large company. The job carries standard health insurance benefits. In 2012, the company likely paid somewhere around $12,350 per year for healthcare for this family. Deductibles probably would have totaled about $5,100 per year. The family also would have borne out-of-pocket expenses somewhere around $3,600 per year.

As I walk you through my proposed solutions, I will return frequently to this hypothetical family to estimate the impact of my proposed changes on their healthcare costs.

Remember, healthcare insurance costs are really *wages*. It is money the employee earns that is siphoned off into the great American healthcare black hole without the employee's permission. The insurance premiums your employer pays on your behalf is money that was generated by your work. What if you could decide how much of that went toward your take-home pay, and how much went to the healthcare industry? The next time you find yourself in the annual meeting to discuss next year's health benefits, look to your right and left. You and your fellow employees are the ones paying for healthcare, not the anonymous insurance company executives or their shareholders.

When one of your fellow employees gets cancer and a doctor wants that person to receive $200,000 of experimental treatments, ask yourself, "Is it fair for the rest of us who work for the same employer to pay for that?" There is no right or wrong answer to this question, but this transfer of money out of your pocket into another employee's healthcare is exactly what happens, minus a lot of overhead siphoned off by the insurance company on top of the treatment costs. (That's not to say employees should make individual healthcare decisions for other employees. But everyone involved in the process should understand exactly what is happening with their money in order to make informed coverage choices.) Some employees will believe such a transfer of money is appropriate, others won't. Employees who think such expenditures for experimental treatments are not worth it should be allowed to form an insurance pool separate from those who would want such treatment expenses approved for themselves.

I contend that you deserve this choice. If you choose, the fruits of your labor could continue to pour into an inefficient and expensive healthcare system. Or, you could choose to take it home and spend it on your family. GIMeC won't like this because GIMeC assumes that only more dollars devoted to healthcare will improve your health.

The elderly of this country should have the same choice. Why let the federal government say how your benefits are divided? The federal government pays a certain amount of money each year to elderly citizens. Part of that money is from Social Security, and part is from Medicare. Elderly citizens of this country deserve the same right to define how much of their government entitlement payments go toward healthcare and how much goes toward living expenses.

Reasonable people could have different preferences of where they draw the line. Some would choose to continue with classic American healthcare benefits. Others would want a minor adjustment. Still others would prefer a significant change in their healthcare approach so they could take home as much money as possible.

I propose that we add two choices to the current list of health insurance alternatives.

The first option, *Family Medicine Care*, will be painful simply because it involves change. Change is stressful, and the transition can be stressful and occasionally inefficient. However, Family Medicine Care shouldn't prove too painful because it will deliver better health at a lower cost.

The second option, *Basic Healthcare*, will be more difficult. Besides involving even more change, it will confront difficult trade-offs head on. I won't beat around the bush in this proposal. It may involve changes that will be too painful for many Americans. That's okay. My proposed changes aren't meant for everybody. Nevertheless, the American path to a difficult solution is through choice, not government mandate.

19 | FAMILY MEDICINE CARE

Family Medicine Care involves taking a population of Americans who believe the vast majority of their healthcare could be provided more cost-effectively by one physician and separating those people into their own insurance pool. People who choose Family Medicine Care agree to the following:

- To make an effort to see the same physician – or at least the home clinic – as much as possible for healthcare needs.
- To not seek ologist care without checking first with your family physician.
- To accept the different practice style of family physicians compared to ologists, specifically:
  - o Family physicians will not order as many tests as ologists, especially in the early stages of symptoms. The corollary to this approach is that a series of useless tests and procedures usually isn't in the best interests of the patient or the greater healthcare system.
  - o Family physicians will take on as much of the patients' care as they are capable of handling. They will refer to an ologist only when the addition of the ologist actually improves your health.

o Family physicians accept that medical science actually cures very little, and the real challenge for many patients is learning to manage and live with chronic diseases. Many times, the best approach is a humble attitude about the limitations of modern medicine.

Other than this one organizational change, which I realize still won't be easy, Family Medicine Care will function like every other healthcare plan in existence in America. All medically necessary care will be provided. Rare diseases and conditions will be investigated, and if found, treated. Standard definitions of "medically necessary" will be used.

People who choose Family Medicine Care will accept a slightly different set of assumptions about healthcare than the POEM assumptions. These new assumptions are:

• *Prevention doesn't save money,* but many patients feel reassured by a lot of prevention from their family physicians. Family Medicine Care patients would receive customary preventive services, except PSA testing because it doesn't work.

• *Family physicians deliver the best health at the lowest cost.* Family Medicine Care patients recognize the best care for most conditions is provided by a single family physician who knows them well. Ologists would become involved only when they add value to a patient's health.

• *Early detection prevents some diseases, but tests and treatments should be done only if there is good evidence to support them.* Family physicians have a different style of managing some health conditions than ologists. An example would be allowing time for non-specific symptoms to mature into a set of symptoms more indicative of a diagnosable disease.

- *More treatments don't equal better care.* Family Medicine Care patients will expect treatments to be offered if there is reasonable proof of effectiveness. Experimental treatments will not be covered.

To make this agreement work, the greater healthcare system must do a better job of meeting the needs of family physicians. For starters, family physicians must be paid for the work they do. A person with a sore throat need not be charged $200 for an office visit just so the family physician can make as much money as an ologist. I won't repeat all of Chapter 8 here, but recall that many services provided by a family physician are not paid by insurance companies or Medicare. If you have five different issues you want to discuss, your family physician should be able to deal with everything in one visit and be compensated fairly for his time. As previously mentioned, it is more cost-effective to deal with several issues in one visit rather than be forced to schedule individual appointments for each problem. In fact, your family physician might even bring up a health issue that you didn't think of, such as checking how long it's been since you had a preventive service appropriate for your age, gender, and other risk factors. Perhaps, for example, you had no intention to discuss bone loss (osteoporosis) testing, but your physician reminds you that it is time for routine testing to start. The physician should be credited for the intellectual work of recognizing the missing healthcare opportunity, explaining the need and rationale to you, and arranging for the appropriate test or treatment. Your family physician shouldn't have to accept a disincentive from the insurance company or Medicare to provide these services.

The Family Medicine Care solution shouldn't be construed as a windfall for family physicians. Frankly, some of them will have to work harder, take on more patient care responsibilities, and challenge themselves not to refer difficult cases to ologists.

Family physicians will be expected to send their patients to other doctors as little as possible. Some proposals for healthcare payment reform mention paying fees to family physicians to coordinate care. That's minor. The crucial change is to pay family physicians to provide *comprehensive* care. The family medicine office practice should be seen as a one-stop healthcare shop. Maybe we should re-label family physicians. Instead of general practitioners, we'll call them "comprehensivists."

Besides not referring as often, family physicians will be expected to provide more hours of coverage for their patients. This may prove difficult, given some of the work and life expectations of young physicians coming down the training pipeline. Generation Y and the millenials may not be willing to work the hours that previous generations did. Even so, if family medicine makes the claim that it can take care of most of the health problems people have, the job can't be done between 8 to 5, Monday through Friday. Face-to-face availability 24/7 is not reasonable, but family physicians should cooperate to provide routine evening and weekend hours. Small independent practices could form networks that pool resources for out-of-hours coverage. Some needs also could be met with email, online chat, or other alternatives. Ideally, needlessly expensive urgent care centers and retail clinics would become obsolete if family physicians met this obligation. For routine visits or non-urgent symptoms, you should still see your personal family physician. But if you develop a sudden worrisome pain or rash, you should be seen quickly by someone at your family physician's office, or by another doctor who shares patient-care responsibilities in a network of family physicians.

Still, there are limitations. Some Americans expect medical care to function like an ATM. The moment they feel a little off, they think they should be able to visit one of a thousand medical ATMs and, within a matter of minutes, have dispensed exactly the amount of healthcare they demanded. While we all understand why many people would find this situation desirable, the attitude itself contributes greatly to unsustainable costs in the healthcare system. Providing that level of convenience only increases the demand for healthcare. We all have aches and pains and other concerns about our health, but there has to be a balance. Family physicians should be available to address their patients' concerns 24/7, but patients shouldn't assume it's appropriate to access this healthcare for every minor symptom or question. There is still no cure for the cold, so it is absolutely appropriate that patients suffer through a common cold taking over-the-counter medications, if any, without formally accessing the healthcare system.

THE FAMILY IMPACT

How would Family Medicine Care affect our imaginary family? Here's how:

Mom: She would probably want to get back on contraception after just having a baby. Her family physician would discuss her options and provide the contraception. Because her family physician will see the new baby regularly, as well, he will be in position to diagnose and treat post-partum depression, if it occurs. Mom will see her family physician for regular Pap smears. When she turns 40, she'll probably start having annual mammograms according to the existing guidelines, if she chooses to after a discussion of the risks and benefits of mammography. She'll also see her family physician for any number of other concerns that arise. She'll be tested for high cholesterol according to standard existing guidelines and receive other customary preventive measures.

Dad: He will see his family physician to determine if he really has high blood pressure. He'll also discuss other concerns, such as his shoulder that aches occasionally, and receive routine preventive care such as cholesterol testing. If his shoulder might benefit from an injection of a corticosteroid, his family physician can provide it. He probably won't need to see the doctor much, especially if his blood pressure turns out to be normal. If he does have high blood pressure, his family physician will make the diagnosis and treat it according to existing guidelines. Minor concerns may even be addressed through other communication mechanisms, such as e-mail.

Baby: She will see her family physician for all routine check ups and immunizations. Fevers, coughs, rashes, and other common baby concerns will also be diagnosed and treated by her family physician. Because mom is seeing the same family physician, appointments may be shared and a few trips saved each year.

Child: He will also see his family physician for routine preventive care and immunizations. His asthma will be treated by his family physician, including the rare times he needs to be hospitalized. The other minor calamities of childhood will be managed by his family physician, such as cuts and injuries on the soccer field. There will be no need to transition to another physician when he becomes a teenager.

Uncle: He will have all of his chronic diseases cared for by one family physician. Referrals to ologists will be kept to a minimum. His family physician will ask for the referral only when she feels the ologist will actually add value to Uncle's health. The payment system will be reformed to encourage the family physician and the Uncle to spend time several times per year visiting about Uncle's health, if that's what he wants. All of the chronic diseases and new concerns could be addressed at the one visit. The Uncle will walk out of the family physician's office with all necessary prescriptions and tests, saving perhaps a dozen trips to other doctors and greatly reducing the potential for medical errors.

Each of the chronic diseases will be managed according to standard existing guidelines, except perhaps in a few instances where the guidelines for one condition conflict with the guidelines for another. The family physician will be in the best position to make those judgment calls.

Aunt: She will see her family physician for all routine preventive care, which will continue in spite of the recent cancer diagnosis. This aspect of her care will be similar to Mom, except that at age 60, additional routine testing should start for diseases like osteoporosis (weak bones). She will not need to continue seeing her oncologist at this point. Any standard monitoring for a recurrence of cancer, such as blood work or CAT scans, can be done by the family physician. The Aunt will visit her oncologist again only if one of these tests indicates the cancer has returned. Visits to address preventive concerns or new issues could be combined with regular post-cancer visits.

Grandmother: She will receive all routine care from her family physician, including treatment for her heart failure. Treatment would continue according to existing guidelines throughout the remainder of her life. Episodes where her heart failure flares up and requires a visit to the emergency room with a subsequent admission to the hospital also will be managed by her personal family physician. If she qualifies for care that requires devices to be implanted to extend her life, a cardiologist will be asked to assist in that decision-making process because, in this and similar instances, the cardiologist would add value to her care. A cardiovascular surgeon would probably implant the device.

Great-Grandmother: She will be seen by her family physician both in the office and at the assisted living center, as appropriate. Occasional hospitalizations will be almost unavoidable, and her family physician will care for her in that setting, as well. All chronic diseases will be treated according to existing guidelines and continued for the rest of her natural life. Her moderate Alzheimer's disease will limit her ability to make decisions, so an ongoing conversation with her family will occur to ensure her wishes are honored. If the family desires aggressive care in the face of serious illness, that decision will be followed. If the family desires more of a comfort care approach, that decision will be followed.

END RESULT

For employed families who choose Family Medicine Care, their total healthcare costs – those paid by their employer combined with their own expenses – will decrease by approximately 20 percent, or $4,210 in 2012. This will result in lower co-pays for some insured items and more take-home pay. The ratio of these two payouts – co-pays versus take home pay – will depend on how the employee or employer would want to divvy up the savings. If all of these savings went to take-home pay, it would result in $351 more per month. (Details on how I calculated this estimate are in the Appendix.)

A similar trade-off could occur for elderly Americans who receive Social Security and Medicare benefits. The average elderly couple in America receives about $47,600 per year from the taxpayers through the federal government from these two programs: $24,000 from Social Security and $23,600 from Medicare in 2012 ($33,800 per year in annual medical costs if out-of-pocket expenses and supplemental insurance are included). This money could be treated like the cafeteria plans common in the workplace. By choosing to spend less on healthcare by choosing the Family Medicine Care plan, more of the money set aside for the elderly couple could be directed to Social Security payments instead.

Therefore, for a couple on Medicare who chooses Family Medicine Care, their total healthcare costs would decrease by approximately $4,720 in 2012 ($6,760 if the other costs are included). This would increase their monthly Social Security check by about $393 per month—from an average in 2012 of $2,000 per month to $2,393 per month ($563 per month of increased income if the other costs are included).

This extra income could be used to reduce their stress by relieving some of their budget concerns. Perhaps they could afford to move into a safer retirement community. They might feel the satisfaction of helping their grandchildren with college expenses. They could join a local YMCA or inexpensive health club and start exercising regularly. They could buy healthier foods. People can improve their health in many ways that have nothing to do with the healthcare system.

20 | BASIC HEALTHCARE

Before I offer the specifics of the next solution, let me be very clear about one thing. What follows will be a radical departure from healthcare options currently available. It will involve discussion of difficult truths and difficult trade-offs. Also, the ideas I present haven't been vetted by or endorsed by my family physician colleagues. Some will agree with me; I'm sure some won't.

Regardless, people should have a fresh option they've never before had – to be able to drastically transfer their resources away from the healthcare industry to other aspects of their lives that also hold potential to improve their health and well-being. This plan is for people who believe good health doesn't come from just pills and MRIs. This plan is for people who believe their lives are healthier if they have secure jobs, live in safe neighborhoods, and don't have to live from paycheck to paycheck.

Basic Healthcare will succeed where other plans have failed because it will directly attack the root causes of inefficient expensive American healthcare – risk avoidance and runaway costs.

MEDICAL NECESSITY

Every commercially available health insurance plan contains language to explain its benefits as something like all "medically necessary" care. The contract between an insurance company and a policyholder is that any medical care will be provided – no matter how costly the care (within certain total limits) or rare the benefit. Policyholders carry these expectations with them into their doctors' offices.

Basic Healthcare will entail a different set of expectations appropriate for people who can agree to the following:

- *Participants in Basic Healthcare voluntarily accept less aggressive healthcare in return for less expensive healthcare.*

- *Some tests and treatments recommended by GIMeC won't be appropriate for Basic Healthcare patients*, either because the risk of the condition is too rare to be justifiable, or more commonly, because there is no proof that identifying the risk early will make a difference later. The medical directors of the Basic Healthcare plan will develop diagnostic and treatment guidelines to set this level of risk similar to the subconscious level of risk that Americans accept in their daily lives. In other words, the risk accepted by foregoing rarely beneficial tests or treatments will approximate the risk of injury or death we accept by driving a car.

- *Before a doctor recommends a certain test or treatment, a minimal level of proof in the scientific literature must support the benefit of the intervention in question.* Expert opinion by a group of ologists, without solid scientific evidence to back it up, will not serve as justification to order tests or treatments. Exceptions could be made for rare, life-threatening diseases that, by virtue of their rarity, have little research to inform physicians on the best options.

However, minimal proof doesn't mean physicians are limited only to FDA-approved indications. Many high-quality, published articles describe uses for drugs and devices that haven't gone through the formal FDA approval process.

- *Some tests or treatments that could possibly benefit a person won't be provided because they aren't cost-effective.* The medical directors of the Basic Healthcare plan – with the cooperation of a panel of non-medical representatives that includes other members of the Basic Healthcare plan – will be responsible for setting these limits.

- *When making decisions for their patients, doctors will take the general approach of: "when in doubt, don't."*

- *Immediate needs take precedence over future needs.*

- *Life means more than being kept alive by machines; quality of life matters.*

- *Many treatments physicians offer their patients don't save lives; they delay death.* If God wants to miraculously heal an individual, He doesn't need machines to do it.

- *Experimental treatments will not be covered.*

People who choose Basic Healthcare do so with the understanding that the Family Medicine Care assumptions apply, with the following additions:

- *Early detection doesn't prevent much, and some proven interventions only rarely make a difference.* Approaches to prevention would be adjusted to accept a level of subconscious risk. Examples would include less frequent Pap smear testing, and adjustments to diagnostic and treatment goals for high cholesterol. Doctors and patients would allow time for vague symptoms to mature before some tests are ordered or treatments begun.

- *An ounce of prevention costs a ton of money.*
- *Ologist care also needs limits.* The ologists' decision-making also would be constrained by cost considerations.

BASIC HEALTHCARE – IMPACT ON THE FAMILY

Mom: Her immediate post-delivery care would not be affected. After that, some of the routine care would change. She would continue having Pap smears, but only about every three years or so. Routine cholesterol testing would begin when she turns 50, unless there is a strong family history or other risk factor that greatly increases her risk of heart disease. If she had a hysterectomy for any reason other than cancer, she would not need any more pelvic exams or Pap smears unless a symptom appeared that required investigation. She wouldn't have routine mammograms until age 50, and only every other year afterward. She would receive basic mammograms only, no routine ultrasounds or MRIs.

Baby: There would be no major differences compared to existing standards. Well baby visits would include less routine education by the doctor because, in most cases, the evidence shows it does not improve the baby's health. In other words, the visit would be less of a long speech by the physician and more of a chance for the parents to discuss their concerns. Additional educational resources such as websites could be provided.

Child: There would be no major differences compared to existing standards. Some routine later immunizations may be skipped, such as the 24-year old tetanus shot. Stricter rules to discourage the over-diagnosis of ADHD would also be put in place.

Dad: The definition of high blood pressure requiring treatment would probably rise to a pressure more like 160/100. Blood pressure goals could vary depending on the medications required to achieve a certain pressure. For example, if generic drugs costing pennies per pill can get his pressure below 140/90, then that goal may be acceptable. If patented drugs costing several dollars per pill are required, the goal might creep up to 160/100. He would be tested less often for high cholesterol, and the levels at which he would receive drugs would be raised so that both testing and treatments are more cost-effective.

Aunt: She would receive some follow up of her cancer with tests like CAT scans, but not for long. Further follow-up of her cancer will be triggered by symptoms suggesting the cancer has recurred. She may be tested for high cholesterol in a narrow range of years, maybe 55 to 70, depending on other risk factors.

Uncle: He would receive treatment for his chronic diseases but with a less aggressive approach. The lone exception would be treatments shown to make a big difference in keeping him out of the hospital. Some asymptomatic screening tests may not be offered because his several chronic diseases decrease his life expectancy, which make these interventions less cost-effective for him compared to a healthier population. In some cases, however, the presence of chronic diseases makes routine testing more cost-effective.

Grandmother: She would receive most of the chronic medications for her heart failure similar to standard care. She probably wouldn't receive expensive implantable devices to treat abnormal heart rhythms. The concept of sudden cardiac death would be seen as a preferred alternative to a lingering and painful death. She probably wouldn't be eligible for a heart transplant; it wouldn't be cost-effective. As her heart continues to weaken over the coming years, measures to keep her as comfortable as possible would be provided.

Great-Grandmother: She probably wouldn't receive drugs for Alzheimer's disease because these treatments are not cost-effective, except in very narrow circumstances. Alzheimer's drugs are barely effective in the first place and extremely expensive. Her high blood pressure treatment would be less aggressive. Should she develop something like a routine skin cancer (basal cell cancer), it wouldn't be treated because it would have no impact on her life expectancy and would not cause significant symptoms. She wouldn't receive routine mammograms or cholesterol testing and treatment. If she suddenly quit breathing or her heart stopped beating, she wouldn't be resuscitated. She would receive a complete array of treatments to keep her as comfortable as possible.

To provide a more thorough description of the specifics of a Basic Healthcare plan, more examples are given in the Appendix.

REASSURANCES

A few other important things will be missing with Basic Healthcare. An army of accountants will not keep watch at the bedsides of sick patients, ready and waiting to pull the plug the moment the patient crosses some cost threshold. A few patients will always become suddenly ill and rack up thousands of dollars per day in hospital and doctors' charges.

Unavoidably, some patients have one-thing-after-another hospitalizations. One example is a person with breathing trouble who is diagnosed with pneumonia. Treatment is started, and while they're in the hospital – in spite of appropriate treatment – fluid collects in their lungs that requires them to be put on a breathing machine. A few days later they have a heart attack, then develop a blood clot in the leg, a secondary infection on top of their first infection, the intestines stop working, and so forth. Each of these events is treatable, but sometimes patients develop one complication on top of another. Basic Healthcare will continue to treat each of these conditions as they arise, as long as they are reasonably fixable.

If you have a heart attack on Basic Healthcare, you will receive aggressive care, including expensive procedures such as stent placements and bypass surgery. Those are indeed expensive, but they are also effective and cost-effective if provided to the right patients. If you have a bad case of pneumonia, you will be put on a breathing machine and given expensive antibiotics. If you are in a car wreck and require a long hospitalization and follow-up rehabilitation, you will receive it. If your are seen in an emergency room for abdominal pain and there is more than a sliver of a chance something is seriously wrong, all the expensive tests emergency physicians commonly order will be covered.

As well, doctors will not receive bonuses to deny appropriate healthcare. Basic Healthcare patients who felt they were denied a needed test like an MRI won't have to worry that the doctor made that decision because he received a 20 percent kickback for denying the expensive test. This could become a little tricky, I acknowledge, since doctors respond to incentives like anyone else. A system of accountability must be implemented for participating doctors to make medical decisions consistent with the general principles of Basic Healthcare so no one tries to cheat the system. A supportive culture for physicians who provide Basic Healthcare would go a long way toward insuring that the system isn't abused.

On a positive note, the financial burden carried by families under the current healthcare system would be greatly reduced under Basic Healthcare. Since fewer expensive tests and treatments will be ordered, those that are provided could come with reasonable co-pays. Co-pays for visits to a family physician and other routine tests will also be reasonable.

GOVERNANCE

I won't spend an inordinate amount of time covering the operational details of a Basic Healthcare plan. That's beyond the scope of this book. Operational details will vary by state, in any case, because the power to regulate medical practice and insurance is different in each. But as medical research continues to invent new tests and treatments, the administrators of a Basic Healthcare plan will continue to have to make decisions about which they should add to the benefit package.

What defines a test or treatment as cost-effective? We shouldn't fixate on a specific number, as long as it is one that is agreed upon by the people who sign up for Basic Healthcare. Britain uses a specific number range, currently about £30,000 per year of life extended. That translates to about $50,000, depending on the exchange rate. This is in line with cost-effectiveness ranges used in the Netherlands and parts of Canada.[1]

As a starting point for a baseline number of cost-effectiveness, I suggest using the average amount of money an American household earns per year in work outside the home. That amount was $49,445 in 2010,[2] which is remarkably similar to the cost-effective thresholds found in the rest of the developed world. If this approach is agreeable, the cut-off value will naturally rise with wages and serve as a consistent benchmark for many years.

Equally important, we must have an oversight panel that includes members of the general public, preferably individuals who are members of the Basic Healthcare plan. The perspective of non-physicians will always be crucial. Doctors can become parochial in their thinking, just like any other group of people with similar backgrounds. The benefits package of a Basic Healthcare plan must reflect a common-sense approach understandable to just about anyone. I don't expect lay people on an oversight panel to become medical experts; the doctors on the panel will handle those duties. The role of non-physician members is to keep the doctors grounded.

CHANGING YOUR MIND

What if you signed up for Basic Healthcare, became gravely sick, then changed your mind?

First, I would hope that most people sign up for Basic Healthcare not because they view it as a way to generate a little more take-home pay, but because they have underlying ethical and spiritual beliefs causing them to be humble about their expectations of the healthcare system.

Second, Basic Healthcare should have fairly aggressive approaches to dealing with patients who want unproven, aggressive medical care the moment they face a life-threatening disease. Patients will always have the right to switch health insurance plans, but the rest of the patients in the Basic Healthcare insurance pool shouldn't bear the burden of patients who demand care not provided by the plan. If, for example, a person developed an incurable cancer but demanded still more rounds of chemotherapy beyond those covered by Basic Healthcare, that person should pay for all additional care from that time forward. If he dies without paying any of the costs while alive, his estate should remain liable for any expenses the deceased left unpaid.

All European countries wrestle with this dilemma when their wealthier citizens want services not covered by national healthcare plans. In Britain, the phenomenon is called topping up. Britain's NHS is still trying to decide if NHS facilities can be used for these extra services, for example infusion centers to administer chemotherapy that isn't supplied by the NHS. Otherwise, those services would have to be provided completely apart from NHS facilities.

This problem might prove more complicated than you think. For instance, what if a patient had a severe allergic reaction to a chemotherapy drug not covered by a Basic Healthcare plan that was given in a private medical facility? The drug isn't covered, but allergic reactions are. A viable Basic Healthcare plan should err on the side of categorizing any possible reactions to an unapproved treatment as part of the cost of that treatment, which the patient will be completely responsible for paying.

While this may sound harsh, the system needs strict boundaries. Otherwise, there would be too much temptation to "game" Basic Healthcare, which would completely undermine its effectiveness.

END RESULT

The overall cost of healthcare would eventually decrease about 20% further than Family Medicine Care for people who choose Basic Healthcare. This would result in about $4,210 more per year of personal income for a family of four for a grand total of $8,420 more personal income (Family Medicine plus Basic Healthcare changes). For a couple on Medicare, it would mean about $4,720 more per year for a grand total of $9,440 per year for Basic Healthcare ($13,520 if the out-of-pocket expenses and supplemental insurance costs are included). This would translate to a total of $787 per month in extra income--from an average in 2012 of $2,000 per month to $2,787 per month ($3,127 total income per month if the other costs are included).

21 | FINAL THOUGHTS

Not long ago, I saw a young woman who had a breast lump. She was 19 years old and wanted to join the Air Force. In her routine physical, the Air Force doctor felt the lump in her breast and told her she had to have it cleared before she could join. Uninsured, she came to the urgent care clinic at the county hospital where I work. The lump was easy to find. It had the consistency of soft rubber, like a grape-sized piece of Jello in the middle of her breast. Cancers are usually very hard. She had no family history of breast or ovarian cancer. I concluded this lump was nothing more than a variant of normal breast tissue. I ordered no tests. I didn't try to biopsy it. I patted her on the shoulder and told her not to worry; she didn't have breast cancer.

Was I a bad doctor? There is no right or wrong answer to this question. Nineteen-year-old women can have breast cancer; it's just extremely rare. For her, the likelihood was even lower because the lump did not feel like cancer and she had no unusual family history of breast cancer. Still, low likelihood does not mean zero likelihood.

Sending her through the breast industry diagnostic mill would have exposed her to risk, as well. There was at least a small chance a radiologist would report something suspicious in a mammogram and recommend a biopsy, which would start a cascade of procedures that could physically harm her: a lifetime of extra mammograms and the attendant radiation exposure (ironically increasing her chance of developing breast cancer), a risk of infection from the biopsy itself (including the rare but nasty staph infections of the flesh-eating variety), possible misinterpretation of the biopsy as cancerous when it was benign, followed by more unnecessary surgery, chemotherapy, and radiation treatment, all of which have harmful side effects, including death.

As I pondered which course of action was in her best interest, I faced a mental fork in the road with possible, though rare, bad outcomes on either side. The leave-her-alone-and-reassure-her path included a very slim chance that I would leave a cancer in her breast to spread throughout her body and ultimately kill her. The order-a-mammogram path included a very rare chance that a subsequent procedure would cause complications that injured or killed her. The risk of harm on either path was certainly less than the subconscious risk we accept every day.

I also knew that no existing medical research answers this question. We completely lack sophisticated estimates or measures of the competing risks to help me choose the safest path. Given the lack of evidence or guidance, I had to do what other doctors do dozens of times a day – make an educated guess on the best course of action for my patient.

I shouldered a tiny amount of risk by making my decision. If breast cancer is found in her a few years from now, she certainly could decide to sue me. Such a case probably would be settled out of court, and my malpractice insurance company would pay a lot of money. I would have to report it to my state medical board, write a report to the board, and possibly appear at a hearing. My personal malpractice insurance premiums likely would increase. Whenever I applied for privileges at a hospital or wanted to switch insurance companies in the future, I would have to re-live the story of this lawsuit.

Yet, my duty is to my patient, and I expect myself to make decisions only in my patient's best interest. In my mind, I practiced medicine like a good family physician should. I understood her concern from her perspective. I learned what I needed about her background and family history. I performed a thorough examination of her breasts. Drawing on all my years of medical training, my comfort with uncertainty, and a large dose of common sense, I reached the conclusion that, in the delicate balance of competing risks, it was in her best interest to do nothing. (Although, knowing the legal system and the expectations of many patients, I did say I would order a mammogram if she really wanted one, but that I didn't think it was necessary. She and her mother agreed it was unnecessary. The patient even said she thought it was stupid that she had to see me in the first place, and I agreed.) As a family physician, I concluded that what she needed most was reassurance that she didn't have cancer and permission to move on to the next exciting stage of her life. She could do without a litany of scans, repeat scans, sonograms, needles, and knives.

Was I a bad doctor? Your own answer to this question plays a large role in determining the cost of your healthcare. I don't claim to have the final answer of which pathway was the best. The truth is, no one knows. But patients who can choose non-aggressive approaches whenever possible should enjoy the lower healthcare costs resulting from this attitude.

BACK TO GIMeC

For America ever to have reasonably affordable healthcare, the relationship between doctors and patients must change. The current relationship between doctors and the American public – that all possible healthcare services be provided no matter how rare the benefit or expensive the service – is unsustainable. Until we accept this reality, healthcare costs will continue to rise faster than personal incomes, and soon a family's health insurance expenditures will surpass the combined cost of food and shelter. The great American healthcare irony – we spend the most but get the least – will only grow worse.

GIMeC is extraordinarily successful at convincing Americans that good health is dispensed by bottles of pills and expensive machines. Their propaganda works because people hear what they want to hear; they can live their lives however they want, but some test, pill, procedure, or scan will save them from their human frailties. It's an alluring message neither heard nor believed in the rest of the world. GIMeC delivers on this promise once in a while, but at a huge cost we can no longer afford.

We've witnessed four decades of politicians tinkering with healthcare finances, and it hasn't worked. Healthcare costs have continued to outpace general inflation by around 3 percent per year over the last three decades, and healthcare inflation shows no sign of slowing down. Something radical has to happen. We can achieve real healthcare reform only if we stop focusing on how healthcare is paid and turn our attention to which services should be provided.

Recall that the spiraling cost of healthcare played a significant role in the decline of the American automobile industry. It also has caused millions of lower wage earners to lose their healthcare coverage. It has caused millions of people who still have insurance to skip prescribed medicines because of higher deductibles and co-pays. The high cost of healthcare has made America less healthy.

For American healthcare to become more affordable, it first must become less aggressive. American physicians order too many tests and treatments of little or no proven benefits. Even some of the beneficial interventions are enormously expensive. We need fewer aggressive preventive efforts, especially for young adults and the elderly. We need narrower definitions of chronic disease, and doctors must be slower to label people who feel fine as having a chronic disease. A lifetime of medications, usually expensive, follows chronic disease diagnoses. Doctors must establish higher thresholds to start multi-thousand dollar diagnostic work-ups for people with symptoms that aren't severe. We must be willing to back off on some aggressive care as people enter the twilight of their life.

Health and wellness should be understood to derive more from having supportive relationships, developing quality friendships, choosing balanced meals, not overeating, and staying active. Personal responsibility for these choices will be expected.

Again, the relationship between doctors and patients must change. Frankly, doctors' jobs will become more difficult. The new relationship must be one in which doctors balance the needs of not only their patients in their offices or hospitals, but also all other patients in the healthcare system. It is intellectually and emotionally much easier for doctors to order a multitude of tests and procedures than it is to say, "I don't think a mammogram is necessary."

I am not insistent on the specific details of the two healthcare options I proposed. I spelled out some specifics to be sure the solutions weren't just abstractions. The average person should have an understanding of what their choices might include. Of course, I couldn't cover every detail, and I realize that other things may need to change, such as tort (malpractice) and insurance laws, which vary by state, in order to implement some of my suggestions. But in the meantime, many of my solutions can be written into insurance contracts now, without waiting for federal and state governments to enact new legislation.[1] However, I have no delusions that my proposed changes will come quickly or easily.

To me, a better healthcare system is a simple issue of fairness. If a person agrees to one of the approaches I proposed, she will get something out of it: lower costs provided in a family medicine-based system. If she chooses Basic Healthcare, she will get very low-cost healthcare by accepting only a small amount of risk. Those savings from the formal healthcare system then can be applied to other aspects of her life, which could improve her family's health. She could stop living paycheck to paycheck and enjoy a little financial cushion at the end of each month. She could buy a newer car that doesn't break down four times a year. She could buy a gym membership and exercise more regularly. She could move to a safer neighborhood. Whatever she chooses. Now, finally, it's her money.

My proposals will work where managed care failed for two simple reasons: they're honest and transparent, and they take into account the core issues driving healthcare inflation – risk and cost. The new rules would put the positives and negatives on the table in plain sight for everyone. Much of the blame for the high administrative healthcare costs in the U.S. rests with conflicting incentives between the different stakeholders. Ologists want to order expensive tests and procedures; insurance companies that run the company health plans are instructed by the large employers to discourage expensive tests. Doctors earn more if a patient stays in a hospital longer; hospitals are paid a flat rate for the hospitalization. An army of more than a million workers in the U.S. exists to do almost nothing but take part in these daily turf battles. If we can get all the stakeholders on the same page and align their incentives, administrative costs should drop precipitously until they match the rest of the developed world.

My plan dispenses with the tension that existed in managed care between patients and their family physicians, who were given the ignoble epithet of "gatekeeper" in that era. The family physician office will be well supported by the entire healthcare system, and therefore become the easiest and most convenient place for patients to access healthcare. Most healthcare needs will be met at the family medicine clinic, creating little reason to go to other facilities. Family physicians will be paid for all of their time like the ologists; therefore, more medical students will want to become family physicians, and a larger supply of family physicians will build the capacity to become the convenient first choice of patients. Patients will not have to wander around from ER to urgent care center to ologist to receive the majority of their care.

When will policymakers know they have appropriately reformed the payment rules for doctors? When more than half of American medical students beat down the doors trying to enter family medicine residencies.

Should my suggestions be adopted, medical ethics will become more like a European or Canadian model. Doctors there have always provided services in the best interest of the individual patient in their office, balanced against the needs of the greater system. Their realities are different from most American doctors. Most of these doctors work in systems that have yearly fixed budgets, so difficult choices have to be made. If they can do it, so can we.

In the rest of the developed world, citizens know their healthcare is rationed. As bad as that word might sound to American ears, remember those countries have better health at a lower cost than us, and their citizens are happier with their healthcare systems. Perhaps another way to look at my proposals is that I am suggesting a segment of the American population voluntarily enroll in a more European-style approach to healthcare.

In the past, when we've tried to talk about setting reasonable limits, the demagogues crawled out of the woodwork with silly claims, *a la* the "death panels." Such an approach should not and could not be forced upon privately insured Americans. In our present dire straits, however, I believe we have achieved a critical mass of Americans willing to take a chance to achieve the goal of more affordable healthcare. If just one-third of American adults desired a radical change in their healthcare expenses, perhaps a significant number of them would feel Family Medicine Care or Basic Healthcare meets their needs.

It is absolutely imperative that people who would consider signing up for one of these healthcare options think about their healthcare dollars in a different way. Most Americans view the healthcare premiums paid on their behalf to an insurance company as the insurance company's money. That insurance money belongs to you, your co-workers, and maybe even your company's retirees. Every time $200,000 is spent on the healthcare of one individual, $200,000 is taken out of the collective pockets of your friends, neighbors, and co-workers. We must balance the needs of the individuals and the group. In the two choices I proposed, I essentially laid out two different places that a line could be drawn between the needs of the individual and the needs of the group. It is not an impossible task.

I see rural Americans as perhaps the first group to take the plunge and sign up for one of the two solutions. Rural Americans are comfortable with having the vast majority of their care provided by family physicians. A colleague of mine who practices in the small town of Coleman, Texas, told me about a man who likely had a skin cancer on his face. The physician recommended the man travel 150 miles to the city to have a plastic surgeon cut it off. The physician felt some generic medico-legal pressure to send the patient with a facial cancer to an ologist. The man replied, "I don't need to go to Abilene, Doc. I'm sure you can do it." My colleague cut out the skin cancer. The man healed just fine.

Another family physician colleague has a grandfather in Comanche, Texas. The old man was having some potentially serious health issues, and she tried to convince him to travel more than 100 miles to see an ologist or have some expensive test performed. Her grandfather would have nothing of it. When warned that he could die if he did not follow his physician granddaughter's advice, the man replied, "That's OK, honey. Somethin's gonna getcha."

Medicare pays less money to rural Americans than urban Americans.[2] The total volume of physician services is about 40 percent lower for rural than urban Americans.[2] Fewer hospital beds and more family physicians, not other differences in the populations, account for this difference. Rural Americans could make a great argument that they deserve higher Social Security payments since they cost Medicare less.

Basic Healthcare is for people who humbly accept that, eventually, "somethin's gonna getcha." It's for people who don't fret that they might wind up with a scar, and who would rather not fuss about the minor physical setbacks in life. They'll see a doctor the day they can't walk. Until then, they'll get on with their day and not expect the healthcare system to make their lives or bodies perfect.

THE LOOMING MEDICARE CRISIS

I apologize for what I'm about to do. Like a hypocrite, I must now adopt the strategy of one of the targets of my wrath.

I've complained about the media playing upon people's fears. However, we actually do face a looming and unavoidable demographic reality that should scare you into action. For Medicare, the healthcare crisis is just beginning. The first baby boomers began to retire in 2008 at age 62, and the onslaught began when they turned 65 in 2011. The initial wave of new

Medicare beneficiaries will continue unabated for the next three decades.[3]

Number of Medicare Beneficiaries

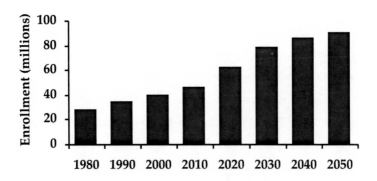

By 2030, we will have just two workers for every retiree.[3] How in the world do we imagine these workers can earn enough to support their families in addition to carrying half of a retired person's entire living expenses, including healthcare? Analysts at the Urban Institute recently estimated that a 56-year old couple will pay $140,000 in Medicare taxes per person over their work lives, but will receive $430,000 of benefits (adjusted for inflation to represent constant 2011 dollars). This is unsustainable welfare.

It just isn't possible for workers to support their families and retirees under current levels of benefits. This particular disaster will affect us much sooner than global warming.

IMPLEMENTING THE CHANGES

I have no delusions that any of my proposed changes will be rapidly accepted by the American public. My proposals may be too blunt for American ears. At a minimum, they run counter to decades of GIMeC misinformation and propaganda. Healthcare is hugely complicated, and the many special interests profiting off the current system will not accept these proposals willingly. I do, however, have a few thoughts on how my proposals might see the light of day.

One employer (or a coalition of employers) willing to try a completely different approach to healthcare might be enough. Simply offer employees my two healthcare options, start small, and be patient enough to let the plans mature over time. The employer shouldn't force its employees to enroll in one of my proposed healthcare options, and it should be willing not to see savings for a few years. The plan will need time to grow the infrastructure to make the vision a reality. Specifically, it requires a critical mass of family physicians available to provide the kind of comprehensive services needed to realize all the potential efficiencies.

I have no idea how many Americans would take the plunge and enroll in one of the proposed choices, nor do I know the distribution of interest in the two choices. In the early days, physicians will see patients from traditional plans, as well as patients in the new plans. This will be hard to sustain. If interest in the new plans grows, the future that makes the most sense to me is that patients and doctors committed to Basic Healthcare will become completely separate entities from traditional healthcare delivery systems. They might resemble the Kaiser

Permanente system, with its own hospitals, clinics, and other healthcare services.

The plans will have to evolve as new technologies become available, even if federal research dollars start to move away from finding miracles to finding methods to make healthcare more efficient. Guidelines for cost-effectiveness will have to change as the economy changes.

Patients also will form a crucial part of the governance of the health plans. There will be appeals processes if a patient thinks she should receive an expensive test or treatment. Overall, transparency of these difficult trade-offs is paramount.

FINAL THOUGHTS

America does not need a nationalized health plan. It would not work anyway because the politicians are not willing to make difficult decisions on a consistent basis. If you don't believe this, just look at our national debt, look at what our Iraq veterans faced when they came home to substandard conditions at Walter Reed Army Hospital, look at how Medicare and the comparative effectiveness initiative are forbidden to consider healthcare costs in their deliberations.

If my proposals intrigue you, talk to your employer. Go to my website, www.healthscareonline.com to learn more and respond. If you are on Medicare or Medicaid, talk to your U.S. Representative or Senator. Advocate for current federal regulations to change enough to allow at least some of these innovations to see the light of day. Demand new choices that have never been offered before.

I have offered solutions to provide people with healthcare choices based on the true driving forces of outrageous healthcare costs: risk and cost. Government-run programs may work in other nations, but they don't fit our individualistic culture. We should allow people to take responsibility for their health and to make the healthcare choices that fit their own values and lives. Real choice in healthcare – that's the American way.

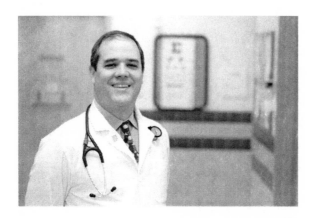

Dr. Richard Young is a family physician, educator, and researcher at America's largest family medicine program, the John Peter Smith Hospital family medicine residency in Fort Worth, TX. Among other duties, Dr. Young turns recent medical school graduates into family physicians. He also teaches students still in medical school, and every now and then convinces one of them to become a family physician.

Dr. Young serves on Commissions, Task Forces, and the Board of the Texas Academy of Family Physicians. He is also the Director of Research for the JPS family medicine department, and has published dozens of studies in the medical literature over a wide range of topics. You can follow Dr. Young at his blog American Health Scare at *www.healthscareonline.com*.

APPENDIX

OTHER EXAMPLES OF THE BASIC HEALTHCARE PLAN

COST-EFFECTIVENESS

Doctors will make medical decisions based on cost-effectiveness in three ways.

First, they will determine appropriate testing and treatment based on published cost-effectiveness analyses. There are hundreds, if not thousands, of these studies readily available.

Second, technologies can be cost-effective for some people and not others. For example, a study might determine it is cost-effective to treat a 65-year-old woman with high blood pressure, diabetes, and high cholesterol with a statin, but it's not cost-effective to treat a 40-year-old man with only elevated cholesterol. Cost-effectiveness guidelines will be continuously updated to reflect new understandings of disease risk and current drug prices.

Third, diagnostic and treatment decisions are often subjective and nebulous. Even though there may be thousands of cost-effectiveness studies, there are tens of thousands of scenarios for which no good cost-effectiveness studies can guide decisions. Doctors therefore must be protected by the legal and regulatory systems when they make judgment calls factoring in risk and cost. (In other words, they should not get sued for malpractice or punished by state medical boards for taking cost-effectiveness into consideration when deciding on a course of treatment.)

For example, imagine a middle-aged woman who comes into a family medicine clinic and reports abdominal pain with the following details: The pain was worse yesterday, but it's pretty much gone today. She ate lunch without difficulty, had no fever, and experienced no pain when the doctor pressed on her belly. At this point the doctor should be able to conclude that there is a tiny chance that an $800 CAT scan could find something bad in her, but the chance is so remote it would not be cost-effective to order the test. There are no cost-effectiveness studies exploring this specific scenario.

The patient understands when she leaves the clinic that no further testing is indicated, because of the remote – but not zero – possibility of the test finding anything. Even if the next day she feels worse and is later discovered to have a ruptured appendix, or months later is found to have ovarian cancer, her doctor's past decision was justified based on their relationship under Basic Healthcare.

For most medical encounters, patients won't perceive much of a difference. They will still see their doctors for various problems; their doctors will still order tests and prescribe treatments; and many expensive treatments will still be offered. The primary difference will be in the provision of marginal, unproven treatments. Some critics of American healthcare believe that waste accounts for 30 to 50 percent of healthcare spending and is primarily caused by failing to adopt evidence-based care.[1] Basic Healthcare will make explicit attempts to curb this marginal care.

CHOLESTEROL

There will be no cholesterol testing for young adults without some extraordinary family history of heart attacks at a young age. There is no proof that cholesterol testing and treatment saves lives (or even reduces symptoms) in this population.

If a person develops symptoms, such as certain kinds of chest pain, that suggest cholesterol blockage in the arteries of the heart, appropriate testing will be provided. If blockage is found, then treatment with appropriate procedures and medications (statins, for the most part) will be provided. There is little point to starting treatment earlier.

POTENTIALLY LIFE-THREATENING SYMPTOMS

People who go to an ER with chest pain would be treated mostly the same as now for the first few hours. Heart attacks and other life-threatening conditions can be the cause of chest pain and should be appropriately ruled out in most patients. Nevertheless, the risk of heart disease causing chest pain is highly unusual in young people. Protocols to evaluate very low-risk patients with chest pain would be developed to facilitate efficient utilization of medical tests and other ER resources. Of course, on some occasions a young person with chest pain would receive a few reassuring tests and be discharged from the ER, then suffer a heart attack or even die from another disease in his chest in the days or weeks after leaving the ER. The risk of this occurring would be similar or less than the risk he already accepts driving his car each year.

CANCER TREATMENT

The diagnosis and initial treatment of cancers would not change much, as long as there is reasonable proof that a recommended treatment will actually improve the quality of life (or life expectancy) of a person with a certain type of cancer. Experimental treatments would not be covered.

Some changes will occur in treatment and follow up of the person with cancer after the initial course of treatment. There is a universal assumption in GIMeC that it is necessary to order loads of follow-up tests after the initial cancer treatment is finished. I'm referring to things such as CAT scans every three months for five years after the initial round of treatment, even though by all accounts the cancer is gone. A few cancers exist for which there is some proof that aggressive testing after the initial treatment actually improves the health of those who were tested, although uncertainty remains as to which tests are the most important.[2] Other studies find no difference between aggressive and less aggressive testing after the initial cancer treatment.[3] For most cancers, there is no evidence either way. Because one of the underlying principles of Basic

Healthcare is *"when in doubt, don't,"* doctors will err on the side of not ordering tests and treatments in uncertain clinical cases.

Some testing will have to occur after the initial treatment to verify whether the cancer was cured. This piece of information will drive what happens next – more treatment or not. I acknowledge the psychological benefit a person receives from having some testing to ensure the cancer is gone. There is a compromise between no follow-up testing and extensive testing. However, after the initial round of post-treatment testing, people in Basic Healthcare must accept the approach that, if they're feeling pretty much status quo after the recovery from the cancer treatment, no further testing will routinely occur. At this point, the need to see an oncologist on a regular basis also ends. New symptoms that might indicate a cancer recurrence would be appropriately investigated, though.

SYMPTOMS THAT PROBABLY AREN'T LIFE-THREATENING
Basic Healthcare members also accept the premise that vague symptoms suggesting non-life-threatening conditions will not be aggressively tested at the first visit. Doctors will allow time for the symptoms to develop into a pattern more suggestive of a particular disease before extensive testing is performed. Many times, symptoms fall into typical patterns over time, which further reduces the need for extensive testing. Basic Healthcare members acknowledge there will rarely be cases where a mild or vague symptom not investigated aggressively initially will eventually lead to the discovery of a condition that theoretically could have been caught and treated earlier.

Say, for example, a middle-aged woman tells her doctor she has a new symptom of dizziness. The doctor asks lots of questions and examines her and tells her that everything checks out. It's probably the result of an inner ear infection that should clear up in a few weeks. Over the next several months, the dizziness comes and goes but never interferes with her life, and she really doesn't think much of it. A year after the original report of the dizziness, it has grown much worse. It's more constant, and some of her family tells her that she has started to walk a little funny.

Now she returns to her doctor with this new information. The doctor appropriately orders a CAT scan of her head, which reveals a large brain tumor. The tumor is removed, but the recovery period is rocky. The woman is left deaf on one side and has profound weakness on the other, to the point where she can barely walk. Basic Healthcare participants acknowledge cases like this will rarely occur, and they agree with the assertion that earlier detection of the tumor would not have necessarily changed the outcome.

PERSISTENT VEGETATIVE STATE
Basic Healthcare probably will include specific provisions to withdraw life-sustaining care for patients in a persistent vegetative state or other forms of severe brain injury or disease.

Imagine a motorcyclist crashes his bike and sustains a severe blow to the head and other internal injuries. He is unconscious and sustains fractures and internal injuries. Under Basic Healthcare, he would receive all aggressive diagnostic and treatment measures. Many people in this scenario fully recover. Unfortunately, no test can determine in the first few days of hospitalization who will wake up and who won't.

For the severe cases in which the patient remains unconscious, feeding tubes are commonly placed in the stomach or upper intestine. Liquid artificial nutrition is dripped through tubes to provide energy, vitamins, and water. Now, it's just a matter of waiting and hoping for the best. It takes weeks, and maybe a few months, to develop a good idea of which patients will have a meaningful recovery.

Suppose three months have passed since the original injury, and the motorcyclist is still in a vegetative state. Most of his brain is dead, including the parts that contain memory, feelings, and emotions. The only part of his brain left alive is the brainstem – the primitive part that controls basic body functions such as breathing and body temperature. To an observer, he might seem to have some awareness of his surroundings. At times his eyes are open. His eyes might move around occasionally. He may occasionally make grunting sounds. But otherwise, he just lies there 24 hours a day.

Nursing home care for a patient like this would cost at least $100,000 a year and probably more. Under Basic Healthcare, after a three-month observation period, if the man is still in a persistent vegetative state, the artificial feeding would cease, and he would be allowed to die naturally. He wouldn't feel hunger or thirst. The part of the brain that perceives and interprets those feelings is dead.

Has he been denied a chance of some meaningful recovery? It is extremely rare, but the answer is, yes. There have been a few reported cases of people who have been in a vegetative state for several years who miraculously woke up one day. Basic Healthcare would deny them that chance. Why? Because it isn't cost-effective.

As radical as this must sound to some people, I don't think this scenario differs much from the approach some Alzheimer's centers take with patients with an advanced case of that disease. These centers go through great pains to feed their patients by mouth. As the forgetfulness of Alzheimer's worsens, patients literally forget how to chew and swallow. Alzheimer's centers take the attitude that the inability of patients to eat on their own defines the terminal condition of the disease. They are given all necessary comfort measures, but feeding tubes are not placed.

ELIMINATING DEFENSIVE MEDICINE

Basic Healthcare is the plan that really cuts to the heart of frivolous lawsuits. What exactly defines "frivolous"? For a patient with chest pain, the truth of the situation is there is no question a doctor could ask, body part he could examine, or test he could run in the office to prove with 100 percent certainty the pain wasn't coming from her heart. The science of medicine has not figured out how to quickly diagnose which patient with chest pain is actually having a heart attack, short of an extensive work up. If the patient who reported mild chest pain for six months left my office with no tests ordered and died in her sleep three weeks later and I was sued, would that lawsuit be frivolous? A lot of doctors would say yes; a lot of lawyers would say no.

Because doctors are human, we will continue to make mistakes. I am in no way advocating that doctors should be released from their duty to diagnose and treat obvious diseases. The problem is, after a patient has died, the reason for the symptom becomes obvious. Before that, it is often not so simple.

Many clinical prediction rules have been validated by high-quality research. Examples include clinical information to predict which patients with injuries to an ankle[4] or knee[5] might actually have a fracture, or which patients are at higher risk of dying of pneumonia[6] or dying in the ICU.[7] The problem for doctors is none of these prediction rules can absolutely rule out the worst case scenario. Guidelines can predict patients who pose LOW risk for a bad outcome, but cannot predict those who are at NO risk. For example, the ankle injury rules are highly accurate at predicting who has increased risk for an ankle fracture. Several studies have shown that if ERs applied these rules to their patients with ankle injuries, those with no risk factors have a 99 percent chance of not having a fracture.[4, 8, 9]

That's great for one of the 99 percent. Maybe not so great if you fall in the 1 percent group. Under the current legal system, if ER physicians appropriately apply and interpret these validated ankle rules, but the patient later turns out to have a fracture and claims to suffer from chronic ankle pain, the patient could sue the doctor and hospital, and almost certainly money would change hands.

Under Basic Healthcare, that would not happen. A person in Basic Healthcare understands and agrees that the doctor will exercise judgment based on reasonable probabilities to decide who needs further testing and who needs treatments. Validated clinical decision rules will be used whenever possible. The Basic Healthcare participant accepts that on rare occasions the doctor will be wrong, but as long as the information available to the doctor on the first day of symptoms suggested a low-risk situation, the patient accepts a tiny risk of long-term injury or death because of this approach. The patient also agrees not to sue if something bad happens. In other words, if doctors use the prediction rules and guidelines appropriately, the patient would be exposed to no more risk than the subconscious risk many Americans face every day.

ADMINISTRATIVE COSTS

The administrative costs of Basic Healthcare will be far less than commercial health insurance plans. Fewer tests and treatments will occur to which administrators can add overhead. There will be no need for armies of quality overlords and disease managers. These activities will happen at the level of the family physician's medical practice. Basic Healthcare will require fewer employees to review prior authorization requests for expensive procedures because fewer will be ordered in the first place. More importantly, the doctors, patients, and insurance people will be much more aligned in the expectations of services that should be provided.

One other reality I must disclose is that people who sign up for Basic Healthcare may or may not be able to continue seeing their current doctors. For

Basic Healthcare to thrive, it will be crucial that all doctors on the plan – both family physicians and ologists – agree to the overall philosophical and ethical foundations of it. To keep administrative costs down, the leaders of the Basic Healthcare plan must trust the participating doctors to make decisions in the spirit of Basic Healthcare. These leaders should not waste the health plan's money on an army of nurses and medical directors charged with looking over the shoulders of the participating doctors. I predict an extensive interview process will occur before doctors are included in the plan.

SUPPORTING DATA FOR COST ESTIMATES

MEDICARE COSTS
Average Medicare costs per person per year were obtained from the Centers for Medicare and Medicaid Services (CMS) website.[10] The latest figures available at the time of access were for 2004. Those estimates were inflated by other expenditure data from CMS through 2012.[11] I assumed an annual percent change of 5.2 percent per year from 2009 through 2012.

SOCIAL SECURITY COSTS
Average Social Security payments were obtained from the U.S. Census Bureau through 2010.[12] The annual cost of living increase for 2011 and 2012 assumed no increase in 2011 and a 3.6% increase in 2012. My estimate is similar, though slightly higher, to an estimate generated in 2008 for the Minnesota House of Representatives.[4]

HOUSEHOLD INCOME
Household income estimates were obtained from the U.S. Census Bureau for 2006.[13] The annual cost of living increase for 2009 to 2012 was averaged and used to project 2009 to 2012 at 3.2 percent per year.

PERSONAL HEALTH INSURANCE COSTS
Average health insurance and healthcare costs for a hypothetical family of four were obtained from the Milliman Company for 2011: $19,393 in total healthcare costs, of which $11,385 was paid by the employer, $4,728 was paid by the employee as a payroll deduction, and $3,280 in out-of-pocket expenses.[14] Milliman estimates are in line with previous estimates from sources such as the Kaiser Family Foundation.[15] I inflated the 2011 numbers by 8.5% to generate 2012 estimates, which comes from the Society of Human Resource Managers.

COST SAVINGS ESTIMATES
For Family Medicine Care, I used the experience of Quad Graphics and the Geisinger Healthcare System[16] and applied their annual savings to the per capita and per family estimates obtained from other sources. I assumed an annual savings of 20 percent compared to existing health plans.

For Basic Healthcare, I assumed a further 20 percent decrease in the annual healthcare costs for the two groups.

FURTHER EXPLANATION FOR THE COST SAVINGS ESTIMATES

Overall estimates of "waste" in healthcare tend to run in the 30 to 50 percent range.[1] My Basic Healthcare proposal gives a total savings estimate of 40 percent, which falls in the middle of that range. My proposals differ from other statements about reducing waste and inefficiency in that they provide much more detail about what exactly will be cut: care with no solid proof of its effectiveness, care that is only marginally effective, care that is effective but costs too much, and excess administrative costs.

Other published estimates show similar overall trends. One study estimated savings in a slightly different way:[17]

Policy Option	National Savings over 10 years (billions of dollars)
Establishing a Center for Medical Effectiveness and Health Care Decision Making	$368
Instituting Medicare episode-of-care payment	$229
Strengthening primary care	$194
Limiting federal tax exemptions for premium contributions	$131
Resetting benchmark rates for Medicare Advantage plans	$50
Instituting competitive bidding between traditional Medicare and private plans	$104
Applying Medicare provider-payment methods and rates to all payers	$122
Limiting payment updates in high-cost areas	$158
Total	**$1,356**

I did not include cost savings estimates that I did not believe would actually save money, such as prevention efforts and electronic health record systems. I also believe that these authors underestimate the savings from establishing a well-supported family physician workforce. My proposals would reduce costs further than these estimates because it would eliminate services beyond these estimates and achieve lower costs for other goods, such as drugs.

Another author listed potential savings in U.S. healthcare by comparing similar cost categories in other developed countries.[18] I inflated the 2006 estimates to 2009, which gives the following results:

Purpose of Expenditures	Difference between Actual and Expected Expenditures ($ billion per year)
Total health care spending	$788
Outpatient care	$534
Inpatient care	$49
Drugs and nondurables	$120
Administrative costs	$111

This estimate reinforces the assumption that the real driving forces in healthcare costs are the intensity and pricing of services, not just administrative costs.

Other sources estimate similar savings patterns as above.[19, 20] In the interest of space, I will not cover them here. Other categories for potential savings not listed in the Tables include changes in chronic disease care.

MORE ON ADMINISTRATIVE COSTS

Clearly, reducing administrative costs is an imperative of healthcare reform. The costs become more ridiculous as the insurance pool of customers gets smaller. Administrative costs of private insurance are estimated to consume 25-40 percent of the premium dollar in the individual market, 15-25 percent in the small business market, and 5-15 percent in companies with 50 or more employees.[21]

Another way to look at insurance administrative costs is that they consume about 14 percent of the gross revenues of doctors' medical practices, 8 percent of hospitals' gross revenue, and 11 percent of private insurers' gross revenue.[22] All of these cover just the costs of shuffling paper and generating bills. Furthermore, doctors' offices spend 27 percent of their gross revenue on administration, hospitals 21 percent, and insurance companies 10 percent.[22] Some administrative structure is necessary in each of these locations, but those percentages are excessive.

The cost of generating a bill in the rest of the commercial world – think of the fees credit cards charge the merchants – is more like 3 percent. Why the difference? The fundamental problem is the infighting that occurs between healthcare system stakeholders who have been pitted against each other. For example, the doctors' duty in relation to patients is to order lots of tests and treatments. The insurance company is required by the employer, who coincidentally pays said insurance company, to minimize premium costs. Thus is born an army of people who do nothing but question the decisions of doctors. A tremendous amount of time and effort is wasted at insurance companies, doctors' offices, and hospitals' administrative offices in this game of preauthorizing/denying/appealing requests for expensive healthcare.

If all three parties were on the same page as to what the relationship is between doctors and patients who sign up for Family Medicine Care or Basic Healthcare, almost all of these paper pushers could disappear. Looked at another way, if all administrative costs in the healthcare system constitute 25 percent of total costs (about $625 billion in 2009), and the cost of financial transactions between the parties was reduced to 3 percent without all the oversight and marketing, that leaves a 22 percent savings, ideally just in administrative costs. Even if 10 percent of the claims at that point were unnecessary or fraudulent, the healthcare system would still come out 12 percent ahead of the current situation.

TRIANGULATING THE ESTIMATES

If people agreed to the tenets of Basic Healthcare, their healthcare costs would decrease by about 40 percent. From the perspective of the overall healthcare costs by GDP, this means costs would drop from about 17.3 percent of GDP to 10.4 percent of GDP, which would put our total costs in the same realm as the overall average cost of healthcare in the rest of the developed world.[23] In other words, Basic Healthcare would approximate the style and costs of a European healthcare system for the citizens of the U.S. who would volunteer to enroll in that plan.

There are numerous details I have not covered. I hope to work with other interested people, including potential patients and their employers, to develop the master list of services that should be covered under the two plans, and which patients should be eligible to receive those services. Most of all, I look forward to helping make healthcare more affordable for all Americans.

REFERENCES

Chapter 1

1. Screening for breast cancer: U.S. Preventive services task force recommendation statement. *Ann Intern Med.* Nov 17 2009;151(10):716-726, W-236.

2. CNN. Mammogram debate grows. [online]. 2009 Nov 18 [cited 2009 Nov 29]. Available from: http://www.cnn.com/video/#/video/health/2009/11/18/gupta.more.mammo.debat e.cnn.

3. Woolf SH, Lawrence RS. Preserving scientific debate and patient choice: lessons from the Consensus Panel on Mammography Screening. National Institutes of Health. *JAMA.* Dec 17 1997;278(23):2105-2108.

4. Jatoi I, Baum M. American and European recommendations for screening mammography in younger women: a cultural divide? *BMJ.* Dec 4 1993;307(6917):1481-1483.

5. NHS Breast Screening Programme. [online]. [cited 2009 Nov 30]. Available from: http://cancerscreening.org.uk/breastscreen/.

6. Ringash J. Preventive health care, 2001 update: screening mammography among women aged 40-49 years at average risk of breast cancer. *CMAJ.* Feb 20 2001;164(4):469-476.

7. The Royal College of Australian General Practitioners. Preventive activities over the lifecycle – adults. [online]. 2009 [cited 2009 Nov 30]. Available from: http://www.racgp.org.au/Content/NavigationMenu/ClinicalResources/RACGPG uidelines/TheRedBook/Red_book7_Adult_Chart.pdf.

8. THE BOARDS OF TRUSTEES FEDERAL HOSPITAL INSURANCE AND FEDERAL SUPPLEMENTARY MEDICAL INSURANCE TRUST FUNDS. ASDSA. 2008 ANNUAL REPORT OF THE BOARDS OF TRUSTEES OF THE FEDERAL HOSPITAL INSURANCE AND FEDERAL SUPPLEMENTARY MEDICAL INSURANCE TRUST FUNDS [online]. 2008 Mar 25 [cited 2009 Jul 31]. Available from: http://www.cms.hhs.gov/reportstrustfunds/downloads/tr2008.pdf.

9. Jacobs LR. 1994 all over again? Public opinion and health care. *N Engl J Med.* May 1 2008;358(18):1881-1883.

10. Roehr B. One in three people in the US want to see "radical change" in health care. *BMJ.* May 24 2008;336(7654):1150.

11. Emanuel EJ, Fuchs VR. Who really pays for health care? The myth of "shared responsibility". *JAMA.* Mar 5 2008;299(9):1057-1059.

12. Kaiser Family Foundation. Employer Health Benefits 2009 Annual Survey. [online]. 2009 Sep 15 [cited 2010 June 6]. Available from: http://www.kff.org/insurance/ehbs091509nr.cfm.

13. Gruber J. Universal health insurance coverage or economic relief--a false choice. *N Engl J Med.* Jan 29 2009;360(5):437-439.

14. Arvantes J. Obama Stresses Need for Primary Care, Calls for Physician Payment Changes. AAFP News Now [online]. [cited June 17, 2009]. Available from: http://www.aafp.org/online/en/home/publications/news/news-now/professional-issues/20090617obama-ama.html.

15. Griswold D. GM's woes homemade, not imported. Cato Institute [online]. 2005 June 26 [cited 2008 Aug 25]. Available from: http://www.freetrade.org/node/378.

16. McAlinden S. Boom Gone to Bust? The CAW/UAW Labor Deals in Light of Market Restructuring. [online]. [cited 2009 Apr 1]. Available from: <http://auto21.ca/uploads/2008_Conference/Outlook_MCALINDEN_040608.pdf>.

17. Post-Katrina Stress, Heart Problems Linked. Tulane University [online]. [cited 2009 May 17]. Available from: http://tulane.edu/research/discovery/story-katrina-heart-attacks.cfm.

18. Tanner L. Experts say Americans getting too many medical tests, maybe even President Obama. [online]. 2010 Mar 12 [cited 2010 Mar 19]. Available from: http://www.startribune.com/lifestyle/87450557.html.

19. Djulbegovic M, Beyth RJ, Neuberger MM, et al. Screening for prostate cancer: systematic review and meta-analysis of randomised controlled trials. *BMJ*. 2010;341:c4543.

20. Centers for Medicare and Medicaid Services. Decision Memo for Screening Computed Tomography Colonography (CTC) for Colorectal Cancer (CAG-00396N). [online]. 2009 May 12 [cited 2010 March 19]. Available from: https://www.cms.hhs.gov/mcd/viewdecisionmemo.asp?from2=viewdecisionmemo.asp&id=220&.

21. Bluemke DA, Achenbach S, Budoff M, et al. Noninvasive coronary artery imaging: magnetic resonance angiography and multidetector computed tomography angiography: a scientific statement from the american heart association committee on cardiovascular imaging and intervention of the council on cardiovascular radiology and intervention, and the councils on clinical cardiology and cardiovascular disease in the young. *Circulation*. Jul 29 2008;118(5):586-606.

22. Brenner DJ, Hall EJ. Computed tomography--an increasing source of radiation exposure. *N Engl J Med*. Nov 29 2007;357(22):2277-2284.

23. Harkin T. Op-ed contributor: shifting America from sick care to genuine wellness. Yahoo! News [online]. 2009 Jun 25 [cited 2009 Jun 26]. Available from: http://news.yahoo.com/s/ynews/20090625/ts_ynews/ynews_ts408.

24. Oberlander J. Learning from failure in health care reform. *N Engl J Med*. Oct 25 2007;357(17):1677-1679.

25. Truffer CJ, Keehan S, Smith S, et al. Health spending projections through 2019: the recession's impact continues. *Health Aff (Millwood)*. 2010;29(3):1-8.

26. Ginsburg PB. High and rising health care costs: Demystifying U.S. health care spending. Robert Wood Johnson Foundation [online]. 2008 Oct [cited 2009 May 11]. Available from: http://www.rwjf.org/pr/product.jsp?id=35368.

27. Gilmer TP, Kronick RG. Hard Times And Health Insurance: How Many Americans Will Be Uninsured By 2010? *Health Aff (Millwood)*. May 28 2009.

28. Crutsinger M. Experts: deficit may bring on crisis. *Fort Wort Star-Telegram*. October 17, 2009, 2009;A: 13.

29. The World Factbook: France. Central Intelligence Agency [online]. [cited 2009 Aug 12]. Available from: https://www.cia.gov/library/publications/the-world-factbook/geos/fr.html.

30. OECD Health Data 2009 - Frequently Requested Data. Organization for Economic Co-operation and Development [online]. [cited 2009 Jul 14]. Available from: http://www.oecd.org/document/16/0,3343,en_2649_34631_2085200_1_1_1_1,00.html.

31. Pear R. Health Care Cost Increase Is Projected for New Law. [online]. 2010 Apr 23 [cited 2010 May 29]. Available from: http://www.nytimes.com/2010/04/24/health/policy/24health.html?scp=1&sq=p ear percent20april percent2024 percent20health percent20spending percent20actuary&st=cse.

32. Starfield B, Shi L, Grover A, Macinko J. The effects of specialist supply on populations' health: assessing the evidence. *Health Aff (Millwood)*. Jan-Jun 2005;Suppl Web Exclusives:W5-97-W95-107.

Chapter 2

1. Barnes B. Mickey Mantle Obituary. [online]. [cited 2009 May 21]. Available from: http://www.baseball-almanac.com/deaths/mickey_mantle_obituary.shtml.

2. The Mick: the official Mickey Mantle website. [online]. [cited 2009 May 21]. Available from: http://qsigroup.com/clients/mickeymantle/mmf.html.

3. Christopher and Dana Reeve Foundation. [online]. [cited 2009 May 21]. Available from: http://www.christopherreeve.org/site/c.ddJFKRNoFiG/b.4048063/k.BDDB/Ho me.htm.

4. Landau E. Many studies great news for mice, not so much for humans. CNN News.com [online]. 2010 Jun 8 [cited 2010 Jun 10]. Available from: http://www.cnn.com/2010/HEALTH/06/08/mice.rats.studies/index.html.

5. Grady D. In Study, Hormone Reduced Appetite in Mice NYTimes.com [online]. 2005 Nov 11 [cited 2009 Jun 29]. Available from: http://query.nytimes.com/gst/fullpage.html?res=9B01E4D9123EF932A25752C1 A9639C8B63&sec=health.

6. Bakalar N. Hibernating Mice May Someday Save Humans. [online]. [cited April 26, 2005]. Available from: http://www.nytimes.com/2005/04/26/health/26mice.html?pagewanted=print& position=.

7. Blakeslee S. Spinal Shocks Ease Parkinson's in Mice *New York Times.* March 19, 2009.

8. Altman L. Team Creates Rat Heart Using Cells of Baby Rats. NYTimes.com [online]. 2008 Jan 14 [cited 2009 Jun 29]. Available from: http://www.nytimes.com/2008/01/14/health/14heart.html.

9. Brody JE. Health Sleuths Assess Homocysteine as Culprit. *New York Times.* June 13, 2000.

10. Toole JF, Malinow MR, Chambless LE, et al. Lowering homocysteine in patients with ischemic stroke to prevent recurrent stroke, myocardial infarction, and death: the Vitamin Intervention for Stroke Prevention (VISP) randomized controlled trial. *JAMA*. Feb 4 2004;291(5):565-575.

11. Lewis SJ, Ebrahim S, Davey Smith G. Meta-analysis of MTHFR 677C->T polymorphism and coronary heart disease: does totality of evidence support causal role for homocysteine and preventive potential of folate? *BMJ*. Nov 5 2005;331(7524):1053.

12. Kuhlman J. The president's first annual physical exam as president. [online]. 2010 Feb 28 [cited 2010 Aug 21]. Available from: http://www.whitehouse.gov/sites/default/files/rss_viewer/potus_med_exam_feb2010.pdf.

13. Brody JE. Know Your Numbers and Improve Your Odds *New York Times*. June 28, 2005.

14. Mishori R. Who gets sick in America--and why. *Parade*. Vol June 28, 2009 ed.:8,10.

15. Kaye R. Dying Iowa voter grills candidates on health care. CNNHealth.com [online]. 2008 Jan 3 [cited 2009 Oct 5]. Available from: http://www.cnn.com/2008/HEALTH/01/03/dying.voter/.

16. Schwitzer D. Unhealthy Advocacy: Journalists and Health Screening Tests. Poynter Online.com [online]. 2007 May 15 [cited 2009 Aug 20]. Available from: http://www.poynter.org/column.asp?id=101&aid=123044.

17. Epstein R. How other countries judge malpractice. *The Wall Street Journal*. June 30, 2009.

18. Studdert DM, Mello MM, Gawande AA, et al. Claims, errors, and compensation payments in medical malpractice litigation. *N Engl J Med*. May 11 2006;354(19):2024-2033.

19. Anderson GF, Hussey PS, Frogner BK, Waters HR. Health spending in the United States and the rest of the industrialized world. *Health Aff (Millwood)*. Jul-Aug 2005;24(4):903-914.

20. USA Spends More Per Capita on Health Care Than Other Nations, Study Finds. Medical News Today [online]. 2005 Jul 13 [cited 2009 Jul 12]. Available from: http://www.medicalnewstoday.com/articles/27348.php.

21. Bodenheimer T. High and rising health care costs. Part 3: the role of health care providers. *Ann Intern Med*. Jun 21 2005;142(12 Pt 1):996-1002.

22. Kane C. Medical Liability Claim Frequency: A 2007-2008 Snapshot of Physicians. [online]. 2010 [cited 2010 Aug 21]. Available from: http://www.ama-assn.org/ama1/pub/upload/mm/363/prp-201001-claim-freq.pdf.

23. Budetti PP. Market justice and US health care. *JAMA*. Jan 2 2008;299(1):92-94.

24. Truffer CJ, Keehan S, Smith S, et al. Health spending projections through 2019: the recession's impact continues. *Health Aff (Millwood)*. 2010;29(3):1-8.

25. Karvounis N, Mahar M. The Managed Care Roller Coaster. The Century Foundation [online]. 2008 Jul 17 [cited 2009 Oct 20]. Available from: http://takingnote.tcf.org/2008/07/the-managed-car.html.

26. Mahar M, Karvounis N. The managed care roller coaster. The Health Care Blog [online]. 2008 Jul 16 [cited 2009 Jun 20]. Available from: http://www.thehealthcareblog.com/the_health_care_blog/2008/07/the-managed-car.html.

27. Biles B, Pozen J, Guterman S. The Continuing Cost of Privatization: Extra Payments to Medicare Advantage Plans Jump to $11.4 Billion in 2009. The Commonwealth Fund [online]. 2009 May [cited 2009 Jun 12]. Available from: http://www.commonwealthfund.org/Content/Publications/Issue-Briefs/2009/May/The-Continuing-Cost-of-Privatization.aspx.

28. Bodenheimer T. High and rising health care costs. Part 2: technologic innovation. *Ann Intern Med.* Jun 7 2005;142(11):932-937.

29. Reinhardt UE, Hussey PS, Anderson GF. U.S. health care spending in an international context. *Health Aff (Millwood).* May-Jun 2004;23(3):10-25.

30. Collins S, Nuzum R, Rustgi S, Mika S, Schoen C, Davis K. *How Health Care Reform Can Lower the Costs of Insurance Administration*: The Commonwealth Fund; July 2009.

31. Woolhandler S, Himmelstein DU. The deteriorating administrative efficiency of the U.S. health care system. *N Engl J Med.* May 2 1991;324(18):1253-1258.

32. *Bringing Better Value: Recommendations to Address the Costs and Causes of Administrative Complexity in the Nation's Healthcare System* Healthcare Administrative Simplification Coalition July 2009.

33. Hollander C. A High Performance Health System for the United States: An Ambitious Agenda for the Next President. Commonwealth Fund [online]. 2007 Nov 15 [cited 2009 Apr 28]. Available from: http://www.commonwealthfund.org/Content/Publications/Fund-Reports/2007/Nov/A-High-Performance-Health-System-for-the-United-States--An-Ambitious-Agenda-for-the-Next-President.aspx.

34. Moses H, 3rd, Dorsey ER, Matheson DH, Thier SO. Financial anatomy of biomedical research. *JAMA.* Sep 21 2005;294(11):1333-1342.

35. Alexander GC, Stafford RS. Does comparative effectiveness have a comparative edge? *JAMA.* Jun 17 2009;301(23):2488-2490.

36. Selker HP, Wood AJ. Industry influence on comparative-effectiveness research funded through health care reform. *N Engl J Med.* Dec 31 2009;361(27):2595-2597.

37. Woolf SH, Johnson RE. The break-even point: when medical advances are less important than improving the fidelity with which they are delivered. *Ann Fam Med.* Nov-Dec 2005;3(6):545-552.

38. Gray BH, Gusmano MK, Collins SR. AHCPR and the changing politics of health services research. *Health Aff (Millwood).* Jan-Jun 2003;Suppl Web Exclusives:W3-283-307.

39. Turner EH, Matthews AM, Linardatos E, Tell RA, Rosenthal R. Selective publication of antidepressant trials and its influence on apparent efficacy. *N Engl J Med*. Jan 17 2008;358(3):252-260.

40. Brody H. *Hooked: Ethics, the medical profession, and the pharmaceutical industry*. Lanham, MD: Rowman & LIttlefield Publishing Group; 2007.

41. Relman AS, Angell M. America's other drug problem: how the drug industry distorts medicine and politics. *New Repub*. Dec 16 2002;227(25):27-41.

42. Campbell EG. Doctors and drug companies--scrutinizing influential relationships. *N Engl J Med*. Nov 1 2007;357(18):1796-1797.

43. Lenzer J. Watching over the medical device industry. *BMJ*. 2009;338:b2321.

44. Dhruva SS, Bero LA, Redberg RF. Strength of study evidence examined by the FDA in premarket approval of cardiovascular devices. *JAMA*. Dec 23 2009;302(24):2679-2685.

45. Emanuel EJ, Fuchs VR. The perfect storm of overutilization. *JAMA*. Jun 18 2008;299(23):2789-2791.

46. Kamerow D. Yankee Doodling. Our perfectly designed US healthcare system. *BMJ*. 2008;337:a2702.

47. Nielson N. We must protect guidelines against undue influence. *American Medical News*. April 27, 2009, 2009: 20.

48. Moynihan R. Court hears how drug giant Merck tried to "neutralise" and "discredit" doctors critical of Vioxx. *BMJ*. 2009;338:b1432.

49. Unsales' reps divert docs from high-cost drugs. MSNBC.com [online]. [cited 2008 March 3]. Available from: http://www.msnbc.msn.com/id/23436690.

50. Landers S. Medical schools, teaching hospitals help drive local economies. amednews.com [online]. 2009 2009 Oct 27 [cited 2009 Nov 3]. Available from: http://www.ama-assn.org/amednews/2009/10/26/prsd1027.htm.

51. Campbell EG. The future of research funding in academic medicine. *N Engl J Med*. Apr 9 2009;360(15):1482-1483.

52. Kaiser Family Foundation. *Trends in health care costs and spending*. Kaiser Family Foundation [online]. 2007 Sep [cited 2007 Nov 6]. Available from: http://www.kff.org/insurance/upload/7692.pdf.

53. Reinhardt UE, Hussey PS, Anderson GF. Cross-national comparisons of health systems using OECD data, 1999. *Health Aff (Millwood)*. May-Jun 2002;21(3):169-181.

54. Why healthcare costs are rising. *Family Practice Management*. (June 2002):28.

55. Anderson GF. From 'soak the rich' to 'soak the poor': recent trends in hospital pricing. *Health Aff (Millwood)*. May-Jun 2007;26(3):780-789.

56. Bennett J. The Other Credit Crunch. Newsweek [online]. 2008 Nov 4 [cited 2010 Aug 21]. Available from: http://www.newsweek.com/2008/11/23/the-other-credit-crunch.html.

57. Cholesterol drug use rising rapidly in young. MSNBC.com [online]. [cited 2007 October 30]. Available from: http://www.msnbc.msn.com/id/21534447/.

58. Kolata G. Cancer society, in shift, has concerns on screenings. NYTimes.com [online]. 2009 Oct 21 [cited 2009 Oct 22]. Available from: http://www.nytimes.com/2009/10/21/health/21cancer.html?_r=1&scp=1&sq=scr eenings&st=cse.

59. Wennberg DE, Fisher ES, Goodman DC, Skinner JS, Bronner KK, Sharp SM. Taking care of patients with severe chronic disease: the Dartmouth atlas of health care 2008. The Dartmouth Institute for Health Policy and Clinical Practice Center for Health Policy Research [online]. 2008 [cited 2009 May 2]. Available from: http://www.dartmouthatlas.org/atlases/2008_Chronic_Care_Atlas.pdf.

60. A controlled trial to improve care for seriously ill hospitalized patients. The study to understand prognoses and preferences for outcomes and risks of treatments (SUPPORT). The SUPPORT Principal Investigators. *JAMA.* Nov 22-29 1995;274(20):1591-1598.

61. National Institutes of Health. Health economics: NIH research priorities for health care reform. [online]. [cited 2010 Aug 18]. Available from: http://commonfund.nih.gov/pdf/2010May10_11_Health_Econ_Meeting_Summ ary.pdf.

Chapter 3

1. Stange KC, Ferrer RL. The paradox of primary care. *Ann Fam Med.* Jul-Aug 2009;7(4):293-299.

2. Starfield B, Shi L, Grover A, Macinko J. The effects of specialist supply on populations' health: assessing the evidence. *Health Aff (Millwood).* Jan-Jun 2005;Suppl Web Exclusives:W5-97-W95-107.

3. Task Force 1 Writing Group, Green L, Graham R, et al. Task Force 1. Report of the Task Force on Patient Expectations, Core Values, Reintegration, and the New Model of Family Medicine. *Ann Fam Med.* 2004;2(Supplement 1):S33-S50.

4. Almond SC, Summerton N. Diagnosis in General Practice. Test of time. *BMJ.* 2009;338:b1878.

5. Rosser WW. Approach to diagnosis by primary care clinicians and specialists: is there a difference? *J Fam Pract.* Feb 1996;42(2):139-144.

6. Katerndahl DA, Wood R, Jaen CR. A method for estimating relative complexity of ambulatory care. *Ann Fam Med.* Jul-Aug 2010;8(4):341-347.

7. Pham HH, Alexander GC, O'Malley AS. Physician consideration of patients' out-of-pocket costs in making common clinical decisions. *Arch Intern Med.* Apr 9 2007;167(7):663-668.

8. Jarvis J. Health-screening businesses are attracting more consumers. *Fort Worth Star-Telegram.* July 4, 2009: 1B,7B.

9. Screening for Abdominal Aortic Aneurysm. U.S. Preventive Services Task Force [online]. 2005 Feb [cited 2009 Oct 25]. Available from: http://www.ahrq.gov/CLINIC/USPSTF/uspsaneu.htm.

10. Andriole GL, Crawford ED, Grubb RL, 3rd, et al. Mortality results from a randomized prostate-cancer screening trial. *N Engl J Med.* Mar 26 2009;360(13):1310-1319.

11. Schroder FH, Hugosson J, Roobol MJ, et al. Screening and prostate-cancer mortality in a randomized European study. *N Engl J Med.* Mar 26 2009;360(13):1320-1328.

12. Djulbegovic M, Beyth RJ, Neuberger MM, et al. Screening for prostate cancer: systematic review and meta-analysis of randomised controlled trials. *BMJ.* 2010;341:c4543.

13. Haas GP, Delongchamps N, Brawley OW, Wang CY, de la Roza G. The worldwide epidemiology of prostate cancer: perspectives from autopsy studies. *Can J Urol.* Feb 2008;15(1):3866-3871.

14. Stark JR, Mucci L, Rothman KJ, Adami HO. Screening for prostate cancer remains controversial. *BMJ.* 2009;339:b3601.

15. Schwartz LM, Woloshin S, Fowler FJ, Jr., Welch HG. Enthusiasm for cancer screening in the United States. *JAMA.* Jan 7 2004;291(1):71-78.

16. Lee JM. Screening and informed consent. *N Engl J Med.* Feb 11 1993;328(6):438-440.

17. Salzmann P, Kerlikowske K, Phillips K. Cost-effectiveness of extending screening mammography guidelines to include women 40 to 49 years of age. *Ann Intern Med.* Dec 1 1997;127(11):955-965.

18. Eddy DM. Screening for breast cancer. *Ann Intern Med.* Sep 1 1989;111(5):389-399.

19. American Cancer Society. Overview: Breast Cancer: How Many Women Get Breast Cancer? http://www.cancer.org/docroot/CRI/content/CRI_2_2_1X_How_many_people_get_breast_cancer_5.asp?sitearea=. Accessed October 11, 2009.

Chapter 4

1. Wennberg DE, Fisher ES, Goodman DC, Skinner JS, Bronner KK, Sharp SM. Taking care of patients with severe chronic disease: the Dartmouth atlas of health care 2008. The Dartmouth Institute for Health Policy and Clinical Practice Center for Health Policy Research [online]. 2008 [cited 2009 May 2]. Available from: http://www.dartmouthatlas.org/atlases/2008_Chronic_Care_Atlas.pdf.

2. Risks and benefits of screening for intracranial aneurysms in first-degree relatives of patients with sporadic subarachnoid hemorrhage. *N Engl J Med.* Oct 28 1999;341(18):1344-1350.

3. Vernooij MW, Ikram MA, Tanghe HL, et al. Incidental findings on brain MRI in the general population. *N Engl J Med.* Nov 1 2007;357(18):1821-1828.

4. Greenfield S, Rogers W, Mangotich M, Carney MF, Tarlov AR. Outcomes of patients with hypertension and non-insulin dependent diabetes mellitus treated by different systems and specialties. Results from the medical outcomes study. *JAMA.* Nov 8 1995;274(18):1436-1444.

5. Carey TS, Garrett J, Jackman A, McLaughlin C, Fryer J, Smucker DR. The outcomes and costs of care for acute low back pain among patients seen by primary care practitioners, chiropractors, and orthopedic surgeons. The North Carolina Back Pain Project. *N Engl J Med.* Oct 5 1995;333(14):913-917.

6. Winslow CM, Kosecoff JB, Chassin M, Kanouse DE, Brook RH. The appropriateness of performing coronary artery bypass surgery. *JAMA.* Jul 22-29 1988;260(4):505-509.

7. Winslow CM, Solomon DH, Chassin MR, Kosecoff J, Merrick NJ, Brook RH. The appropriateness of carotid endarterectomy. *N Engl J Med.* Mar 24 1988;318(12):721-727.

8. Brook RH. Health policy and public trust. *JAMA.* Jul 9 2008;300(2):211-213.

9. I also don't take credit for coining this phrase. I read it a long time ago and can't find the reference.,.

10. Hatziandreu E, Hadler S, Brown R, et al. The cost and benefits of childhood immunization. [online]. 1994 [cited Available from: http://gateway.nlm.nih.gov/MeetingAbstracts/ma?f=102211769.html.

11. Bodenheimer T. High and rising health care costs. Part 1: seeking an explanation. *Ann Intern Med.* May 17 2005;142(10):847-854.

12. Prevention for a healthier America: investments in disease prevention yield significant savings, stronger communities. [online]. 2008 [cited Available from: http://healthyamericans.org/reports/prevention08/.

13. Hutchison BG, Stoddart GL. Cost-effectiveness of primary tetanus vaccination among elderly Canadians. *CMAJ.* Dec 15 1988;139(12):1143-1151.

14. Miller MA, Sutter RW, Strebel PM, Hadler SC. Cost-effectiveness of incorporating inactivated poliovirus vaccine into the routine childhood immunization schedule. *JAMA.* Sep 25 1996;276(12):967-971.

15. Lieu TA, Ray GT, Black SB, et al. Projected cost-effectiveness of pneumococcal conjugate vaccination of healthy infants and young children. *JAMA.* Mar 15 2000;283(11):1460-1468.

16. Shepard CW, Ortega-Sanchez IR, Scott RD, 2nd, Rosenstein NE. Cost-effectiveness of conjugate meningococcal vaccination strategies in the United States. *Pediatrics.* May 2005;115(5):1220-1232.

17. Ho KK, Anderson KM, Kannel WB, Grossman W, Levy D. Survival after the onset of congestive heart failure in Framingham Heart Study subjects. *Circulation.* Jul 1993;88(1):107-115.

18. Carrier ER, Reschovsky JD, Mello MM, Mayrell RC, Katz D. Physicians' fears of malpractice lawsuits are not assuaged by tort reforms. *Health Aff (Millwood).* Sep 2010;29(9):1585-1592.

Chapter 5

1. Poll: Many worried about paying for health care--nearly one in four fear losing coverage in the next year. MSNBC.com [online]. 2009 Jun 18 [cited 2009 Jul 28]. Available from: http://www.cnbc.com/id/31424267.

2. AFL-CIO. 2008 Health Care for America Survey. [online]. [cited 2009 Jul 25]. Available from: http://www.aflcio.org/issues/healthcare/survey/2008results.cfm.

3. Himmelstein DU, Warren E, Thorne D, Woolhandler S. Illness and injury as contributors to bankruptcy. *Health Aff (Millwood)*. Jan-Jun 2005;Suppl Web Exclusives:W5-63-W65-73.

4. Himmelstein DU, Thorne D, Warren E, Woolhandler S. Medical bankruptcy in the United States, 2007: results of a national study. *Am J Med*. Aug 2009;122(8):741-746.

5. Dranove D, Millenson ML. Medical bankruptcy: myth versus fact. *Health Aff (Millwood)*. Mar-Apr 2006;25(2):w74-83.

6. Heriot G. Misdiagnosed--A medical-bankruptcy study doesn't live up to its billing. Nationalreviewonline [online]. 2005 Feb 11 [cited 2009 Apr 18]. Available from:
http://www.nationalreview.com/comment/heriot200502110735.asp.

7. Nelson P. AARP Peddles Medical Bankruptcy Myth to New Extremes Center of the American Experiment [online]. 2008 Sep 5 [cited 2009 May 14]. Available from: http://www.statehousecall.org/aarp-peddles-medical-bankruptcy-myth-to-new-extremes.

8. Herbert B. It's not just the uninsured. . *New York Times*2007.

9. 2010 Milliman Medical Index. Milliman [online]. [cited 2010 Oct 1]. Available from:
http://publications.milliman.com/periodicals/mmi/pdfs/milliman-medical-index-2010.pdf.

10. Health insurance premiums have more than doubled since 1996. *Research News*. Vol 338. Agency for Healthcare Research and Quality; 2008:25.

11. King J. Help Move U.S. Health System to Primary Care Base. [online]. 2008 Jan 18 [cited 2008 Jan 18]. Available from:
http://www.aafp.org/online/en/home/publications/news/news-now/opinion/20080118presmsgescan.mem.html?aafpvlogin=7225722&aafpvpw=&URL_success=http percent3A percent2F percent2Fwww.aafp.org percent2Fonline percent2Fen percent2Fhome percent2Fpublications percent2Fnews percent2Fnews-now percent2Fopinion percent2F20080118presmsgescan.mem.html.

12. Reinhardt UE, Hussey PS, Anderson GF. U.S. health care spending in an international context. *Health Aff (Millwood)*. May-Jun 2004;23(3):10-25.

13. Blumenthal D. Employer-sponsored insurance--riding the health care tiger. *N Engl J Med*. Jul 13 2006;355(2):195-202.

14. Ginsburg PB. High and rising health care costs: Demystifying U.S. health care spending. Robert Wood Johnson Foundation [online]. 2008 Oct [cited 2009 May 11]. Available from:
http://www.rwjf.org/pr/product.jsp?id=35368.

15. OECD Health Data 2009 - Frequently Requested Data. Organization for Economic Co-operation and Development [online]. [cited 2009 Jul 14]. Available from:
http://www.oecd.org/document/16/0,3343,en_2649_34631_2085200_1_1_1_1,00.html.

16. Borger C, Smith S, Truffer C, et al. Health spending projections through 2015: changes on the horizon. *Health Aff (Millwood).* Mar-Apr 2006;25(2):w61-73.

17. Trapp D. CBO: Medicare and medicaid spending growth unsustainable. *American Medical News.* Vol Chicago: American Medical Association; 2007:10.

18. Iglehart JK. Budgeting for change--Obama's down payment on health care reform. *N Engl J Med.* Apr 2 2009;360(14):1381-1383.

19. Emanuel EJ. Cost savings at the end of life. What do the data show? *JAMA.* Jun 26 1996;275(24):1907-1914.

20. Bodenheimer T, Fernandez A. High and rising health care costs. Part 4: can costs be controlled while preserving quality? *Ann Intern Med.* Jul 5 2005;143(1):26-31.

21. Emanuel EJ, Emanuel LL. The economics of dying. The illusion of cost savings at the end of life. *N Engl J Med.* Feb 24 1994;330(8):540-544.

22. Jha AK, Chan DC, Ridgway AB, Franz C, Bates DW. Improving safety and eliminating redundant tests: cutting costs in U.S. hospitals. *Health Aff (Millwood).* Sep-Oct 2009;28(5):1475-1484.

23. Bodenheimer T. High and rising health care costs. Part 3: the role of health care providers. *Ann Intern Med.* Jun 21 2005;142(12 Pt 1):996-1002.

24. Mello MM, Chandra A, Gawande AA, Studdert DM. National costs of the medical liability system. *Health Aff (Millwood).* Sep 2010;29(9):1569-1577.

25. Morris L. Combating fraud in health care: an essential component of any cost containment strategy. *Health Aff (Millwood).* Sep-Oct 2009;28(5):1351-1356.

26. Gottlieb DJ, Zhou W, Song Y, Andrews K, Skinner J, Sutherland J. Prices don't drive regional Medicare spending variations. *Health Aff (Millwood).* 2010;29(3):1-7.

27. Gold MR. Geographic variation in Medicare per capita spending: Should policy-makers be concerned? Robert Wood Johnson Foundation [online]. Research Synthesis Report No. 6 [cited 2009 Aug 1]. Available from: http://www.rwjf.org/files/research/RWJF percent20Medicare percent20SYNTHESIS percent20July04.pdf.

28. Lucas FL, Sirovich BE, Gallagher PM, Siewers AE, Wennberg DE. Variation in cardiologists' propensity to test and treat: is it associated with regional variation in utilization? *Circ Cardiovasc Qual Outcomes.* May;3(3):253-260.

29. Sutherland JM, Fisher ES, Skinner JS. Getting past denial--the high cost of health care in the United States. *N Engl J Med.* Sep 24 2009;361(13):1227-1230.

30. Baicker K, Chandra A. Medicare spending, the physician workforce, and beneficiaries' quality of care. *Health Aff (Millwood).* 2004;Suppl Web Exclusives:W184-197.

31. Starfield B, Shi L, Grover A, Macinko J. The effects of specialist supply on populations' health: assessing the evidence. *Health Aff (Millwood).* Jan-Jun 2005;Suppl Web Exclusives:W5-97-W95-107.

32. Bodenheimer T. High and rising health care costs. Part 2: technologic innovation. *Ann Intern Med.* Jun 7 2005;142(11):932-937.

33. Anderson GF. Medicare and chronic conditions. *N Engl J Med.* Jul 21 2005;353(3):305-309.

34. Hawryluk M. Managing multiple conditions. *American Medical News.* December 1, 2003: 5-6.

35. Peikes D, Chen A, Schore J, Brown R. Effects of care coordination on hospitalization, quality of care, and health care expenditures among Medicare beneficiaries: 15 randomized trials. *JAMA.* Feb 11 2009;301(6):603-618.

36. Geyman JP. Disease management: panacea, another false hope, or something in between? *Ann Fam Med.* May-Jun 2007;5(3):257-260.

37. Krause DS. Economic effectiveness of disease management programs: a meta-analysis. *Dis Manag.* Apr 2005;8(2):114-134.

38. Eddy DM, Schlessinger L, Kahn R. Clinical outcomes and cost-effectiveness of strategies for managing people at high risk for diabetes. *Ann Intern Med.* Aug 16 2005;143(4):251-264.

39. Orszag PR, Ellis P. Addressing rising health care costs--a view from the Congressional Budget Office. *N Engl J Med.* Nov 8 2007;357(19):1885-1887.

40. Abelson R. An Insurer's New Approach to Diabetes. [online]. 2010 Apr 13 [cited 2010 Apr 16]. Available from: http://www.nytimes.com/2010/04/14/health/14diabetes.html.

41. Tynan A, Christianson J. Consumer-directed health plans: mixed employer signals, complex market dynamics. 2008(119).

42. Singer P. Why We Must Ration Health Care *New York Times Magazine.* Vol.

43. Rosen H, Saleh F, Lipsitz S, Rogers SO, Jr., Gawande AA. Downwardly mobile: the accidental cost of being uninsured. *Arch Surg.* Nov 2009;144(11):1006-1011.

44. Hasan O, Orav EJ, Hicks LS. Insurance status and hospital care for myocardial infarction, stroke, and pneumonia. *J Hosp Med.* Jun 10.

45. Wilper AP, Woolhandler S, Lasser KE, McCormick D, Bor DH, Himmelstein DU. Health insurance and mortality in US adults. *Am J Public Health.* Dec 2009;99(12):2289-2295.

46. Herring AA, Woolhandler S, Himmelstein DU. Insurance status of U.S. organ donors and transplant recipients: the uninsured give, but rarely receive. *Int J Health Serv.* 2008;38(4):641-652.

47. Wilper A, Woolhandler S, Himmelstein D, Nardin R. Impact of insurance status on migraine care in the United States: a population-based study. *Neurology.* Apr 13;74(15):1178-1183.

48. U.S. Census Bureau. Median Household Income by State: 1984 to 2009. [online]. [cited 2011 Apr 7]. Available from: http://www.census.gov/hhes/www/income/data/historical/household/H08_2009.xls.

49. Medical Expenditure Panel Survey. [online]. [cited 2011 May 25]. Available from: <http://www.meps.ahrq.gov/mepsweb/>.

50. U.S. Census Bureau. National Health Expenditures-Summary, 1960 to 2006, and Projections, 2007 to 2017. [online]. [cited 2011 May 25]. Available from: http://www.census.gov/compendia/statab/tables/09s0124.pdf.

Chapter 6

1. Cordani D, Kang J. Cigna president letter regarding liver transplant tragedy. Medical News Today [online]. 2007 Dec 26 [cited 2009 Jun 27]. Available from: http://www.medicalnewstoday.com/articles/92696.php.

2. Hennessy-Fiske M. Tough calls in transplant case. *Los Angeles Times*2007.

3. Behrens Z. Northridge Teen Dies Because Health Insurance Would Not Pay. [online]. 2007 Dec 21 [cited 2010 Mar 9]. Available from: http://laist.com/2007/12/21/northridge_teen.php.

4. Chang A. Bereaved family to sue insurer after dispute over liver transplant. Approval came too late for teen. *Boston Globe*. December 21, 2007, 2007.

5. Family sues insurer who denied teen transplant. [online]. 2007 [cited Available from: http://www.msnbc.com/id/22357873.

6. Family Attorney Says He'll Sue Insurance Company That Initially Denied 17-Year-Old Girl a Liver Transplant. FoxNews.com [online]. 2007 Dec 22 [cited 2009 Jun 13]. Available from: http://www.foxnews.com/story/0,2933,317809,00.html.

7. Wise J. Age for starting cervical cancer screening in England will not be lowered. *BMJ*. 2009;338:b2583.

8. Sims J. Judge orders baby off life-support. . Toronto Sun [online]. [cited 2011 Feb 18]. Available from: http://www.torontosun.com/news/canada/2011/02/18/17322476.html.

9. Dubinski K. Baby Joseph flown to U.S. hospital. Toronto Sun [online]. [cited 2011 Mar 13]. Available from: http://www.torontosun.com/news/canada/2011/03/13/17601961.html.

10. Delamothe T. How the NHS measures up. *BMJ*. Jun 28 2008;336(7659):1469-1471.

11. Kmietowicz Z. NHS reforms have produced "only limited benefits so far". *BMJ*. 2008;337:1327.

12. Coombes R. The NHS debate. *BMJ*. 2008;337:a628.

13. Black N. "Liberating the NHS"--another attempt to implement market forces in English health care. *N Engl J Med*. Sep 16 2010;363(12):1103-1105.

14. Feest TG, Rajamahesh J, Byrne C, et al. Trends in adult renal replacement therapy in the UK: 1982-2002. *QJM*. Jan 2005;98(1):21-28.

15. Aaron H. Financing Health Care with Limited Resources. Brookings Institute [online]. 2004 Oct 7 [cited 2009 Jul 27]. Available from: http://www.brookings.edu/views/speeches/20041007aaron.pdf.

16. Farrington K, Rao R, Stenkamp R, Ansell D, Feest T. All patients receiving renal replacement therapy in the United Kingdom in 2005 (chapter 4). *Nephrol Dial Transplant*. Aug 2007;22 Suppl 7:vii30-50.

17. Laurance J. Dialysis shortage exposes failings of NHS. *The Independent*. January 14, 2003, 2003.

18. Blank L, Peters J, Lumsdon A, et al. Regional differences in the provision of adult renal dialysis services in the UK. *QJM*. Mar 2005;98(3):183-190.

19. Hines S, Moss A, McKenzie J. Prolonging Life or Prolonging Death: Communication's Role in Difficult Dialysis Decisions *Health Communication*. 1997;9:369-388.

20. Bruton F. A tale of 2 sickbeds: health care in U.K. vs. U.S. [online]. 2008 [cited Available from: www.msnbc.msn.com/id/26794291.

21. Collins SR, Kriss J, Doty M, Rustgi S. Losing Ground: How the Loss of Adequate Health Insurance Is Burdening Working Families—Findings from the Commonwealth Fund Biennial Health Insurance Surveys, 2001–2007. [online]. 2008 [cited Available from: http://www.commonwealthfund.org/Content/Publications/Fund-Reports/2008/Aug/Losing-Ground--How-the-Loss-of-Adequate-Health-Insurance-Is-Burdening-Working-Families--8212-Finding.aspx.

22. Matthys J, De Meyere M, van Driel ML, De Sutter A. Differences among international pharyngitis guidelines: not just academic. *Ann Fam Med*. Sep-Oct 2007;5(5):436-443.

23. Froom J, Culpepper L, Grob P, et al. Diagnosis and antibiotic treatment of acute otitis media: report from International Primary Care Network. *BMJ*. Mar 3 1990;300(6724):582-586.

24. Soares HP, Kumar A, Daniels S, et al. Evaluation of new treatments in radiation oncology: are they better than standard treatments? *JAMA*. Feb 23 2005;293(8):970-978.

25. Kumar A, Soares HP, Balducci L, Djulbegovic B. Treatment tolerance and efficacy in geriatric oncology: a systematic review of phase III randomized trials conducted by five National Cancer Institute-sponsored cooperative groups. *J Clin Oncol*. Apr 1 2007;25(10):1272-1276.

26. Djulbegovic B, Kumar A, Soares HP, et al. Treatment success in cancer: new cancer treatment successes identified in phase 3 randomized controlled trials conducted by the National Cancer Institute-sponsored cooperative oncology groups, 1955 to 2006. *Arch Intern Med*. Mar 24 2008;168(6):632-642.

27. Kumar A, Soares H, Wells R, et al. Are experimental treatments for cancer in children superior to established treatments? Observational study of randomised controlled trials by the Children's Oncology Group. *BMJ*. Dec 3 2005;331(7528):1295.

28. Detailed List of all Indicators--Clinical Domain - Secondary Prevention in Coronary Heart Disease (CHD) [online]. [cited 2009 Jun 13]. Available from: http://www.dhsspsni.gov.uk/qof-indicators.pdf.

29. Wald DS. Problems with performance related pay in primary care. *BMJ*. Sep 15 2007;335(7619):523.

30. Williams B, Poulter NR, Brown MJ, et al. British Hypertension Society guidelines for hypertension management 2004 (BHS-IV): summary. *BMJ*. Mar 13 2004;328(7440):634-640.

31. The Seventh Report of the Joint National Committee on Prevention, Detection, Evaluation, and Treatment of High Blood Pressure (JNC 7) National

Heart Lung and Blood Institite--National Institutes of Health [online]. [cited 2009 Jun 13]. Available from: http://www.nhlbi.nih.gov/guidelines/hypertension/.

32. Mayor S. Can NICE guidance be given more clout? *BMJ.* Jul 22 2006;333(7560):170.

33. Kmietowicz Z. NICE hears appeals over dementia drugs. *BMJ.* Jul 22 2006;333(7560):165.

34. Horton R. NICE vindicated in UK's High Court. *Lancet.* Aug 18 2007;370(9587):547-548.

35. Dyer C. Appeal Court rules that NICE procedure was unfair. *BMJ.* May 10 2008;336(7652):1035.

36. Hawkes N. Why is the press so nasty to NICE? *BMJ.* 2008;337:a1906.

37. Dyer C. High court rejects challenge to NICE guidelines on chronic fatigue syndrome. *BMJ.* 2009;338:b1110.

38. Dyer C. High court rules that NICE process lacked transparency. *BMJ.* 2009;338:b772.

39. Coombes R. Review strengthens patients' right to NICE approved drugs. *BMJ.* 2008;337:a660.

40. Kmietowicz Z. Professors call for review of way cancer drugs in NHS are rationed after last ruling from NICE. *BMJ.* 2008;337:a1450.

41. Lipid modification. National Institute for Health and Clinical Excellence [online]. [cited 2009 Apr 22]. Available from: http://www.nice.org.uk/nicemedia/pdf/CG067NICEGuideline.pdf.

42. Third Report of the Expert Panel on Detection, Evaluation, and Treatment of High Blood Cholesterol in Adults (Adult Treatment Panel III). National Heart Lung and Blood Institute--National Institutes of Health [online]. [cited 2009 Jun 13]. Available from: http://www.nhlbi.nih.gov/guidelines/cholesterol/index.htm.

43. Thorpe KE, Howard DH, Galactionova K. Differences in disease prevalence as a source of the U.S.-European health care spending gap. *Health Aff (Millwood).* Nov-Dec 2007;26(6):w678-686.

44. OECD Health Data 2009 - Frequently Requested Data. Organization for Economic Co-operation and Development [online]. [cited 2009 Jul 14]. Available from: http://www.oecd.org/document/16/0,3343,en_2649_34631_2085200_1_1_1_1,00.html.

45. Liu K, Moon M, Sulvetta M, Chawla J. International infant mortality rankings: a look behind the numbers. *Health Care Financ Rev.* Summer 1992;13(4):105-118.

46. Sachs BP, Fretts RC, Gardner R, Hellerstein S, Wampler NS, Wise PH. The impact of extreme prematurity and congenital anomalies on the interpretation of international comparisons of infant mortality. *Obstet Gynecol.* Jun 1995;85(6):941-946.

47. Wegman ME. Infant mortality: some international comparisons. *Pediatrics.* Dec 1996;98(6 Pt 1):1020-1027.

48. Davis K, Shoen C, Shoenbaum S, et al. Mirror, mirror on the wall: an international update on the comparative performance of American health care. [online]. 2007 [cited Available from: www.commonwealthfund.org/.../Mirror--Mirror-on-the-Wall--An-International-Update-on-the-Comparative-Perform.

49. Avendano M, Glymour MM, Banks J, Mackenbach JP. Health disadvantage in US adults aged 50 to 74 years: a comparison of the health of rich and poor Americans with that of Europeans. *Am J Public Health*. Mar 2009;99(3):540-548.

50. Anderson GF, Reinhardt UE, Hussey PS, Petrosyan V. It's the prices, stupid: why the United States is so different from other countries. *Health Aff (Millwood)*. May-Jun 2003;22(3):89-105.

51. Bodenheimer T. High and rising health care costs. Part 2: technologic innovation. *Ann Intern Med*. Jun 7 2005;142(11):932-937.

52. U.S. kids prescribed more anti-psychotic drugs. [online]. 2008 [cited Available from: http://www.msnbc.msn.com/id/24455621/.

53. Wang YR, Alexander GC, Stafford RS. Outpatient hypertension treatment, treatment intensification, and control in Western Europe and the United States. *Arch Intern Med*. Jan 22 2007;167(2):141-147.

54. Schroeder SA, Sandy LG. Specialty distribution of U.S. physicians--the invisible driver of health care costs. *N Engl J Med*. Apr 1 1993;328(13):961-963.

55. Kmietowicz Z. Prime minister promises a more personal NHS. *BMJ*. Sep 29 2007;335(7621):631.

56. Forrest CB. Primary care in the United States: primary care gatekeeping and referrals: effective filter or failed experiment? *BMJ*. Mar 29 2003;326(7391):692-695.

57. Valderas JM, Starfield B, Forrest CB, Sibbald B, Roland M. Ambulatory care provided by office-based specialists in the United States. *Ann Fam Med*. Mar-Apr 2009;7(2):104-111.

58. Starfield B, Shi L, Macinko J. Contribution of primary care to health systems and health. *Milbank Q*. 2005;83(3):457-502.

59. Heath I. The blind leading the blind. *BMJ*. Sep 15 2007;335(7619):540.

60. Sullivan F, Butler C, Cupples M, Kinmonth AL. Primary care research networks in the United Kingdom. *BMJ*. May 26 2007;334(7603):1093-1094.

61. Bindman AB, Forrest CB, Britt H, Crampton P, Majeed A. Diagnostic scope of and exposure to primary care physicians in Australia, New Zealand, and the United States: cross sectional analysis of results from three national surveys. *BMJ*. Jun 16 2007;334(7606):1261.

62. Beasley JW, Hankey TH, Erickson R, et al. How many problems do family physicians manage at each encounter? A WReN study. *Ann Fam Med*. Sep-Oct 2004;2(5):405-410.

63. Tai-Seale M, McGuire TG, Zhang W. Time allocation in primary care office visits. *Health Serv Res*. Oct 2007;42(5):1871-1894.

64. Reid TR. *The healing of America: a global quest for better, cheaper, and fairer health care*. New York: The Penguin Press; 2009.

65. Mooney H. General practice consultations rose by two thirds in 13 years. *BMJ*. 2009;339:594.

66. Sawicki PT, Bastian H. German health care: a bit of Bismarck plus more science. *BMJ.* 2008;337:a1997.

67. Hampton T. 7-country survey of patients: US adults most unhappy with health care. *JAMA.* Dec 19 2007;298(23):2730-2731.

68. Shea KK, Holmgren A, Osborn R, Schoen C. Health system performance in selected nations: a chartpack. Commonwealth Fund [online]. 2007 May [cited 2009 May 15]. Available from: http://www.commonwealthfund.org/usr_doc/Shea_hltsysperformanceselected nations_chartpack.pdf.

69. Singer P. Why We Must Ration Health Care *New York Times Magazine.* Vol.

70. Cole A. More spending on the NHS has led to highest satisfaction rates in 25 years. *BMJ.* 2009;338:315.

71. Spence D. The American Crisis. *BMJ.* 2009;338:464.

72. Grimes G. Wondering physician. [online]. 2009 [cited Available from: http://gilgrimes.blogspot.com.

73. Klein R. Rationing in the NHS. *BMJ.* May 26 2007;334(7603):1068-1069.

Chapter 7

1. Weeks WB, Wallace AE. Long-term financial implications of specialty training for physicians. *Am J Med.* Oct 1 2002;113(5):393-399.

2. Bodenheimer T. Primary care--will it survive? *N Engl J Med.* Aug 31 2006;355(9):861-864.

3. Phillips RL, Dodoo M, Petterson SM, et al. What Influences Medical Student & Resident Choices? [online]. 2009 [cited Available from: http://www.josiahmacyfoundation.org/documents/pub_grahamcenterstudy.p df.

4. 2005-2010 Texas State Health Plan. . Statewide Health Coordinating Council [online]. 2004 [cited Available from.

5. Code Red: The Critical Condition of Health Care in Texas. [online]. 2006 [cited Available from.

6. Felland L, Hurley R, Kemper N. Safety net hospital emergency departments: creating safety valves for non-urgent care. [online]. 2008 [cited Available from: http://www.hschange.org/CONTENT/983/.

7. Steinbrook R. Health care reform in Massachusetts--expanding coverage, escalating costs. *N Engl J Med.* Jun 26 2008;358(26):2757-2760.

8. Woolhandler S, Himmelstein DU. Grim prognosis for massachusetts reform. *Health Aff (Millwood).* Mar-Apr 2009;28(2):604-605; author reply 605.

9. Truffer CJ, Keehan S, Smith S, et al. Health spending projections through 2019: the recession's impact continues. *Health Aff (Millwood).* 2010;29(3):1-8.

10. Starfield B, Shi L, Macinko J. Contribution of primary care to health systems and health. *Milbank Q.* 2005;83(3):457-502.

11. Shi L, Macinko J, Starfield B, Wulu J, Regan J, Politzer R. The relationship between primary care, income inequality, and mortality in US States, 1980-1995. *J Am Board Fam Pract.* Sep-Oct 2003;16(5):412-422.

12. Campbell RJ, Ramirez AM, Perez K, Roetzheim RG. Cervical cancer rates and the supply of primary care physicians in Florida. *Fam Med.* Jan 2003;35(1):60-64.

13. Ferrante JM, Gonzalez EC, Pal N, Roetzheim RG. Effects of physician supply on early detection of breast cancer. *J Am Board Fam Pract.* Nov-Dec 2000;13(6):408-414.

14. Cooper RA. States with more physicians have better-quality health care. *Health Aff (Millwood).* Jan-Feb 2009;28(1):w91-102.

15. Baicker K, Chandra A. Medicare spending, the physician workforce, and beneficiaries' quality of care. *Health Aff (Millwood).* 2004;Suppl Web Exclusives:W184-197.

16. Parchman ML, Culler S. Primary care physicians and avoidable hospitalizations. *J Fam Pract.* Aug 1994;39(2):123-128.

17. Kravet SJ, Shore AD, Miller R, Green GB, Kolodner K, Wright SM. Health care utilization and the proportion of primary care physicians. *Am J Med.* Feb 2008;121(2):142-148.

18. Paulus RA, Davis K, Steele GD. Continuous innovation in health care: implications of the Geisinger experience. *Health Aff (Millwood).* Sep-Oct 2008;27(5):1235-1245.

19. Arvantes J. Geisinger Health System Reports That PCMH Model Improves Quality, Lowers Costs. [online]. 2010 May 26 [cited 2010 May 27]. Available from: http://www.aafp.org/online/en/home/publications/news/news-now/practice-management/20100526geisinger.html.

20. Arvantes J. Health Care Reform Roundtable Discussion at White House Focuses on Primary Care Solutions. [online]. [cited 2009 Aug 20]. Available from: http://www.aafp.org/online/en/home/publications/news/news-now/government-medicine/20090819deparle-rndtbl.html.

21. Larson EB. Group Health Cooperative--one coverage-and-delivery model for accountable care. *N Engl J Med.* Oct 22 2009;361(17):1620-1622.

22. Porter S. AAFP, IBM team up to pitch family medicine. AAFP News Now [online]. 2006 [cited Available from: http://www.aafp.org/online/en/home/publications/news/news-now/professional-issues/20060815aafpibm.html.

23. Bodenheimer T. North Carolina medicaid: a fruitful payer-practice collaboration. *Ann Fam Med.* Jul-Aug 2008;6(4):292-294.

24. Heneghan C, Glasziou P, Thompson M, et al. Diagnostic strategies used in primary care. *BMJ.* 2009;338:b946.

25. Pham HH, Alexander GC, O'Malley AS. Physician consideration of patients' out-of-pocket costs in making common clinical decisions. *Arch Intern Med.* Apr 9 2007;167(7):663-668.

26. Laing BY, Bodenheimer T, Phillips RL, Jr., Bazemore A. Primary care's eroding earnings: is congress concerned? *J Fam Pract.* Sep 2008;57(9):578-583.

Chapter 8

1. New Report Takes In-depth Look at Reasons Behind Low Level of Student Interest in Family Medicine. AAFP News Now [online]. 2009 Sep 2 [cited 2009 Sep 4]. Available from: http://www.aafp.org/online/en/home/publications/news/news-now/resident-student-focus/20090902nrmp-report.html.

2. Phillips JP, Weismantel DP, Gold KJ, Schwenk TL. Medical student debt and primary care specialty intentions. *Fam Med.* Oct 2010;42(9):616-622.

3. Weeks WB, Wallace AE, Wallace MM, Welch HG. A comparison of the educational costs and incomes of physicians and other professionals. *N Engl J Med.* May 5 1994;330(18):1280-1286.

4. French HE. *Regulating doctors' fees: competition, benefits, and controls under medicare.* Lanham, MD: AEI Press; 1991.

5. Nicholson S. Medical career choices and rates of return. Cornell University and NBER [online]. 2006 [cited 2009 Aug 12]. Available from: http://new.oberlin.edu/arts-and-sciences/departments/economics/index.dot.

6. 1997 Documentation Guidelines for Evaluation and Management Services. In: Centers for Medicare and Medicaid Services, ed.

7. Hawryluk M. E&M guidelines still don't work; panel says dump 'em. *American Medical News.* Vol Chicago: American Medical Association.

8. Medicare physician payment: Time to act on E&M mess. *American Medical News.* Vol Chicago: American Medical Association.

9. Moore KJ, Felger TA, Larimore WL, Mills TL, Jr. What every physician should know about the RUC. *Fam Pract Manag.* Feb 2008;15(2):36-39.

10. Goodson JD. Unintended consequences of resource-based relative value scale reimbursement. *JAMA.* Nov 21 2007;298(19):2308-2310.

11. Bodenheimer T, Berenson RA, Rudolf P. The primary care-specialty income gap: why it matters. *Ann Intern Med.* Feb 20 2007;146(4):301-306.

12. Newhouse JP. Medicare spending on physicians - no easy fix in sight. *N Engl J Med.* May 3 2007;356(18):1883-1884.

13. Hsiao WC, Dunn DL, Verrilli DK. Assessing the implementation of physician-payment reform. *N Engl J Med.* Apr 1 1993;328(13):928-933.

14. Arvantes J. Senate hearing links physician payment rates to primary care shortages. AAFP News Now [online]. 2008 [cited Available from: www.aafp.org/news-now/government-medicine/20080219helphearing.html.

15. Arvantes J. MedPAC Members Characterize RBRVS System as Subjective, 'Deeply Flawed'. AAFP News Now [online]. 2009 Nov 3 [cited 2009 Nov 29]. Available from.

16. Bodenheimer T. Primary care--will it survive? *N Engl J Med.* Aug 31 2006;355(9):861-864.

17. Iglehart JK. Medicare, graduate medical education, and new policy directions. *N Engl J Med.* Aug 7 2008;359(6):643-650.

18. Woo B. Primary care--the best job in medicine? *N Engl J Med.* Aug 31 2006;355(9):864-866.

19. Ostbye T, Yarnall KS, Krause KM, Pollak KI, Gradison M, Michener JL. Is there time for management of patients with chronic diseases in primary care? *Ann Fam Med.* May-Jun 2005;3(3):209-214.

20. Newbell BJ. Coding nonsense, NOS. *Fam Pract Manag.* Oct 2005;12(9):82.

21. Wachter RM, Goldman L. The hospitalist movement 5 years later. *JAMA.* Jan 23-30 2002;287(4):487-494.

22. Were MC, Li X, Kesterson J, et al. Adequacy of hospital discharge summaries in documenting tests with pending results and outpatient follow-up providers. *J Gen Intern Med.* Sep 2009;24(9):1002-1006.

23. Smith PC, Westfall JM, Nichols RA. Primary care family physicians and 2 hospitalist models: comparison of outcomes, processes, and costs. *J Fam Pract.* Dec 2002;51(12):1021-1027.

24. Lindenauer PK, Rothberg MB, Pekow PS, Kenwood C, Benjamin EM, Auerbach AD. Outcomes of care by hospitalists, general internists, and family physicians. *N Engl J Med.* Dec 20 2007;357(25):2589-2600.

25. Bodenheimer T. Coordinating care--a perilous journey through the health care system. *N Engl J Med.* Mar 6 2008;358(10):1064-1071.

26. Starfield B, Shi L, Macinko J. Contribution of primary care to health systems and health. *Milbank Q.* 2005;83(3):457-502.

27. Cardiovascular Disease: Certification Examination Blueprint. American Board of Internal Medicine [online]. [cited 2009 Oct 14]. Available from: http://www.abim.org/pdf/blueprint/card_cert.pdf.

Chapter 9

1. Brenner DJ, Hall EJ. Computed tomography--an increasing source of radiation exposure. *N Engl J Med.* Nov 29 2007;357(22):2277-2284.

2. Vetter VL, Elia J, Erickson C, et al. Cardiovascular monitoring of children and adolescents with heart disease receiving medications for attention deficit/hyperactivity disorder [corrected]: a scientific statement from the American Heart Association Council on Cardiovascular Disease in the Young Congenital Cardiac Defects Committee and the Council on Cardiovascular Nursing. *Circulation.* May 6 2008;117(18):2407-2423.

3. Pediatricians nix heart tests for ADHD drugs. MSNBC.com [online]. [cited 2008 Jul 29]. Available from: http://www.msnbc.msn.com/id/25919551.

Chapter 10

1. Third Report of the Expert Panel on Detection, Evaluation, and Treatment of High Blood Cholesterol in Adults (Adult Treatment Panel III). National Heart Lung and Blood Institute--National Institutes of Health [online]. [cited 2009 Jun 13]. Available from: http://www.nhlbi.nih.gov/guidelines/cholesterol/index.htm.

2. Guidelines for the Diagnosis and Management of Asthma. [online]. July 2007 [cited Available from: http://www.nhlbi.nih.gov/guidelines/asthma/.

3. Guidelines and resources. [online]. November 2008 [cited Available from: http://www.goldcopd.com/GuidelinesResources.asp.

4. The Seventh Report of the Joint National Committee on Prevention, Detection, Evaluation, and Treatment of High Blood Pressure (JNC 7) National Heart Lung and Blood Institite--National Institutes of Health [online]. [cited

2009 Jun 13]. Available from:
http://www.nhlbi.nih.gov/guidelines/hypertension/.

5. Grodstein F, Stampfer MJ, Manson JE, et al. Postmenopausal estrogen and progestin use and the risk of cardiovascular disease. *N Engl J Med.* Aug 15 1996;335(7):453-461.

6. Grodstein F, Manson JE, Colditz GA, Willett WC, Speizer FE, Stampfer MJ. A prospective, observational study of postmenopausal hormone therapy and primary prevention of cardiovascular disease. *Ann Intern Med.* Dec 19 2000;133(12):933-941.

7. The Coronary Drug Project. Initial findings leading to modifications of its research protocol. *JAMA.* Nov 16 1970;214(7):1303-1313.

8. The Coronary Drug Project. Findings leading to discontinuation of the 2.5-mg day estrogen group. The coronary Drug Project Research Group. *JAMA.* Nov 5 1973;226(6):652-657.

9. Hulley S, Grady D, Bush T, et al. Randomized trial of estrogen plus progestin for secondary prevention of coronary heart disease in postmenopausal women. Heart and Estrogen/progestin Replacement Study (HERS) Research Group. *JAMA.* Aug 19 1998;280(7):605-613.

10. Grady D, Herrington D, Bittner V, et al. Cardiovascular disease outcomes during 6.8 years of hormone therapy: Heart and Estrogen/progestin Replacement Study follow-up (HERS II). *JAMA.* Jul 3 2002;288(1):49-57.

11. Scherer FM. The pharmaceutical industry--prices and progress. *N Engl J Med.* Aug 26 2004;351(9):927-932.

12. Acute low back problems in adults: assessment and treatment. Acute Low Back Problems Guideline Panel. Agency for Health Care Policy and Research. *Am Fam Physician.* Feb 1 1995;51(2):469-484.

13. Gray BH, Gusmano MK, Collins SR. AHCPR and the changing politics of health services research. *Health Aff (Millwood).* Jan-Jun 2003;Suppl Web Exclusives:W3-283-307.

14. Jensen MC, Brant-Zawadzki MN, Obuchowski N, Modic MT, Malkasian D, Ross JS. Magnetic resonance imaging of the lumbar spine in people without back pain. *N Engl J Med.* Jul 14 1994;331(2):69-73.

15. Deyo RA, Nachemson A, Mirza SK. Spinal-fusion surgery - the case for restraint. *N Engl J Med.* Feb 12 2004;350(7):722-726.

16. Carragee EJ. The increasing morbidity of elective spinal stenosis surgery: is it necessary? *JAMA.* Apr 7 2010;303(13):1309-1310.

17. Sessions SY, Detsky AS. Incorporating economic reality into medical education. *JAMA.* Sep 15 2010;304(11):1229-1230.

18. Nguyen TH, Randolph DC, Talmage J, Succop P, Travis R. Long-term Outcomes of Lumbar Fusion Among Workers' Compensation Subjects: An Historical Cohort Study. *Spine (Phila Pa 1976).* Aug 23 2010.

19. Deyo RA, Mirza SK, Turner JA, Martin BI. Overtreating chronic back pain: time to back off? *J Am Board Fam Med.* Jan-Feb 2009;22(1):62-68.

20. Chou R, Qaseem A, Snow V, et al. Diagnosis and treatment of low back pain: a joint clinical practice guideline from the American College of

Physicians and the American Pain Society. *Ann Intern Med.* Oct 2 2007;147(7):478-491.

21. Landers S. New guidelines on back pain seen as collaborative effort. *American Medical News.* Vol Chicago, IL: American Medical Association; 2007:29-30.

22. Carman KL, Maurer M, Yegian JM, et al. Evidence that consumers are skeptical about evidence-based health care. *Health Aff (Millwood).* Jul;29(7):1400-1406.

Chapter 11

1. Singer N. In push for cancer screening, limited benefits. *New York Times.* July 17, 2009.

2. Doll R, Peto R, Boreham J, Sutherland I. Mortality in relation to smoking: 50 years' observations on male British doctors. *BMJ.* Jun 26 2004;328(7455):1519.

3. Fiscella K, Franks P. Cost-effectiveness of the transdermal nicotine patch as an adjunct to physicians' smoking cessation counseling. *JAMA.* Apr 24 1996;275(16):1247-1251.

4. Stapleton JA, Lowin A, Russell MA. Prescription of transdermal nicotine patches for smoking cessation in general practice: evaluation of cost-effectiveness. *Lancet.* Jul 17 1999;354(9174):210-215.

5. Cromwell J, Bartosch WJ, Fiore MC, Hasselblad V, Baker T. Cost-effectiveness of the clinical practice recommendations in the AHCPR guideline for smoking cessation. Agency for Health Care Policy and Research. *JAMA.* Dec 3 1997;278(21):1759-1766.

6. Javitz HS, Swan GE, Zbikowski SM, et al. Cost-effectiveness of different combinations of bupropion SR dose and behavioral treatment for smoking cessation: a societal perspective. *Am J Manag Care.* Mar 2004;10(3):217-226.

7. Song F, Raftery J, Aveyard P, Hyde C, Barton P, Woolacott N. Cost-effectiveness of pharmacological interventions for smoking cessation: a literature review and a decision analytic analysis. *Med Decis Making.* Sep-Oct 2002;22(5 Suppl):S26-37.

8. Barendregt JJ, Bonneux L, van der Maas PJ. The health care costs of smoking. *N Engl J Med.* Oct 9 1997;337(15):1052-1057.

9. Eddy DM. Screening for breast cancer. *Ann Intern Med.* Sep 1 1989;111(5):389-399.

10. Mandelblatt J, Saha S, Teutsch S, et al. The cost-effectiveness of screening mammography beyond age 65 years: a systematic review for the U.S. Preventive Services Task Force. *Ann Intern Med.* Nov 18 2003;139(10):835-842.

11. Salzmann P, Kerlikowske K, Phillips K. Cost-effectiveness of extending screening mammography guidelines to include women 40 to 49 years of age. *Ann Intern Med.* Dec 1 1997;127(11):955-965.

12. Kerlikowske K, Salzmann P, Phillips KA, Cauley JA, Cummings SR. Continuing screening mammography in women aged 70 to 79 years: impact on life expectancy and cost-effectiveness. *JAMA.* Dec 8 1999;282(22):2156-2163.

13. Goldman L, Weinstein MC, Goldman PA, Williams LW. Cost-effectiveness of HMG-CoA reductase inhibition for primary and secondary prevention of coronary heart disease. *JAMA*. Mar 6 1991;265(9):1145-1151.

14. Prosser LA, Stinnett AA, Goldman PA, et al. Cost-effectiveness of cholesterol-lowering therapies according to selected patient characteristics. *Ann Intern Med*. May 16 2000;132(10):769-779.

15. Cost-effectiveness of intensive glycemic control, intensified hypertension control, and serum cholesterol level reduction for type 2 diabetes. *JAMA*. May 15 2002;287(19):2542-2551.

16. Grima DT, Thompson MF, Sauriol L. Modelling cost effectiveness of insulin glargine for the treatment of type 1 and 2 diabetes in Canada. *Pharmacoeconomics*. 2007;25(3):253-266.

17. Neeser K, Lubben G, Siebert U, Schramm W. Cost effectiveness of combination therapy with pioglitazone for type 2 diabetes mellitus from a German statutory healthcare perspective. *Pharmacoeconomics*. 2004;22(5):321-341.

18. Patel A, MacMahon S, Chalmers J, et al. Intensive blood glucose control and vascular outcomes in patients with type 2 diabetes. *N Engl J Med*. Jun 12 2008;358(24):2560-2572.

19. Bruno G, Biggeri A, Merletti F, et al. Low incidence of end-stage renal disease and chronic renal failure in type 2 diabetes: a 10-year prospective study. *Diabetes Care*. Aug 2003;26(8):2353-2358.

20. Ray KK, Seshasai SR, Wijesuriya S, et al. Effect of intensive control of glucose on cardiovascular outcomes and death in patients with diabetes mellitus: a meta-analysis of randomised controlled trials. *Lancet*. May 23 2009;373(9677):1765-1772.

21. Gerstein HC, Miller ME, Byington RP, et al. Effects of intensive glucose lowering in type 2 diabetes. *N Engl J Med*. Jun 12 2008;358(24):2545-2559.

22. Larson EB. Group Health Cooperative--one coverage-and-delivery model for accountable care. *N Engl J Med*. Oct 22 2009;361(17):1620-1622.

23. Parchman ML, Culler S. Primary care physicians and avoidable hospitalizations. *J Fam Pract*. Aug 1994;39(2):123-128.

24. Goodman DC, Grumbach K. Does having more physicians lead to better health system performance? *JAMA*. Jan 23 2008;299(3):335-337.

25. Clarke PM, Gray AM, Briggs A, Stevens RJ, Matthews DR, Holman RR. Cost-utility analyses of intensive blood glucose and tight blood pressure control in type 2 diabetes (UKPDS 72). *Diabetologia*. May 2005;48(5):868-877.

26. Elliott WJ, Weir DR, Black HR. Cost-effectiveness of the lower treatment goal (of JNC VI) for diabetic hypertensive patients. Joint National Committee on Prevention, Detection, Evaluation, and Treatment of High Blood Pressure. *Arch Intern Med*. May 8 2000;160(9):1277-1283.

27. Heath I. An open letter to the Prime Minister. *BMJ*. Feb 16 2008;336(7640):360.

28. Shea KK, Holmgren A, Osborn R, Schoen C. Health system performance in selected nations: a chartpack. [online]. 2007 [cited Available from:
http://www.commonwealthfund.org/usr_doc/Shea_hltsysperformanceselect ednations_chartpack.pdf.

Chapter 12

1. Loose change: the price of expensive cancer drugs. *Fort Worth Star-Telegram.* July 13, 2008.

2. Minkoff NB. Colorectal cancer: complexities and challenges in managed care. *J Manag Care Pharm.* Aug 2007;13(6 Suppl C):S27-29.

3. Kolata G, Pollack A. Costly Cancer Drug Offers Hope, but Also a Dilemma. NYTimes.com [online]. 2008 July 6 [cited 2009 Aug 11]. Available from: http://www.nytimes.com/2008/07/06/health/06avastin.html?_r=1.

4. Ioannidis JP, Karassa FB. The need to consider the wider agenda in systematic reviews and meta-analyses: breadth, timing, and depth of the evidence. *BMJ.* 2010;341:c4875.

5. Johnson A. Insurer Plays Judge on Cancer Care. The Wall Street Journal [online]. 2010 Feb 9 [cited 2010 Mar 14]. Available from: http://online.wsj.com/article/SB10001424052748703357104575045261652218880. html.

6. Piccart-Gebhart MJ, Procter M, Leyland-Jones B, et al. Trastuzumab after adjuvant chemotherapy in HER2-positive breast cancer. *N Engl J Med.* Oct 20 2005;353(16):1659-1672.

7. Metcalfe S, Burgess C, Laking G, Evans J, Wells S, Crausaz S. Trastuzumab: possible publication bias. *Lancet.* May 17 2008;371(9625):1646-1648.

8. Hind D, Pilgrim H, Ward S. Questions about adjuvant trastuzumab still remain. *Lancet.* Jan 6 2007;369(9555):3-5.

9. Singer P. Why We Must Ration Health Care *New York Times Magazine.* Vol.

10. Engelberg AB, Kesselheim AS, Avorn J. Balancing innovation, access, and profits--market exclusivity for biologics. *N Engl J Med.* Nov 12 2009;361(20):1917-1919.

11. Nadler E, Eckert B, Neumann PJ. Do oncologists believe new cancer drugs offer good value? *Oncologist.* Feb 2006;11(2):90-95.

12. Zuger A. Rx: Canadian drugs. *N Engl J Med.* Dec 4 2003;349(23):2188-2190.

13. Paris V, Docteur E. Pharmaceutical Pricing and Reimbursement Policies in Canada. Organisation for Economic Co-operation and Development [online]. 2007 Feb 15 [cited 2009 Jul 12]. Available from: http://www.oecd.org/dataoecd/21/40/37868186.pdf.

14. Morgan S, Hurley J. Internet pharmacy: prices on the up-and-up. *CMAJ.* Mar 16 2004;170(6):945-946.

15. Canadian and American health care systems compared. Wikipedia.com [online]. [cited 2008 Jul 10]. Available from: http://en.wikipedia.org/wiki/Canadian_and_American_health_care_systems_c ompared.

16. Tappenden P, Jones R, Paisley S, Carroll C. Systematic review and economic evaluation of bevacizumab and cetuximab for the treatment of metastatic colorectal cancer. *Health Technol Assess.* Mar 2007;11(12):1-128, iii-iv.

17. Garber AM, McClellan MB. Satisfaction guaranteed--"payment by results" for biologic agents. *N Engl J Med.* Oct 18 2007;357(16):1575-1577.

18. Orszag PR, Ellis P. Addressing rising health care costs--a view from the Congressional Budget Office. *N Engl J Med.* Nov 8 2007;357(19):1885-1887.

19. Gillick MR. Medicare coverage for technological innovations--time for new criteria? *N Engl J Med.* May 20 2004;350(21):2199-2203.

20. Tunis SR. Why Medicare has not established criteria for coverage decisions. *N Engl J Med.* May 20 2004;350(21):2196-2198.

21. Hernandez AF, Shea AM, Milano CA, et al. Long-term outcomes and costs of ventricular assist devices among Medicare beneficiaries. *JAMA.* Nov 26 2008;300(20):2398-2406.

22. Neumann PJ, Rosen AB, Weinstein MC. Medicare and cost-effectiveness analysis. *N Engl J Med.* Oct 6 2005;353(14):1516-1522.

Chapter 13

1. Anderson G. Chronic conditions: making the case for ongoing care. [online]. [cited 2009 May 2]. Available from: http://www.fightchronicdisease.com/news/pfcd/documents/ChronicCareChart book_FINAL.pdf.

2. Berenson RA, Horvath J. Confronting the barriers to chronic care management in Medicare. *Health Aff (Millwood).* Jan-Jun 2003;Suppl Web Exclusives:W3-37-53.

3. Diabetes, cholesterol, and anti-obesity drugs top spending. *AHRQ News.* Vol March 2008 ed. Washington, DC: Agency for Healthcare Research and Quality; 2008:18.

4. Tynan A, Draper D. Getting what we pay for: innovations lacking in provider payment reform for chronic disease care. Center for Studying Health System Change [online]. 2008 Jun [cited 2009 May 2]. Available from: http://www.hschange.com/CONTENT/996/.

5. Gerstein HC, Miller ME, Byington RP, et al. Effects of intensive glucose lowering in type 2 diabetes. *N Engl J Med.* Jun 12 2008;358(24):2545-2559.

6. Patel A, MacMahon S, Chalmers J, et al. Intensive blood glucose control and vascular outcomes in patients with type 2 diabetes. *N Engl J Med.* Jun 12 2008;358(24):2560-2572.

7. Duckworth W, Abraira C, Moritz T, et al. Glucose control and vascular complications in veterans with type 2 diabetes. *N Engl J Med.* Jan 8 2009;360(2):129-139.

8. Lehman R, Krumholz HM. Tight control of blood glucose in long standing type 2 diabetes. *BMJ.* 2009;338:b800.

9. Lehman R, Krumholz HM. No to QOF target of <7 percent, again. *BMJ.* 2010;340:437.

10. Pogach L, Aron D. Balancing hypoglycemia and glycemic control: a public health approach for insulin safety. *JAMA.* May 26;303(20):2076-2077.

11. Changes to the Diabetes Recognition Program. [online]. 2010 [cited 2010 May 31]. Available from: http://www.ncqa.org/tabid/1023/Default.aspx.

12. Summary of revisions for the 2009 Clinical Practice Recommendations. *Diabetes Care.* Jan 2009;32 Suppl 1:S3-5.

13. Aron D, Pogach L. Transparency standards for diabetes performance measures. *JAMA.* Jan 14 2009;301(2):210-212.

14. Bruno G, Biggeri A, Merletti F, et al. Low incidence of end-stage renal disease and chronic renal failure in type 2 diabetes: a 10-year prospective study. *Diabetes Care.* Aug 2003;26(8):2353-2358.

15. Ray KK, Seshasai SR, Wijesuriya S, et al. Effect of intensive control of glucose on cardiovascular outcomes and death in patients with diabetes mellitus: a meta-analysis of randomised controlled trials. *Lancet.* May 23 2009;373(9677):1765-1772.

16. Beale S, Bagust A, Shearer AT, Martin A, Hulme L. Cost-effectiveness of rosiglitazone combination therapy for the treatment of type 2 diabetes mellitus in the UK. *Pharmacoeconomics.* 2006;24 Suppl 1:21-34.

17. Cost-effectiveness of intensive glycemic control, intensified hypertension control, and serum cholesterol level reduction for type 2 diabetes. *JAMA.* May 15 2002;287(19):2542-2551.

18. Clarke PM, Gray AM, Briggs A, Stevens RJ, Matthews DR, Holman RR. Cost-utility analyses of intensive blood glucose and tight blood pressure control in type 2 diabetes (UKPDS 72). *Diabetologia.* May 2005;48(5):868-877.

19. Dijkstra RF, Niessen LW, Braspenning JC, Adang E, Grol RT. Patient-centred and professional-directed implementation strategies for diabetes guidelines: a cluster-randomized trial-based cost-effectiveness analysis. *Diabet Med.* Feb 2006;23(2):164-170.

20. Eastman RC, Javitt JC, Herman WH, et al. Model of complications of NIDDM. II. Analysis of the health benefits and cost-effectiveness of treating NIDDM with the goal of normoglycemia. *Diabetes Care.* May 1997;20(5):735-744.

21. Huang ES, Shook M, Jin L, Chin MH, Meltzer DO. The impact of patient preferences on the cost-effectiveness of intensive glucose control in older patients with new-onset diabetes. *Diabetes Care.* Feb 2006;29(2):259-264.

22. The cost-effectiveness of screening for type 2 diabetes. CDC Diabetes Cost-Effectiveness Study Group, Centers for Disease Control and Prevention. *JAMA.* Nov 25 1998;280(20):1757-1763.

23. Ackermann RT, Marrero DG, Hicks KA, et al. An evaluation of cost sharing to finance a diet and physical activity intervention to prevent diabetes. *Diabetes Care.* Jun 2006;29(6):1237-1241.

24. Diabetes Prevention Program Research G. Within-trial cost-effectiveness of lifestyle intervention or metformin for the primary prevention of type 2 diabetes. *Diabetes Care.* Sep 2003;26(9):2518-2523.

25. Eddy DM, Schlessinger L, Kahn R. Clinical outcomes and cost-effectiveness of strategies for managing people at high risk for diabetes. *Ann Intern Med.* Aug 16 2005;143(4):251-264.

26. Herman WH, Hoerger TJ, Brandle M, et al. The cost-effectiveness of lifestyle modification or metformin in preventing type 2 diabetes in adults with impaired glucose tolerance. *Annals of Internal Medicine.* Mar 1 2005;142(5):323-332.

27. Prevention for a healthier America: investments in disease prevention yield significant savings, stronger communities. Trust for America's Health [online]. 2008 July [cited 2009 Apr 27]. Available from: http://healthyamericans.org/reports/prevention08/.

28. Avendano M, Glymour MM, Banks J, Mackenbach JP. Health disadvantage in US adults aged 50 to 74 years: a comparison of the health of rich and poor Americans with that of Europeans. *Am J Public Health.* Mar 2009;99(3):540-548.

29. Thorpe KE, Howard DH, Galactionova K. Differences in disease prevalence as a source of the U.S.-European health care spending gap. *Health Aff (Millwood).* Nov-Dec 2007;26(6):w678-686.

30. Sessions SY, Detsky AS. The "shadow government" in health care. *JAMA.* Dec 22 2010;304(24):2742-2743.

31. Welschen LM, Bloemendal E, Nijpels G, et al. Self-monitoring of blood glucose in patients with type 2 diabetes who are not using insulin: a systematic review. *Diabetes Care.* Jun 2005;28(6):1510-1517.

Chapter 14

1. Kirsch R. Will it be Déjà vu All Over Again?: Renewing the Fight for Health Care for All. [online]. 2003 [cited Available from: http://cthealth.server101.com/renewing_the_fight_for_health_care_for_all.htm.

2. Stanglin D. 'You lie!' makes Yale's list of top quotes of 2009. USAToday.com [online]. 2009 Dec 16 [cited 2010 Jan 18]. Available from: http://content.usatoday.com/communities/ondeadline/post/2009/12/you-lie-makes-yales-list-of-top-quotes-of-2009/1.

3. National health care expenditures. Center for Medicare and Medicaid Services [online]. [cited 2009 Apr 26]. Available from: http://www.cms.hhs.gov/NationalHealthExpendData/downloads/tables.pdf.

4. Blumenthal D. Employer-sponsored health insurance in the United States--origins and implications. *N Engl J Med.* Jul 6 2006;355(1):82-88.

5. Iglehart JK. Reform of the Veterans Affairs heath care system. *N Engl J Med.* Oct 31 1996;335(18):1407-1411.

6. Rubenstein LV, Yano EM, Fink A, et al. Evaluation of the VA's Pilot Program in Institutional Reorganization toward Primary and Ambulatory Care: Part I, Changes in process and outcomes of care. *Acad Med.* Jul 1996;71(7):772-783.

7. Congressional Budget Office. Quality Initiatives Undertaken by the Veterans Health Administration. [online]. 2009 Aug [cited 2009 Aug 23]. Available from: http://cbo.gov/ftpdocs/104xx/doc10453/08-13-VHA.pdf.

8. Unsterile equipment used on Miami veterans. [online]. 2009 [cited March 23, 2009]. Available from: http://www.msnbc.msn.com/id/29842788/ns/health-health_care/.

9. Unsterile equipment used on Miami veterans. MSNBC.com [online]. 2009 Mar 23 [cited 2009 Jul 1]. Available from: http://www.msnbc.msn.com/id/29842788/ns/health-health_care/.

10. VA centers lack proper training in colonoscopies and other tests. *Fort Worth Star-Telegram.* June 16, 2009.

Chapter 15

1. Maron BJ, Gohman TE, Aeppli D. Prevalence of sudden cardiac death during competitive sports activities in Minnesota high school athletes. *J Am Coll Cardiol.* Dec 1998;32(7):1881-1884.

2. Runner dies in Nashville half-marathon. Knoxnews.com [online]. 2009 Apr 25 [cited 2009 Jul 9]. Available from: http://www.knoxnews.com/news/2009/apr/25/runner-dies-nashville-half-marathon/.

3. Manitoba Marathon runner dies. Manitoba Free Press [online]. 2009 Jun 30 [cited 2009 Jul 9]. Available from: http://www.winnipegfreepress.com/local/manitoba-marathon-runner-dies-49499217.html.

4. Redelmeier DA, Greenwald JA. Competing risks of mortality with marathons: retrospective analysis. *BMJ.* Dec 22 2007;335(7633):1275-1277.

5. Cohen JT, Neumann PJ. What's more dangerous, your aspirin or your car? Thinking rationally about drug risks (and benefits). *Health Aff (Millwood).* May-Jun 2007;26(3):636-646.

6. Traffic Safety Facts: 2007 Traffic Safety Annual Assessment - Highlights. National Highway Traffic Safety Administration [online]. 2008 Aug [cited 2009 May 2]. Available from: http://list.nsc.org/defensivedriving/images/uploads/NHTSA_Traffic_Safety_Facts_-_August_2008.pdf.

7. Kraus JF, Peek C, McArthur DL, Williams A. The effect of the 1992 California motorcycle helmet use law on motorcycle crash fatalities and injuries. *JAMA.* Nov 16 1994;272(19):1506-1511.

8. Motor-vehicle safety: a 20th century public health achievement. *MMWR Morb Mortal Wkly Rep.* May 14 1999;48(18):369-374.

9. Statistical information about casualties of the Vietnam War National Archives [online]. [cited 2009 Jun 26]. Available from: http://www.archives.gov/research/vietnam-war/casualty-statistics.html.

10. U.S. Census Bureau. Motor vehicle occupants and nonoccupants killed and injured. [online]. 2012 [cited 2011 Oct 6]. Available from: http://www.census.gov/compendia/statab/2012/tables/12s1106.pdf.

11. Traffic Safety Facts: 2007 Data--Overview. National Highway Traffic Safety Administration [online]. [cited 2009 Jun 26]. Available from: http://www-nrd.nhtsa.dot.gov/Pubs/810993.PDF.

12. Baker SP, O'Neill B, Ginsburg MJ, Li G. *The Injury Fact Book: Second edition*. New York Oxford: Oxford University Press; 1992.

13. Traffic Safety Facts: 2006 data: Speeding. [online]. 2007 [cited 2009]. Available from: http://www-nrd.nhtsa.dot.gov/Pubs/810818.pdf.

14. Nordhoff L. *Motor vehicle collision injuries: mechanisms, diagnosis, and management*. Gaithersburg, MD: Aspen, Inc.; 1996.

15. Redelmeier DA, Tibshirani RJ. Association between cellular-telephone calls and motor vehicle collisions. *N Engl J Med*. Feb 13 1997;336(7):453-458.

16. Cohen JT, Graham JD. A revised economic analysis of restrictions on the use of cell phones while driving. *Risk Anal*. Feb 2003;23(1):5-17.

17. Jacobson PD, Gostin LO. Reducing distracted driving: regulation and education to avert traffic injuries and fatalities. *JAMA*. Apr 14 2010;303(14):1419-1420.

18. Austin RM, McLendon WW. The Papanicolaou smear. Medicine's most successful cancer screening procedure is threatened. *JAMA*. Mar 5 1997;277(9):754-755.

19. Screening for breast cancer: U.S. Preventive services task force recommendation statement. *Ann Intern Med*. Nov 17 2009;151(10):716-726, W-236.

20. Gotzsche PC, Hartling OJ, Nielsen M, Brodersen J, Jorgensen KJ. Breast screening: the facts--or maybe not. *BMJ*. 2009;338:b86.

21. TRAFFIC SAFETY FACTS 2007. In: National Highway Traffic Safety Administration, ed. Washington, D.C.2009: http://www-nrd.nhtsa.dot.gov/Pubs/811002.PDF.

Chapter 16

1. Orzano AJ, Strickland PO, Tallia AF, et al. Improving outcomes for high-risk diabetics using information systems. *J Am Board Fam Med*. May-Jun 2007;20(3):245-251.

2. Brown T. Are electronic health records (EHRs) used for quality by primary care providers for quality?: an ethnographic study. *NAPCRG Annual Meeting*. Vol Rio Grande, Puerto Rico2008.

3. Casalino LP, Dunham D, Chin MH, et al. Frequency of failure to inform patients of clinically significant outpatient test results. *Arch Intern Med*. Jun 22 2009;169(12):1123-1129.

4. Overhage JM, Tierney WM, Zhou XH, McDonald CJ. A randomized trial of "corollary orders" to prevent errors of omission. *J Am Med Inform Assoc*. Sep-Oct 1997;4(5):364-375.

5. Litzelman DK, Dittus RS, Miller ME, Tierney WM. Requiring physicians to respond to computerized reminders improves their compliance with preventive care protocols. *J Gen Intern Med*. Jun 1993;8(6):311-317.

6. O'Connor PJ, Crain AL, Rush WA, Sperl-Hillen JM, Gutenkauf JJ, Duncan JE. Impact of an electronic medical record on diabetes quality of care. *Ann Fam Med*. Jul-Aug 2005;3(4):300-306.

7. Crosson JC, Ohman-Strickland PA, Hahn KA, et al. Electronic medical records and diabetes quality of care: results from a sample of family medicine practices. *Ann Fam Med.* May-Jun 2007;5(3):209-215.

8. Parchman M, Kaissi AA. Are elements of the chronic care model associated with cardiovascular risk factor control in type 2 diabetes? *Jt Comm J Qual Patient Saf.* Mar 2009;35(3):133-138.

9. Koppel R, Metlay JP, Cohen A, et al. Role of computerized physician order entry systems in facilitating medication errors. *JAMA.* Mar 9 2005;293(10):1197-1203.

10. Virapongse A, Bates DW, Shi P, et al. Electronic health records and malpractice claims in office practice. *Arch Intern Med.* Nov 24 2008;168(21):2362-2367.

11. Simon SR, Kaushal R, Cleary PD, et al. Physicians and electronic health records: a statewide survey. *Arch Intern Med.* Mar 12 2007;167(5):507-512.

12. Cutler DM, Feldman NE, Horwitz JR. U.S. adoption of computerized physician order entry systems. *Health Aff (Millwood).* Nov-Dec 2005;24(6):1654-1663.

13. Ash JS, Gorman PN, Seshadri V, Hersh WR. Computerized physician order entry in U.S. hospitals: results of a 2002 survey. *J Am Med Inform Assoc.* Mar-Apr 2004;11(2):95-99.

14. Blumenthal D, Glaser JP. Information technology comes to medicine. *N Engl J Med.* Jun 14 2007;356(24):2527-2534.

15. Pace WD. Registries, databases, and electronic health records in ambulatory care. *Jt Comm J Qual Patient Saf.* May 2009;35(5):247.

16. Roehr B. United States lags far behind 10 other countries in terms of access to primary healthcare services. *BMJ.*339:1051-1052.

17. Evans JP, Dale DC, Fomous C. Preparing for a consumer-driven genomic age. *N Engl J Med.* Sep 16 2010;363(12):1099-1103.

18. Lee C, Morton CC. Structural genomic variation and personalized medicine. *N Engl J Med.* Feb 14 2008;358(7):740-741.

19. Carr G. Biology 2.0. [online]. 2010 Jun 17 [cited 2010 Jun 18]. Available from: http://www.economist.com/node/16349358.

20. Annes JP, Giovanni MA, Murray MF. Risks of presymptomatic direct-to-consumer genetic testing. *N Engl J Med.* Sep 16 2010;363(12):1100-1101.

21. Navigenics--There's DNA. And then there's what you do with it. Navigenics [online]. 2009 May 11 [cited 2009 Jun 5]. Available from: http://www.navigenics.com/.

22. Health and traits. 23andMe [online]. [cited 2009 Jul 9]. Available from: https://www.23andme.com/health/.

23. Chen F. Genomics: lots of press but how much progress? *J Fam Pract.* February 2009 2009;58(2):62-63.

24. McGuire AL, Burke W. An unwelcome side effect of direct-to-consumer personal genome testing: raiding the medical commons. *JAMA.* Dec 10 2008;300(22):2669-2671.

25. Scheuner MT, Sieverding P, Shekelle PG. Delivery of genomic medicine for common chronic adult diseases: a systematic review. *JAMA.* Mar 19 2008;299(11):1320-1334.

26. Anderson JL, Horne BD, Stevens SM, et al. Randomized trial of genotype-guided versus standard warfarin dosing in patients initiating oral anticoagulation. *Circulation.* Nov 27 2007;116(22):2563-2570.

27. Segal J, Brotman D, Emadi A, et al. Outcomes of Genetic Testing in Adults with a History of Venous Thromboembolism. Evidence Report/Technology Assessment No. 180. [online]. 2009 Jun [cited 2010 Oct 25]. Available from: http://www.ahrq.gov/downloads/pub/evidence/pdf/factorvleiden/fvl.pdf.

28. Laurant M, Reeves D, Hermens R, Braspenning J, Grol R, Sibbald B. Substitution of doctors by nurses in primary care. *Cochrane Database of Systemic Reviews.* July 9, 2009 2007(3. Art. No.: CD001271. DOI: 10.1002/14651858.CD001271.pub2.).

29. Mundinger MO, Kane RL, Lenz ER, et al. Primary care outcomes in patients treated by nurse practitioners or physicians: a randomized trial. *JAMA.* Jan 5 2000;283(1):59-68.

30. DeAngelis CD. Nurse practitioner redux. *JAMA.* Mar 16 1994;271(11):868-871.

31. Venning P, Durie A, Roland M, Roberts C, Leese B. Randomised controlled trial comparing cost effectiveness of general practitioners and nurse practitioners in primary care. *BMJ.* Apr 15 2000;320(7241):1048-1053.

32. Hauer KE, Durning SJ, Kernan WN, et al. Factors associated with medical students' career choices regarding internal medicine. *JAMA.* Sep 10 2008;300(10):1154-1164.

33. Holmes D, Tumiel-Berhalter LM, Zayas LE, Watkins R. "Bashing" of medical specialties: students' experiences and recommendations. *Fam Med.* Jun 2008;40(6):400-406.

34. Bowman R. Family Medicine Central. [online]. [cited 2010 Mar 12]. Available from: http://www.unmc.edu/Community/ruralmeded/family_medicine_central.htm.

Chapter 17

1. Alcoholics Anonymous. [online]. [cited 2009 Sep 13]. Available from: http://www.aahistory.com/prayer.html.

2. de Tocqueville A. *Democracy in America.*

3. Glare P, Virik K, Jones M, et al. A systematic review of physicians' survival predictions in terminally ill cancer patients. *BMJ.* Jul 26 2003;327(7408):195-198.

4. Wildman MJ, Sanderson C, Groves J, et al. Implications of prognostic pessimism in patients with chronic obstructive pulmonary disease (COPD) or asthma admitted to intensive care in the UK within the COPD and asthma outcome study (CAOS): multicentre observational cohort study. *BMJ.* Dec 1 2007;335(7630):1132.

5. Wong DT, Knaus WA. Predicting outcome in critical care: the current status of the APACHE prognostic scoring system. *Can J Anaesth.* Apr 1991;38(3):374-383.

6. Rivera-Fernandez R, Vazquez-Mata G, Bravo M, et al. The Apache III prognostic system: customized mortality predictions for Spanish ICU patients. *Intensive Care Med.* Jun 1998;24(6):574-581.

7. Jennett B, Bond M. Assessment of outcome after severe brain damage. *Lancet.* Mar 1 1975;1(7905):480-484.

8. Medical aspects of the persistent vegetative state (2). The Multi-Society Task Force on PVS. *N Engl J Med.* Jun 2 1994;330(22):1572-1579.

9. American Academy of Neurology. Practice parameters: assessment and management of patients in a persistent vegetative state. [online]. 1994 Sep 24 [cited 2010 March 6]. Available from: http://www.aan.com/professionals/practice/pdfs/pdf_1995_thru_1998/1995.45.1015.pdf.

10. Bruera E, Sweeney C. Hydrate or dehydrate. *Support Care Cancer.* May 2001;9(3):139-140.

11. McCann RM, Hall WJ, Groth-Juncker A. Comfort care for terminally ill patients. The appropriate use of nutrition and hydration. *JAMA.* Oct 26 1994;272(16):1263-1266.

12. Grant MD, Rudberg MA, Brody JA. Gastrostomy placement and mortality among hospitalized Medicare beneficiaries. *JAMA.* Jun 24 1998;279(24):1973-1976.

13. Meier DE, Ahronheim JC, Morris J, Baskin-Lyons S, Morrison RS. High short-term mortality in hospitalized patients with advanced dementia: lack of benefit of tube feeding. *Arch Intern Med.* Feb 26 2001;161(4):594-599.

14. Finucane TE, Christmas C, Travis K. Tube feeding in patients with advanced dementia: a review of the evidence. *JAMA.* Oct 13 1999;282(14):1365-1370.

15. Monti MM, Vanhaudenhuyse A, Coleman MR, et al. Willful modulation of brain activity in disorders of consciousness. *N Engl J Med.* Feb 18;362(7):579-589.

Chapter 20

1. van den Hout WB, Peul WC, Koes BW, Brand R, Kievit J, Thomeer RT. Prolonged conservative care versus early surgery in patients with sciatica from lumbar disc herniation: cost utility analysis alongside a randomised controlled trial. *BMJ.* Jun 14 2008;336(7657):1351-1354.

2. U.S. Census Bureau. Income, Poverty, and Health Insurance Coverage in the United States: 2007 and 2010. [online]. [cited Available from: URL to: http://www.census.gov/prod/2011pubs/p60-239.pdf.

Chapter 21

1. Epstein R. How other countries judge malpractice. *The Wall Street Journal.* June 30, 2009.

2. Dor A, Holahan J. Urban-rural differences in Medicare physician expenditures. *Inquiry.* Winter 1990;27(4):307-318.

3. THE BOARDS OF TRUSTEES FEDERAL HOSPITAL INSURANCE AND FEDERAL SUPPLEMENTARY MEDICAL INSURANCE TRUST FUNDS. 2008 ANNUAL REPORT OF THE BOARDS OF TRUSTEES OF THE FEDERAL HOSPITAL INSURANCE AND FEDERAL SUPPLEMENTARY MEDICAL INSURANCE TRUST FUNDS http://www.cms.hhs.gov/reportstrustfunds/downloads/tr2008.pdf. Accessed July 31, 2009.

4. Leonhardt D. A Medicare plan that exempts too many. [online]. 2011 Apr 5 [cited 2011 Jun 6]. Available from: www.nytimes.com/2011/04/06/business/06leonhardt.html.

Appendix

1. Boat TF, Chao SM, O'Neill PH. From waste to value in health care. *JAMA.* Feb 6 2008;299(5):568-571.

2. Jeffery M, HIckey B, Hider P. Follow-up strategies for patients treated for non-metastatic colorectal cancer. *Cochrane Database of Systemic Reviews.* 2008.

3. Rojas M, Telaro E, Russo A, et al. Follow-up strategies for women treated for early breast cancer. *Cochrane Database of Systemic Reviews.* 2008.

4. Stiell IG, McKnight RD, Greenberg GH, et al. Implementation of the Ottawa ankle rules. *JAMA.* Mar 16 1994;271(11):827-832.

5. Stiell IG, Wells GA, Hoag RH, et al. Implementation of the Ottawa Knee Rule for the use of radiography in acute knee injuries. *JAMA.* Dec 17 1997;278(23):2075-2079.

6. Fine MJ, Auble TE, Yealy DM, et al. A prediction rule to identify low-risk patients with community-acquired pneumonia. *N Engl J Med.* Jan 23 1997;336(4):243-250.

7. Rivera-Fernandez R, Vazquez-Mata G, Bravo M, et al. The Apache III prognostic system: customized mortality predictions for Spanish ICU patients. *Intensive Care Med.* Jun 1998;24(6):574-581.

8. Stiell I, Wells G, Laupacis A, et al. Multicentre trial to introduce the Ottawa ankle rules for use of radiography in acute ankle injuries. Multicentre Ankle Rule Study Group. *BMJ.* Sep 2 1995;311(7005):594-597.

9. Bachmann LM, Kolb E, Koller MT, Steurer J, ter Riet G. Accuracy of Ottawa ankle rules to exclude fractures of the ankle and mid-foot: systematic review. *BMJ.* Feb 22 2003;326(7386):417.

10. Personal Health Care Spending by Age Group and Source of Payment, Calendar Year 2004 Centers for Medicare and Medicaid Services [online]. [cited 2009 Jul 26]. Available from: http://www.cms.hhs.gov/NationalHealthExpendData/downloads/2004-age-tables.pdf.

11. CMS National Health Expenditure Data. Centers for Medicare and Medicaid Services [online]. [cited 2012 Jan 2]. Available from: http://www.cms.hhs.gov/NationalHealthExpendData/downloads/tables.pdf.

12. Social Security (OASDI)—Benefits by Type of Beneficiary: 1990 to 2010. U.S. Census Bureau [online]. [cited 2012 Jan 2]. Available from: http://www.census.gov/compendia/statab/2012/tables/12s0545.pdf.

13. Money Income of Households—Percent Distribution by Income Level, Race, and Hispanic Origin, in Constant (2009) Dollars: 1980 to 2009. U.S. Census Bureau [online]. [cited 2010 Mar 12]. Available from: http://www.census.gov/compendia/statab/2010/tables/10s0674.pdf.

14. 2011 Milliman Medical Index. Milliman [online]. [cited 2011 Oct 1]. Available from: http://publications.milliman.com/periodicals/mmi/pdfs/milliman-medical-index-2011.pdf.

15. Claxton G. Employer health benefits 2007 survey. Henry J. Kaiser Family Foundation [online]. [cited 2009 Apr 26]. Available from: http://www.kff.org/insurance/7672/.

16. Paulus RA, Davis K, Steele GD. Continuous innovation in health care: implications of the Geisinger experience. *Health Aff (Millwood)*. Sep-Oct 2008;27(5):1235-1245.

17. Davis K. Slowing the growth of health care costs--learning from international experience. *N Engl J Med.* Oct 23 2008;359(17):1751-1755.

18. Iglehart JK. Budgeting for change--Obama's down payment on health care reform. *N Engl J Med.* Apr 2 2009;360(14):1381-1383.

19. Davis K. Investing in health care reform. *N Engl J Med.* Feb 26 2009;360(9):852-855.

20. Mongan JJ, Ferris TG, Lee TH. Options for slowing the growth of health care costs. *N Engl J Med.* Apr 3 2008;358(14):1509-1514.

21. Collins S, Nuzum R, Rustgi S, Mika S, Schoen C, Davis K. *How Health Care Reform Can Lower the Costs of Insurance Administration*: The Commonwealth Fund; July 2009.

22. *Bringing Better Value: Recommendations to Address the Costs and Causes of Administrative Complexity in the Nation's Healthcare System* Healthcare Administrative Simplification Coalition July 2009.

23. OECD Health Data 2009 - Frequently Requested Data. Organization for Economic Co-operation and Development [online]. [cited 2009 Jul 14]. Available from: http://www.oecd.org/document/16/0,3343,en_2649_34631_2085200 _1_1_1_1,00.html.

CPSIA information can be obtained at www.ICGtesting.com
Printed in the USA
LVOW042018260712

291709LV00002B/6/P

9 780972 600774